Interventional
Computed Tomography

Interventional Computed Tomography

RAINER M. M. SEIBEL, MD, PD &
DIETRICH H. W. GRÖNEMEYER, MD, PD
Directors
Institute of Diagnostic and Interventional Radiology
Medical Computer Science
Private University of Witten/Herdecke
MRI - Mülheim Radiologic Institute, Germany

TRANSLATION BY
PETER A. ROTHSCHILD, MD
Clinical Director
Department of Diagnostic Radiology
RIL-Radiologic Imaging Laboratory
University of California San Francisco

JÜRGEN PLASSMANN, MD
Institute of Diagnostic and Interventional Radiology
Private University of Witten/Herdecke
MRI - Mülheim Radiologic Institute, Germany

AND

HERMANN SEHNERT
Institute of Diagnostic and Interventional Radiology
Private University of Witten/Herdecke
MRI - Mülheim Radiologic Institute, Germany

FOREWORD BY
ALEXANDER R. MARGULIS, MD
Professor and Chairman, Department of Radiology
School of Medicine
University of California San Francisco

BOSTON
BLACKWELL SCIENTIFIC PUBLICATIONS
OXFORD LONDON EDINBURGH MELBOURNE
PARIS BERLIN VIENNA

English edition ©1990 by
Blackwell Scientific Publications Inc.
Editorial Offices:
3 Cambridge Center, Cambridge
  Massachusetts 02142, USA
Osney Mead, Oxford OX2 OEL, England
25 John Street, London WC1N 2BL
  England
23 Ainslie Place, Edinburgh EH3 6AJ
  Scotland
54 University Street, Carlton
  Victoria 3053, Australia

Other Editorial Offices

Arnette SA
2, rue Casimir-Delavigne
75006 Paris
France

Blackwell Wissenschaft
Meinekestraße 4
D-1000 Berlin 15
Germany

Blackwell MZV
Feldgasse 13
A-1238 Wien
Austria

First published 1990

German edition first published 1989
by Blackwell Wissenschaft

Cover design: R. Hübler, D-1000 Berlin
Layout: Goldener Schnitt · Rainer Kusche, D-7573 Sinzheim
Typesetting and Printing: Kieser, D-8902 Neusäß
Binding: Schäffer, D-6718 Grünstadt 1

90 91 92 93 5 4 3 2 1

DISTRIBUTORS

USA and Canada
  Mosby-Year Book, Inc.
  11830 Westline Industrial Drive
  St Louis, Missouri 63146
  (*Orders:* Tel: 800 633–6699)

Australia
  Blackwell Scientific Publications
  (Australia) Pty Ltd
  54 University Street
  Carlton, Victoria 3053
  (*Orders:* Tel: 03 347 0300)

Outside North America and Australia
  Marston Book Services Ltd
  PO Box 87
  Oxford OX2 ODT
  (*Orders:* Tel: 08 65 79 11 55
            Fax: 08 65 79 19 27
            Telex: 83 75 15)

Library of Congress Cataloging-in-Publication Data

Interventionelle Computertomographie. English
  Interventional computed tomography / by Rainer M. M. Seibel
  and Dietrich H. W. Grönemeyer ; translation by Peter A.
  Rothschild, Jürgen Plaßmann and Hermann Sehnert ; foreword by
  Alexander R. Margulis.
     p. cm.
  Translation of: Interventionelle Computertomographie.
  Includes bibliographical references and index.
  ISBN 0-86542-127-7
  1. Radiology, Interventional. 2. Tomography. I. Seibel. Rainer
M. M. II. Grönemeyer, Dietrich H. W.
  RD33.55.I58713   1990
  617' .05--dc20   90-20089
                                                           CIP

British Library Cataloguing in Publication Data

Interventional computed tomography.
  1. Man. Diagnosis. Tomography. Applications of computer systems
  I. Seibel, Rainer M. M. II. Gronemeyer, Dietrich H. W.
  616.0757

ISBN 0-86542-127-7

Foreword

Modern radiology has been moving in the direction of less invasiveness and the advent of cross sectional modalities has made it possible to combine highly informative anatomic images with the possibility of guiding needles, catheters or tubes.

Interventional radiology is one of the most successful offshoots of advances in imaging. It has reduced the need for anesthesia, hospitalization and surgical intervention. Besides the reduction in pain, suffering, length of debility and complications, it also significantly decreases the expenses that would be incurred if the same procedure were to be conducted by traditional surgery.

This particular book will undoubtedly become one of the most important contributions to the field. By combining interventional computed tomography and interventional radiology with so many useful instructions and images, it will help make general interventional radiology directed by CT a routine procedure in every hospital.

The width of scope of this book, covering the entire body including the head, neck, lung, and abdomen as well as the skeleton, is extraordinary. The many highly competent and well recognized leaders in the field of interventional radiology who have contributed chapters make this book a pioneer in the radiology of the future.

Alexander R. Margulis, MD

Preface

It was Wilhelm Conrad Röntgen who first made it possible to look into the human body without surgery. The evolution of diagnostic radiology and radiation therapy progressed quickly and these are now integral parts of modern medicine. More than thirty years ago, with the first bile duct drainage, a new branch of medicine was created: interventional radiology; advances within this field, however, progressed more slowly.

Next and less than twenty years ago, the development of computed tomography ushered in a new era of radiology. Together with sonography and magnetic resonance imaging, computed tomography has made great advances in diagnostic radiology possible. For the first time cross sectional images of the body could be evaluated. Earlier on, Haaga took advantage of the high tissue differentiation to perform diagnostic punctures under CT guidance. High reproducibility and accurate documentation of CT interventional procedures were a prerequisite for the further development of interventional computed tomography. But unlike sonography, computed tomography does not allow for real-time visualization during the interventional procedures. The use of sonography on the other hand is limited by a variety of factors such as air, bones and adipose tissue overlying the area of interest. In addition, there are problems in maintaining a sterile field during interventional procedures. In attempting to localize both needle tips and catheters as well as small lesions CT has a distinct superiority.

Following the development of special needles and probes, it is now possible to perform interventions under CT guidance to within a few millimeters. This allows for interventional procedures in the region of high risk organs, nerves, and vessels. CT is also important in neurolysis and central nervous system interventional procedures, because of the precise control and documentation, which can lower the complication rate.

A new principle is described in this book, simultaneous combination of the computed tomograph with digital fluoroscopy. With this method, it is possible to perform a precise three-dimensional interventional procedure under fluoro with CT control at the same time. For the future it can be expected that interventional procedures under magnetic resonance imaging guidance will gain popularity because of the high tissue differentiation and the three-dimensional presentation. However, further developments and refinement of new materials for instrumentation and shorter examination times are necessary before these interventional procedures will become clinically relevant.

Among the most important obligations of the interventional radiologist are cooperation and interaction with the other clinical disciplines. Cooperation with the surgeons, especially with the vascular surgeons, neurosurgeons, orthopedic surgeons and all oncologic physicians is an important theme of this book. As members of the German pain society (Schmerztherapeutisches Kolloquium, STK), we have been fortunate to develop an excellent cooperation with the anesthesists in the area of pain management. An example of combined therapeutic strategies is in the thoracic sympathetic trunk neurolysis which has had rewarding results.

We have also developed a close cooperation with our anatomist colleagues which has been rewarding for both parties. Accurate anatomical knowledge is a prerequisite for any radiologist performing interventional procedures. Cooperation with our anatomist gave us the possibility to develop new kinds of interventional procedures. This helped us to recognize anatomical structures at risk in advance and to avoid them. For the anatomist such collaboration offered a new clinical aspect to his work.

In using interventional simulation, for the training of fellow doctors and teaching classes, these specimens have been most helpful.

In this book we attempt to demonstrate a great number of possibilities for interventional CT. The results as well as the effects and the side-effects of these techniques are presented in detail. In the first part of the book, we describe diagnostic interventional procedures by way of an atlas. At this stage we have also attempted to explain three-dimensional puncture techniques. In the second and third part of the book, therapeutic interventional procedures (p.e. management of low back pain, CT-guided percutaneous discectomy, tumor therapy) are described accompanied by detailed images. In the third part, new developments are presented which could be useful in future. Even though the book offers detailed information about different interventional procedures, it is essential to learn these techniques at appropriate institutes in the FRG in accordance with the guidelines of the Arbeitsgemeinschaft Interventionelle Radiologie der Deutschen Röntgengesellschaft (Study Group Interventional Radiology of German Roentgen Association).

The performance of therapeutic interventional procedures demand a detailed knowledge of anatomy, pathology and clinical symptomatology. Furthermore the interventional radiologist is responsible for the patient after the interven-

tion. Through optimal cooperation with other medical branches, good post-operative care can be assured for the patient. Our experience has shown an increasing opportunity for CT interventions to be performed on an outpatient basis. In summary, we wholeheartedly embrace this new era of interventional radiology as it is not only cost-efficient but it also provides for improved patient care without further burdening the health care system.

Following on from the good success of the German edition in 1989 we are pleased to publish now this English translation. The text has been adapted and extended. Furthermore, new figures have been added.

We hope that the reader will enjoy this book as well as perform these new procedures.

Mülheim, November 1990

Rainer M. M. Seibel · Dietrich H. W. Grönemeyer

Acknowledgements

Our very special thanks go to Professor Peter A. Rothschild, M.D. (Radiologic Imaging Laboratory, University of San Francisco) as well as to Jürgen Plaßmann, M.D. and Heinz Sehnert (M.K.I., University of Witten/Herdecke), who translated our German text: Grönemeyer-Seibel, Interventionelle Computertomographie, 1989. This was very hard work over a long period for them and we are most grateful for their excellent efforts.

Our thanks also go to the contributors of this book. Their accurate scientific representation of the subject matter and the intensive intradisciplinary cooperation significantly improved our book.

We thank Mr. Hermann Dornhege for the excellent photographs in the book. As photographer for the "Frankfurter Allgemeine Zeitung" he has a keen eye for the photographic material used in this book.

Without the excellent support of our doctors and X-ray technicians and the diligence with which they work at interventional radiology and care for the patients, many things written here would not have been possible.

We thank Mr. Alexander Rummel, the chief X-ray technician for his assistance in the selection and preparation of the photographic material.

We owe special thanks to Mrs. Doris Brinkmeier and Mrs. Cornelia Glaesner for their untiring typing and correction of this work which they performed with great precision and conscientiousness.

An ideal cooperation was developed with Mr. Rainer Kusche when putting together the layout. With him this difficult job became a pleasure. Last but not least we want to say thanks to the Blackwell Wissenschafts-Verlag for the excellent cooperation and the excellent reproduction in this book. Our special thanks to Dr. Axel Bedürftig and his personnel for their great help during the preparation of this text.

We are honoured that Alexander Margulis has written the foreword to the English edition; it is very gratifying for our book to be recommended by such an outstanding scholar.

Mülheim, November 1990

Rainer M. M. Seibel · Dietrich H. W. Grönemeyer

Contents

Chapter 19 Percutaneous neurolysis of the celiac plexus

Chapter 20 CT-guided neurolysis of the presacral and precoccygeal sympathetic trunk

Percutaneous lysis of nerval structures in vascular disorders

Chapter 21 CT-guided thoracic sympathectomy

Chapter 22 CT-guided lumbar sympathetic trunk neurolysis for the treatment of occlusive arterial disease (OAD)

Percutaneous management of fluid collections and urinary diseases

Chapter 23 Percutaneous decompression of the urinary system

Chapter 24 CT-guided antegrade ureter stent

Chapter 25 CT-guided percutaneous thoracic and abdominal abscess drainage

Chapter 26 Drainage techniques in interventional radiology

Chapter 27 CT-guided therapeutic liver procedures

Future outlook

Chapter 28 Interventional magnetic resonance imaging

List of Contributors

Professor *Ingolf P. Arlart*, MD
Ärztlicher Direktor des Zentralen Röntgeninstitutes des Katharinenhospitals der Stadt Stuttgart,
Kriegsbergstraße 60, 7000 Stuttgart

Professor *Wolfgang H. Arnold*, MD
Lehrstuhl Anatomie II, Funktionelle Morphologie der Mundhöhle, Universität Witten/Herdecke,
In den Espeln 5, 5810 Witten 4

Klaus Balzer, MD
Chefarzt der Gefäßchirurgischen Klinik, Ev. Krankenhaus Mülheim, Wertgasse 30,
4330 Mülheim an der Ruhr

Professor *Douglas P. Boyd*, MD
Director of Physic Research Laboratory, University of California San Francisco,
389 Oyster Point Blvd., So. San Francisco, California 94080

Hans-Jürgen Brambs, MD
Universität Heidelberg, Institut für Radiologie, Im Neuenheimer Feld 110, 6900 Heidelberg

Martin Busch, PhD
Institut für Diagnostische und Interventionelle Radiologie, Medizinische
Computer-Wissenschaften, Universität Witten/Herdecke, Schulstraße 10,
4330 Mülheim an der Ruhr

Professor *Gert Carstensen*, MD
Bleichstraße 5, Mülheim an der Ruhr

Hermann Dornhege
Photographer, Kobellstraße 10, 8000 München 2

Thomas Flöter, MD
Präsident des Schmerztherapeutischen Kolloquiums, Praxis für Schmerztherapie, Roßmarkt 23,
6000 Frankfurt/Main

Dietrich H. W. Grönemeyer, MD, PD
Direktor des Instituts für Diagnostische und Interventionelle Radiologie,
Medizinische Computer-Wissenschaften, Universität Witten/Herdecke,
MKI-Mülheimer Krankenhaus Institut, Schulstraße 10, 4330 Mülheim an der Ruhr

Professor *Thomas Grumme*, MD
Direktor der Neurochirurgischen Klinik, Zentralklinikum, Stenglinstraße, 8900 Augsburg

Michael ten Hompel, PhD
Meß- und Regelungstechnik, Fraunhofer Institut Dortmund,
Emil-Figge-Straße, 4600 Dortmund

Werner Jaschke, MD
Institut für Klinische Radiologie, Universität Mannheim, Theodor-Kutzer-Ufer, 6800 Mannheim

Professor *Günter W. Kauffmann*, MD
Direktor der Abteilung Radiodiagnostik, Universität Heidelberg, Im Neuenheimer Feld 110,
6900 Heidelberg

Professor *Leon Kaufman*, MD
Director of RIL-Radiologic Imaging Laboratory,
University of California San Francisco, 400 Grandview Drive, So. San Francisco, California 94080

Professor *Bernhard Kramann*, MD
Universitätsklinik Homburg/Saar, Direktor der Radiologischen Klinik,
Abteilung für Radiodiagnostik, Universität Homburg/Saar, 6650 Homburg/Saar

Dave Kramer, MD
Toshiba America Inc., So. San Francisco

Jürgen Plaßmann, MD
MKI, University of Witten/Herdecke

Deborah Reinking, MD, Anesthesiologist,
518 Tideway Dr., Alameda, California

Götz Richter, MD
Universität Heidelberg, Institut für Radiologie, Im Neuenheimer Feld 110, 6900 Heidelberg

Professor *Peter A. Rothschild*, MD
RIL-Radiologic Imaging Laboratory, Clinical Director, University of California San Francisco,
400 Grandview Drive, So. San Francisco, California 94080

Professor *Hans H. Schild*, MD
Institut für klinische Strahlenkunde, Klinikum der Universität Mainz, Langenbeckstraße 1,
6500 Mainz

Rüdiger Schliffke
Ruhr-Universität Bochum, Wissenschaftlicher Mitarbeiter, Institut für Diagnostische
und Interventionelle Radiologie, Medizinische Computer-Wissenschaften,
Universität Witten/Herdecke, Schulstraße 10, 4330 Mülheim an der Ruhr

Armin M. Schmidt, MD
Institut für Diagnostische und Interventionelle Radiologie, Medizinische Computer-Wissenschaften, Universität Witten/Herdecke, MKI-Mülheimer Krankenhaus Institut, Schulstraße 10,
4330 Mülheim an der Ruhr

Cornelia Sehnert
Universität Düsseldorf, Wissenschaftliche Mitarbeiterin, Institut für Diagnostische
und Interventionelle Radiologie, Medizinische Computer-Wissenschaften,
Universität Witten/Herdecke, Schulstraße 10, 4330 Mülheim an der Ruhr

Rainer M. M. Seibel, MD, PD
Direktor des Instituts für Diagnostische und Interventionelle Radiologie,
Medizinische Computer-Wissenschaften, Universität Witten/Herdecke,
MKI-Mülheimer Krankenhaus Institut, Schulstraße 10, 4330 Mülheim an der Ruhr

Erhard Starck, MD
Leitender Arzt am Institut für Röntgendiagnostik, Städtische Kliniken Kassel,
Zentrum für Radiologie, Mönchebergstraße 43, 3500 Kassel

Professor *Hanfried Weigand*, MD
Chefarzt des Zentralröntgeninstituts, Dr.-Horst-Schmidt-Kliniken, Ludwig-Erhard-Straße 100,
6200 Wiesbaden

Wolfgang R. Werner, MD
Institut für Diagnostische und Interventionelle Radiologie, Medizinische Computer-Wissenschaften, Universität Witten/Herdecke, MKI-Mülheimer Krankenhaus Institut, Schulstraße 10,
4330 Mülheim an der Ruhr

Atlas of Diagnostic Procedures

Chapter 1
Atlas of CT-Guided Biopsies

D.H.W. Grönemeyer, R.M.M. Seibel, W.H. Arnold, B. Kramann, E. Starck

Introduction

Diagnostic interventional procedures have been known since 1851. The earliest reported tumor biopsies were performed in 1851 by Lebert in Paris and in 1853 by Paget in London. The first German publication of an interventional biopsy procedure was in 1912. After this, Martin and Ellis developed a needle aspiration technique in 1925, which is still the basis for most biopsy methods used today.

Fluoroscopy-, sonography-, and CT-guided biopsies are established diagnostic techniques. However, fluoroscopy-guided methods are being replaced more and more by CT guidance. Fine-needle biopsies are most often performed for cytologic and histologic diagnosis in the abdomen, thorax, mediastinum, pelvis, retroperitoneum, bones, brain, joints and lymph nodes. In general, the results thus far with percutaneous aspiration techniques are very good. Success rates for obtaining cytologic diagnosis of higher than 80% have been reported [Zornoza; Pereiras; Macintosh].

CT-, fluoro-, and ultrasonic-guided punctures have been reported in the literature for more than 20 years. In 1967, Nordenström reported the first series of percutaneous fluoro-guided lymph node biopsies. Other publications followed, such as a report by Rüttimann in 1968 of fluoro-guided biopsies of para-iliac lymph nodes. The trans-lumbar and trans-vascular approaches for lymph node biopsy were described in 1969 and 1972 by Lüning et al. In 1976, Göthlin described the trans-peritoneal route.

In 1977, Zornoza et al. reported excellent results in 85% of 109 patients for the cytologic evaluation of intra-peritoneal lymph nodes after fine-needle biopsies. The correct diagnosis was made in 86% of metastatic lesions and in 64% of lymphomas. Pereiras et al. report a correct diagnosis of 81.6% in 49 patients.

In 1979, Macintosh et al. published a study using fine-needle biopsy in 52 patients with a question of metastatic lymph node invasion. 12 biopsies were positive, 35 biopsies were negative. Only two biopsy examinations proved to be false negative.

Detailed descriptions of conventional biopsy techniques can be obtained in current textbooks [1–3] and relevant literature is listed at the end of this chapter. The basic technique of CT-guided biopsies is the same in all organ systems. There is normally no difference in the equipment used for biopsies in different areas. Therefore, in the first 10 chapters the authors have kept short the description of puncture techniques and presented the biopsy procedures as an atlas by organ system with numerous figures. Only for selected organ systems such as thorax and liver are a detailed description and discussion given.

Combined Interventional Procedures

A new method performed at the authors' clinic in Mülheim is the combined interventional procedure. In this technique, a C-arm is placed directly alongside the CT and is used in cases of complicated interventional procedures. By using a rotating fluoroscope and CT, the structure to be punctured can be visualized three-dimensionally and with excellent morphologic differentiation. With this technique, there is the possibility of exact differentiation of anatomic structures, which in many cases is not possible with fluoroscopy alone. Therefore, difficult lesions can be precisely punctured. This is especially helpful in infiltrating processes. Also, with the addition of CT, complications can be detected at an early stage. Interventional procedures, which begin with CT guidance and are followed by fluoroscopy guidance, are described in another chapter (see chapter on drainage techniques).

The detailed and accurate measurement as to size and/or volume of pathological structures, and their distances to the skin, vessels, neural structures, and surrounding organs is only possible by CT or MRI. Also, the density and resolution of abnormal masses are better defined with CT. The major advantages of CT over ultrasound (US) are:

1. Less training is needed to orient the image;
2. The system itself is not moved. Consequently, an exact reproduction of the scan level is possible.

Another advantage is that, when using ultrasound guidance for biopsy, more time is needed to place the transducer over the area of pathology, especially in cases of repeated examinations. On the other hand, the trained examiner with ultrasound has a method at his disposal, which can interactively demonstrate the structures three-dimensionally. This interactive advantage over CT alone is lost by using simultaneous CT and fluorscopy guidance or with MRI which is being used for an increasing number of biopsies.

At the authors' clinic, it is possible to perform diagnostic punctures and therapeutic interventional procedures using an open MRI (see Chapter Interventional MRI). In comparison with flouroscopy and CT, the advantage of MRI is the lack of ionizing radiation and the possibility of imaging in any plane. The lack of ionizing radiation is especially useful in long interventional procedures.

Indications

In most cases of pathologic findings which cannot be clarified by imaging methods such as X-ray, CT, MRI, or sonography and which are more than 0.5 cm in size, a diagnostic fine-needle biopsy should be performed. The accuracy is approximately the same as with bunch biopsy. Most frequently fine-needle biopsies are performed in the thorax and abdomen. With the high accuracy of CT- and also combined CT- and fluoroscopy-guided punctures, almost any structure can be reached accurately by needle. The puncture precision with CT is 1 mm^3. Organs which are affected by breathing should be punctured during breath holding. Furthermore, it is possible by special puncture techniques to reach structures which are located behind or in front of other organs without damaging these organs. For these special procedures, new methods of the three-dimensional puncture technique have been developed (e.g. for the biopsy of the suprarenal gland).

Technique

Normally the patient is positioned in such a way as to enable the best possible access to the lesion. The prone, supine, oblique, or lateral positions can be used. Also, the patient should be made comfortable in this position by using different types of padding and cushions, which

should always be kept at hand. Due to the minimal trauma from a fine-needle biopsy and the use of local anesthesia, premedication is not normally required. The procedure is as follows: first a CT of the region of interest is performed. An intravenous (I.V.) contrast-medium injection is required at those regions where vascular structures (e.g. in the mediastinum) must be demarcated. Then, on the monitor, the puncture angle and depth are determined. The experienced doctor in most cases can transfer the given puncturing angle to the patient. This requires intensive education and a distinctive three-dimensional mental image. Following the measurement on the monitor, the level is marked on the patient with a felt-tip pen using the positioning light. After the distance is measured on the skin using anatomic structures such as ribs, spinous process or muscles (such as the sternocleidomastoid m.), the exact puncture spot is marked. Anatomic cavities such as the orbit can also serve as visible landmarks. After careful injection of local anesthesia with 1% Mepivacaine using a special guide needle from the puncture set (Seibel-Grönemeyer/Interventional-Needle Set, Cook, Inc.), the same guide needle is inserted in the direction of the structure to be biopsied. The puncture should be performed quickly to minimise any puncture pain. Then, the direction of the guide cannula is checked with CT. Through the guide cannula, the puncture needle (which has a cm scale), is introduced in one or several steps into the structure to be punctured. The importance of the scale is such that the distance from the skin level to the structure, which is to be biopsied, can be determined from the needle. Therefore, the examiner knows at all times, by observing the puncture angle and needle depth, the distance from the needle tip to nearby organs, nerves or large blood vessels. The position of the needle tip is accurately documented by using CT.

For 3-D biopsy techniques, where the needle must be inserted obliquely, a rotating fluoroscopy is performed with a C-arm which alternates with CT.

After documenting the needle tip, the inner mandril of the coaxial needle set is removed and a 20 ml syringe is attached. Then, the syringe is fastened to a Cameco syringe-holder. When pulling the pistol-like Cameco handle, a negative pressure is created. Under continuing negative pressure, the puncture is performed in a fan-like pattern using a rotating motion.

For all biopsies, it is important to puncture the margins of the tumors, since necrotic tissue is mainly in the central portion of the tumor. Furthermore, a sufficient amount of material must appear in the syringe for a pathologic diagnosis. The material obtained for pathology is streaked on to glass slides, and the remainder is placed into a formalin solution. A histologic and cytologic diagnosis can be made by the pathologist within 24 hours. When a bacterial infection is suspected or in the case of a suspected superinfection, additional material is placed into a sterile saline solution for microbiologic examination.

A repetition of the biopsy is performed only in the case of insufficient material or where only necrotic material hade been obtained.

When selecting the biopsy needle, the size of the mass and the access route have to be taken into consideration. For a biopsy, the following needles are often used:

1. Coaxial needle: Seibel-Grönemeyer/Interventional-Needle Set (all biopsy needles by Cook, Inc. can be furnished with a cm scale)
2. Vacu-Cut (18 to 22-G, 10 to 20 cm, Angiomed)
3. Cut-Biopsy needle (18 to 21-G, 5 to 40 cm, Angio-med)
4. Rotex needle
5. Westcot needle
6. Turner needle
7. Menghini needle

Complications

Besides large hematomas, seen especially in anticoagulated patients, pneumothorax can occur after lung, liver, or suprarenal biopsies, especially when using a three-dimensional technique. Other authors have reported pancreatitis or fistula formation, and in one case a fatal outcome after pancreatic biopsy. Furthermore, in a few cases suprarenal biopsies have resulted in hypertensive crises from an undiagnosed phaeochromocytoma.

Contraindications

Contraindications to biopsy are patients with anticoagulant therapy or blood-clotting disorders. Prior to each biopsy the clotting status and platelet counts must be determined. For safety reasons the prothrombin value should not be below 50–60%. No other general contraindications are known.

Summary

Fine-needle biopsies of lymph nodes and pathologic organ findings are acknowledged, safe, and accurate methods to obtain excellent histologic and cytologic information about pathologic processes. The CT-guided methods are repro-

ducible and less training is needed to perform these examinations and procedures than with US. Also, it is much easier with CT guidance to puncture the same area in follow-up procedures than with US guidance. The simultaneous combination of CT and fluoroscopy creates an ultrasound-like control, but with trunch more accurate morphologic location, and density differentiation.

The surgical procedures for obtaining a tissue diagnosis, which often result in a longer hospital stay, can be reduced with fine-needle biopsies. An example is the CT-guided lymph node biopsy which can be performed at almost all regions of the body and can avoid the extensive physical and emotional stress of staging-laparotomies in lymphoma patients.

The radiation exposure, especially the genetic significant dose, is low. If in a given finding there is the question of performing surgery or CT-guided interventional procedure, the radiation exposure is minute by comparison with the physical and emotional strain of a surgical procedure.

The minor side-effects and complications of CT- or simultaneous CT- and fluoroscopy-guided procedures make it possible for these methods to be performed on an outpatient basis. Finally, these methods can contribute to cost savings in health services.

Further Reading

1. Athanasoulis Ch.A., Pfister R.C., Greene R.E., Robertson G.H: Interventional Radiology, Philadelphia 1982
2. Castaneda-Zuniga W.R., Tadavarthy S.M.: Interventional Radiology, Baltimore 1988
3. Dandelinger F., Rossi P., Kurdziel J.C., Wallace S.: Interventional Radiology, Stuttgart, New York 1990
4. Günther R.W., Thelen M.: Interventionelle Radiologie, Stuttgart, New York 1988

References

1. Debnam J.W., Staple T.W.: Needle biopsy of bone. Radiol. Clin. North. AM. XIII (1975) 157
2. Debnam J.W., Staple T.W.: Trephine bone biopsy by radiologist. Results of 73 procedures. Radiology 116 (1975) 607
3. deSantos L.A., Lukeman J.W., Wallace S., et al.: Percutaneous needle biopsy in abdominal lymphoma. Amer. J. Roentgenol. 136 (1981) 97
4. Dixon G.D.: Combined CT and fluoroscopic guidance for liver abscess drainage. Amer. J. Roentgenol. 135 (1980) 397
5. Ferrucci J.T. Jr., Wittenberg J., Mueller P.R., et al.: Diagnosis of abdominal malignancy by radiologic fine needle aspiration biopsy. Amer. J. Roentgenol. 134 (1980) 323
6. Ferrucci J.T. Jr., Wittenberg J.: CT biopsy of abdominal tumors. Aids for lesion localization. Radiology 129 (1978) 739

7. Forsgren L., Orell S.: Aspiration cytology in carcinoma of the pancreas. Surgery 73 (1973) 38
8. Franzen S., Giertz G., Zajicek J.: Cytological diagnosis of prostatic tumors by transrectal aspiration biopsy: A preliminary report. Br. J. Urol. 32 (1960) 193
9. Gerzof S.G., Spira R., Robbins A.H.: Percutaneous abscess drainage. Semin. Roentgenol. 16 (1981) 62
10. Goldstein H.M., Zornoza J., Wallace S., et al.: Percutaneous fine needle aspiration biopsy of pancreatic and other abdominal masses. Radiology 123 (1977) 319
11. Göthlin J.H.: Post-lymphographic percutaneous fine needle biopsy of lymph nodes, guided by fluoroscopy. Radiology 120 (1976) 205
12. Göthlin J.A., Rupp N., Rotehberger K.H., et al.: Percutaneous biopsy of retroperitoneal lymph nodes. A multicentric study. Eur. J. Radiol. 1 (1981) 46
13. Haaga J.R., Alfidi R.J.: Precise biopsy localization by computed tomography. Radiology 118 (1976) 603
14. Haaga J.R., Alfidi R.J., Havrilla T.R., et al.: CT detection and aspiration of abdominal abscess. Amer. J. Roentgenol. 128 (1977) 465
15. Haaga J.R., Vanek J.: Computed tomography guided liver biopsy using the Menghini needl. Radiology 133 (1979) 4053
16. Haaga J.R.: New techniques for CT-guided biopsies. Amer. J. Roentgenol. 133 (1979) 633
17. Haaga J.R., Weinstein A.J.: CT-guided percutaneous aspiration and drainage of abscess. Amer. J. Roentgenol. 135 (1980) 1187
18. Hancke S., Holm H.H., Koch F.: Ultrasonically guided percutaneous fine needle biopsy of the pancreas. Surg. Gynecol. Obstet. 140 (1975) 361
19. Hancke S., Pedersen J.F.: Percutaneous puncture of pancreatic cysts guided by ultrasound. Surg. Gynecol. Obstet. 142 (1976) 551
20. Hardy D.C., Murphy W.A., Gilula L.A.: Computed tomography in planning percutaneous bone biopsy. Radiology 134 (1980) 447
21. Holm H.H.; Perderson J.F., Kristensen J.K., et al.: Ultrasonically guided percutaneous puncture. Radiol. Clin. N. Am. 13 (1975) 493
22. Isler R.J., Ferrucci J.T., Wittenberg J., et al.: Tissue core biopsy of abdominal tumors with a 22 gauge cutting needle. Amer. J. Roentgenol. 136 (1981) 725
23. Jaques P.F., Staab E., Richey W., et al.: CT-assisted pelvic and abdominal aspiration biopsy in gynecological malignancy. Radiology 128 (1978) 651
24. Klince T.S., Neal H.S.: Needle aspiration biopsy. A critical appraisal. JAMA 239 (1978) 36
25. Lüning M., Romaniuk P.A.: Technik der paravasalen Punktion kontrastierter iliakaler Lymphknoten nach Rüttimann. Radiol. Diagn. (Berlin) 10 (1969) 361
26. Lüning M., Gastrein P., Vogeler H., et al.: Überprüfung lymphographischer Befunde durch die paravasale Punktion kontrastierter Lymphknoten des Beckens. Dtsch. Gesundheitsw. 27 (1972) 316
27. MacErlean D.P., Bryan P.J., Murphy J.J.: Pancreatic pseudocyst. Management by ultrasonically guided aspiration. Gastrointest. Radiol. 5 (1980) 255
28. Macintosh P.K., Thomson K.R., Barbaric Z.L.: Percutaneous transperitoneal lymph-node biopsy as a means of improving lymphographic diagnosis. Radiology 131 (1979) 647
29. McLoughlin M.J.: CT and percutaneous fine-needle aspiration biopsy in tropical myositis. Amer. J. Roentgenol. 134 (1980) 167
30. Martin H.E., Ellis E.B.: Biopsy by needle puncture and aspiration. Ann. Surg. 92 (1930) 169
31. Mueller P.R., Wittenberg J., Ferrucci J.T. Jr.: Fine needle aspiration biopsy of abdominal masses. Semin. Roentgenol. 16 (1981) 52
32. Nordenström B.: Paraxiphoid approach to the mediastinum for mediastinography and mediastinal needle biopsy: A preliminary report. Invest. Radiol. 2 (1967) 141
33. Pereiras P.V., Meiers W., Kunhardt B., et al.: Fluoroscopically guided thin needle aspiration biopsy of the abdomen and retroperitoneum. Amer. J. Roentgenol. 131 (1978) 197
34. Pereiras R.V., Meiers W., Kunhardt B., et al.: Fluororscopycally guided thin needle aspiration biopsy. Amer. J. roentgenol. 131 (1978) 197
35. Rüttimann A.: Iliac lymph node aspiration biopsy through paravascular approach: Preliminary report. Radiology 90 (1968) 150
36. Sinner W.N., Zajicek J.: Implantation metastasis after percutaneous transthoracic needle aspiration biopsy. Acta Radiol. [Diagn] (Stockh) 17 (1981) 725
37. Smith E.M., Bartrum R.J. Jr., Chang Y.C., et al.: Percutaneous aspiration biopsy of the pancreas under ultrasonic guidance. New Engl. J. Med. 292 (1975) 825
38. Zornoza J., Jonsson K., Wallace S., et al.: Fine needle aspiration biopsy of retroperitoneal lymph nodes and abdominal masses. An updated report. Radiology 125 (1977) 87
39. Zornoza J.: Abdomen. In: Zornoza J. (ed.) Percutaneous Needle Biopsy, Baltimore, 1981, 102–140
40. Zornoza J., Cabanillas F.F., Altoff T.M., et al.: Percutaneous needle biopsy in abdominal lymphoma. Amer. J. Roentgenol. 136 (1981) 97

Chapter 2
Skull

D.H.W. Grönemeyer, R.M.M. Seibel

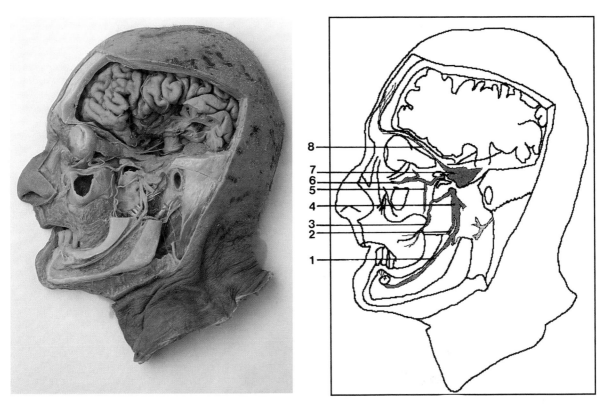

Figs. 2.1. and **2.2.** Plastic imbedded anatomic specimen and diagram of skull. The lateral portion of the cranium has been removed and the trigeminal nerve is well demonstrated. *1* Inferior alveolar n.; *2* lingual n.; *3* buccal n.; *4* otic ganglion; *5* posterior superior alveolar n,; *6* infra-orbital n,; *7* trigeminal ganglion; *8* frontal n.

Figs. 2.3.–2.8. The first CT and MRI investigations in a 72-year old female with trigeminal neuralgias in the entire trigeminal nerve region for the past 26 years. The long-term therapy had involved oral analgesics and psychopharmacologic medication.

Fig. 2.3. Axial MRI (0.064 Tesla) at the level of the first cervical vertebra demonstrates an extensive tumor on the left, lateral to the pharynx. The highly vascular tumor is well shown with the use of Gadolinium-DTPA (Schering).

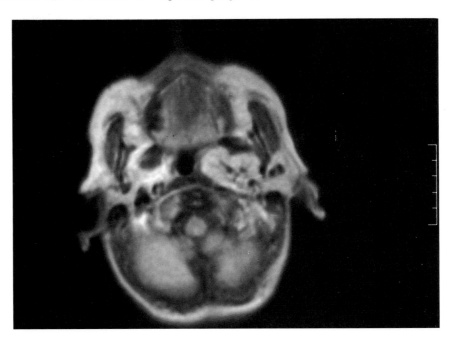

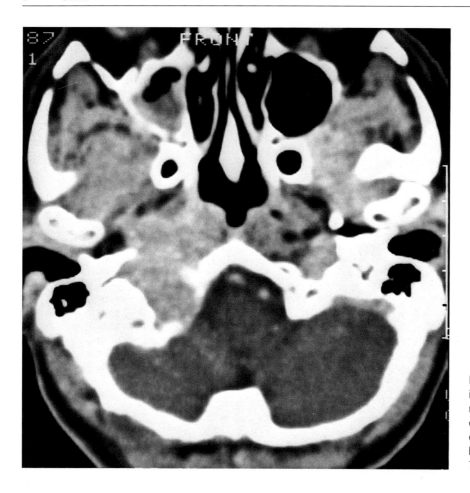

Fig. 2.4. Axial CT. An irregularly demarcated margined mass is identified on the left, that has extended through the skull base over a distance of 7 mm.

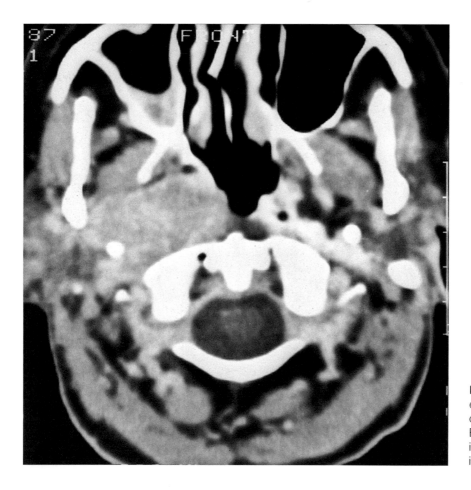

Fig. 2.5. Contrast-enhanced axial CT obtained inferior to Fig. 2.4. Enhancement is identified in this mass which extends into the nasopharynx.

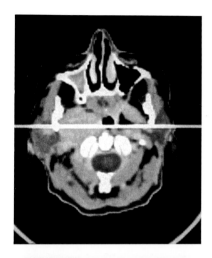

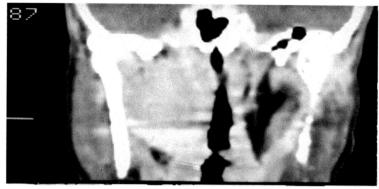

Figs. 2.6. and **2.7.** Coronal and sagittal CT reconstructions. The round-shaped mass can be identified, extending superiorly and destroying the skull base.

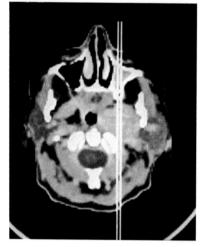

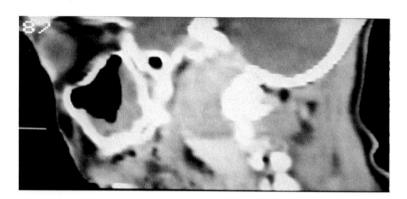

Fig. 2.8. CT-guided biopsy performed using a 20-G Seibel biopsy needle (Cook). The needle was placed to a depth of 8 cm and entered the mass superiorly. Histologic diagnosis was a benign glomus tumor. Six treatments with a solution of 2 ml Scandicaine 1% (local anesthetic), 40 mg Volon A (cortical steroid) and 2 ml oxypolygelatin alternating between peritumoral and intratumoral injections were administered. Each treatment was followed by an interval of 3 weeks. After therapy, the patient was pain-free for the first time in 26 years. Follow-up CT examination showed a reduction in size of the glomus tumor. The patient refused surgical intervention, which was possible due to the decrease in tumor volume after therapy.

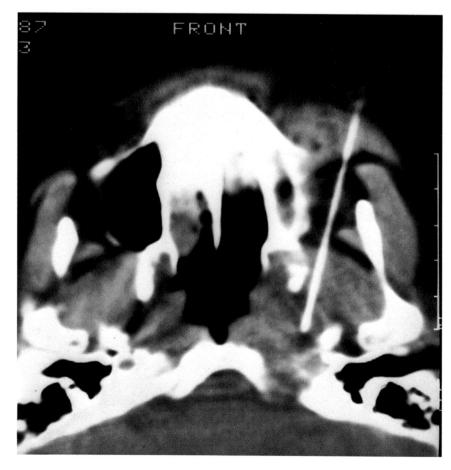

Chapter 3
Neck

D.H.W. Grönemeyer, R.M.M. Seibel

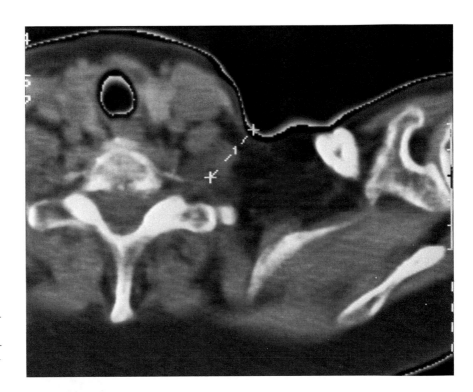

Fig. 3.1. Planning-CT for biopsy of a mass in the region of the upper brachial plexus. The tumor has infiltrated the middle and posterior scalene muscles.

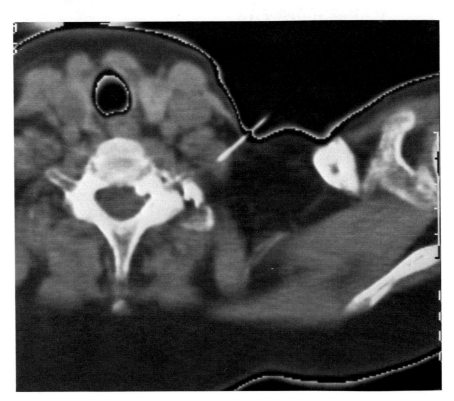

Fig. 3.2. A biopsy was performed on the superior portion of this infiltrating tumor from an anterolateral approach. The histologic diagnosis was breast metastasis.

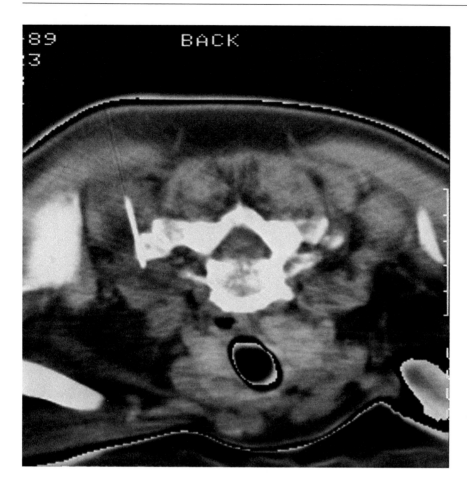

Fig. 3.3. Three-dimensional guided puncture of a mass in the region of the brachial plexus at the C7–T1 level. The needle tip is positioned posterior to the scalene muscle. The biopsy was performed in the prone position. Histologic diagnosis was breast metastasis.

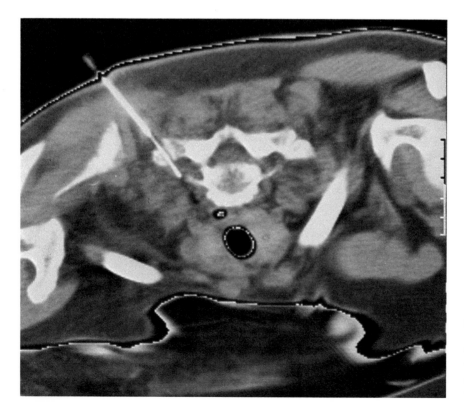

Fig. 3.4. Same patient as in Fig. 2.3. A second aspiration biopsy was performed relatively close to the intervertebral foramen using a 22-G fine needle through a guide needle.

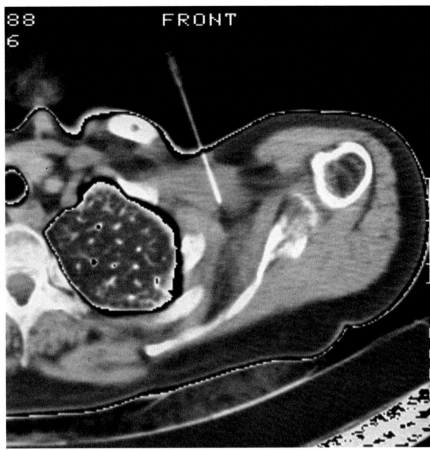

Fig. 3.5. Fine-needle biopsy in the region of the lower brachial plexus from an anterior approach. This patient is a 47-year old female who had received post-operative radiation therapy two years earlier in this area for breast carcinoma. The patient now has shoulder-arm pain and lymphedema. No tumor cells were identified after several extensive aspiration biopsies. The patient then received pain therapy injections using a combination of 40 mg Volon A (cortical steroid) and a mixture of short- and long-acting local anesthetics at 3-week intervals. After five treatments the patient was pain-free and the lymphedema had regressed.

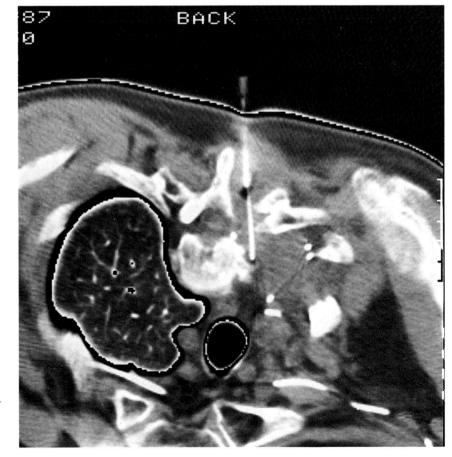

Fig. 3.6. 65-year old patient with a pancoast tumor of the right apex of the lung. This tumor had extended into the adjacent spinal column and upper ribs and infiltrated the brachial plexus within the supraclavicular fossa. Due to the compression of the lower cervical and upper thoracic spinal cord an operative partial resection of the tumor was performed, followed by a combination of radiation and chemotherapy. One year after the operation, the patient had a recurrence of pain. Prior to local tumor therapy a CT-guided histologic biopsy was performed in the region of the paravertebral tumor. A coaxial needle system was used for the biopsy from a posterior approach through the operative scar. Surgical clips are identified around the tumor. The histologic diagnosis was squamous cell carcinoma.

Chapter 4 – Thorax Biopsy
Lung – Pleura – Mediastinum

R.M.M. Seibel, D.H.W. Grönemeyer, H. Weigand

Introduction

Percutaneous puncture of pulmonary pathology was first performed in 1883 by Leyden [4] to obtain bacteria analysis. Three years later Menetrier [5] reported the aspiration of bronchial carcinoma cells. In the mid sixties Dahlgren, Nordenström and Sinner [1, 6] at the Karolinska Institute in Stockholm, performed fine-needle punctures of the lung in a large number of patients. In over 2700 patients with one to three punctures per patient, more than 90% had diagnostic cytology of lung lesions. Benign disease of the lung was found in more than 50% of these patients [9].

Indication

Any rounded intrapulmonary lesion should be considered as potentially malignant and may require biopsy clarification. With a fine-needle biopsy, infiltrates of the lung can be diagnosed. Hilar, mediastinal, and pleural masses are also important indications for percutaneous fine-needle biopsy (Table 4.1.).

Table 4.1. Indication for the percutaneous fine-needle biopsy.

Intrapulmonary focal mass
Lung infiltrates
Intrathoracic space-occupying lesions

Materials and Methods

Techniques

For fine-needle biopsy of the lung we used two techniques:
1. Puncture by rotating fluoroscopy
2. CT-guided puncture.

We performed 306 punctures under rotating fluoroscopy and 338 punctures under CT guidance. CT-guided puncture is the preferred method for central and mediastinal masses as well as for pleural lesions.

In the beginning we used 20-G disposable hypodermic needles and 22-G-Chiba needles. Since 1983 we have performed punctures using either a cutting-biopsy hypodermic needle [7], 10-15 cm long or the biopsy needle developed at the MKI. In the early part of our study we biopsied only peripheral alterations, later we also increasingly punctured central and mediastinal lesions.

Patients

644 patients between 16 and 85 years old with intrapulmonary foci or infiltrates were examined between 1979 and 1989. The average age was 59.6 years. The size of the biopsied lesions fluctuated between 3 mm (Fig. 4.1.) and 17 cm. During the last few years we mainly biopsied smaller lesions. The average diameter of these masses was approximately 1.5 cm.

Localization

226 punctured foci were located at the upper lobe, 201 at the lower lobe and 46 at the middle lobe. 78 infiltrates originated from hilus and could not be assigned to a lobe. 93 tumors were located at the mediastinum. 483 patients were punctured from anterior, 109 from posterior and 52 from a lateral approach.

Technique

Premedication of a patient before carrying out this procedure is unnecessary. The patients must have normal clotting values. Following a discussion of the procedure, the intrapulmonary mass is localized under rotation fluoroscopy or CT. A stylus is then used to mark the optimum approach on the skin. After local anesthesia of the thoracic wall including pleura, the

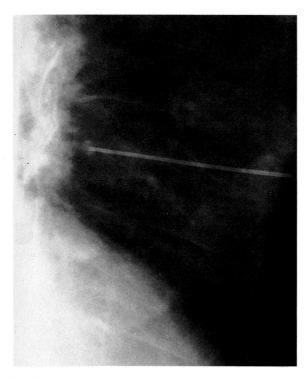

Fig. 4.1. Intrapulmonary focal 3 mm mass in the region of the left hilus. Biopsy with a 20 G-fine needle reveals a tuberculoma.

puncture needle set is introduced into the mass under CT or fluoroscopic control. The puncture point is located at the upper costal edge to avoid bleeding and damage to nerve. A safe position is reached when the needle tip and mandrin are located within the infiltrate: the risk of complication is then extremely low. Every step is documented with CT or by thorax plan films in two planes. The mandrin is then removed and material is obtained from different areas of the mass under rotating needle movements. Continuous aspiration is performed with a 20-ml disposable syringe. A one-hand handle can be used to assist with guiding the needle. It is important to aspirate peripheral areas of the infiltrate because there is frequently only necrotic material in the center. The needle is removed with continuous aspiration. At the end of the procedure a pneumothorax should be excluded. Furthermore, after 24 hours a follow-up X-ray examination of the lung is also performed (Figs. 4.4.–4.7.).

Biopsy Material

Part of the material obtained is smeared on six slides, the remainder is put into a formalin solution(10%). In addition, material can be placed into a suitable culture media for microbiologic examination. The slide preparations can be evaluated by the pathologist on the same day. The formalin preparation is used for histologi-

cal examination. Because the cylinders are often of such high quality, a histologic diagnosis can be made in the majority of cases (Figs. 4.8. to 4.11.).

Results

In 92.1% of the 644 patients, histologic and cytologic diagnoses could be obtained. Only in 7.9% of the cases was the material insufficient. Primary malignant tumors of the lung were found in 63.2% of the patients, metastases of the lung in 14.1% and benign lesions in 14.8% (Table 4.2.). Of the primary malignant tumors of the lung and pleura, the most frequent forms were 35.9% squamous cell carcinomas, 23.8% adenoma carcinomas and 20.9% small cell carcinomas (Table 4.3.).

Table 4.2. Histological results of fine-needle biopsies in 644 patients.

Primary malignant tumors of lung and pleura	63.2%
Lung metastases	14.1%
Benign diseases	14.8%
Material insufficient	7.9%

Table 4.3. Primary malignant tumors of lung and pleura in 407 (63.2%) of the 644 patients.

Squamous cell carcinoma	35.9%
Adenocarcinoma	23.8%
Small cell carcinoma	20.9%
Large-cell carcinoma	10.8%
Alveolar carcinoma	3.4%
Pleura mesothelioma	3.4%
Others	1.8%

By aspiration of lung metastases (Table 4.4.), it was frequently possible to identify the unknown primary tumor or to narrow down the differential diagnosis. An example is the case of a solitary metastasis of 7 mm diameter where the diagnosis of renal cell carcinoma was made. The primary tumor was localized and removed together with the metastasis.

The appearance of round intrapulmonary masses after the removal of a malignant growth is most likely to be a metastatic lesion. An effort should be made to make a histological diagnosis of such masses because they are frequently secondary tumors.

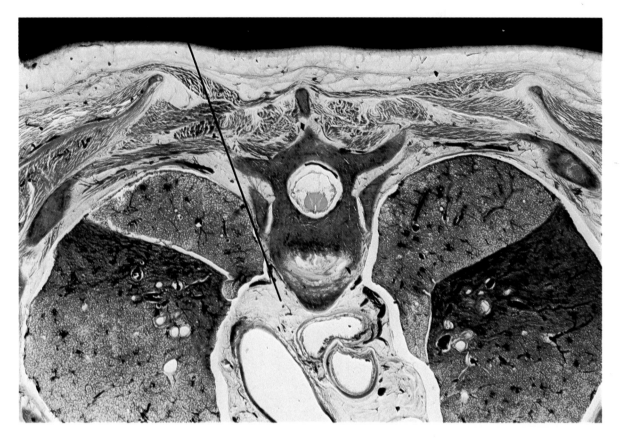

Figs. 4.2. and **4.3.** Anatomic dissection and diagram of the posterior mediastinum at the level of the aortic arch. The needle tip in the simulated puncture is at the level of the retroesophageal lymph node. *1* Trachea; *2* esophagus; *3* aortic arch; *4* lung; *5* retromediastinal tissue; *6* rib; *7* head of rib; *8* intercostal muscles; *9* and *10* iliocostal muscle; *11* medial tract of the back muscles; *12* trapezius muscle.

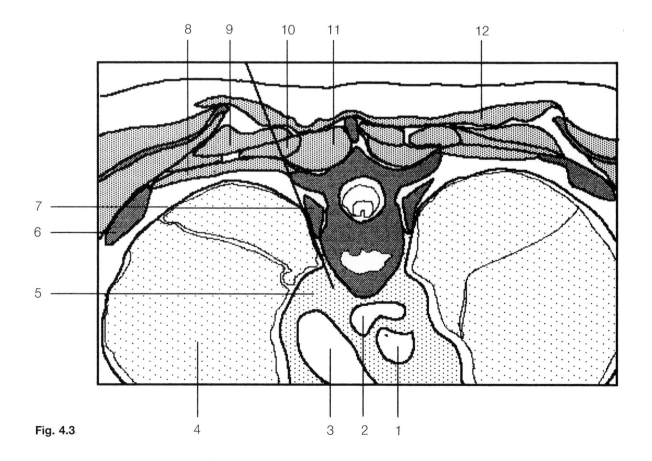

Fig. 4.3

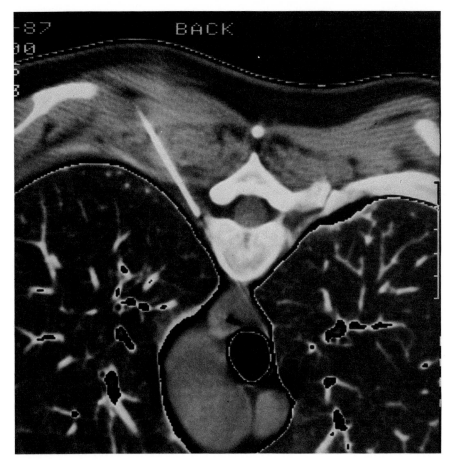

Figs. 4.4.–4.7. 24-year old with dysphagia. CT demonstrates a retroesophageal lymph node about 10 mm in diameter. The anatomic cut (Fig. 4.2.). in the vicinity of the aortic arch and trachea is at a corresponding level to the CT slice. In addition, the azygos vein joins the superior vena cava just below this cut. In the anatomic cut it is not possible to advance the needle into the region of the node without puncturing the lung. However, by using the following technique it is possible to perform the biopsy without a pneumothorax. During CT guidance the needle position is well controlled in each step (Figs. 4.4. and 4.5.). During the advancement of the needle, the pleura is displaced by an injection of local anesthetic ahead of the needle tip. Therefore, using this technique the mediastinum can be biopsied without puncturing the lung. A FNA can be performed after the needle is in the lymph node (Fig. 4.7.). The histologic diagnosis was tuberculosis of the lymph node.

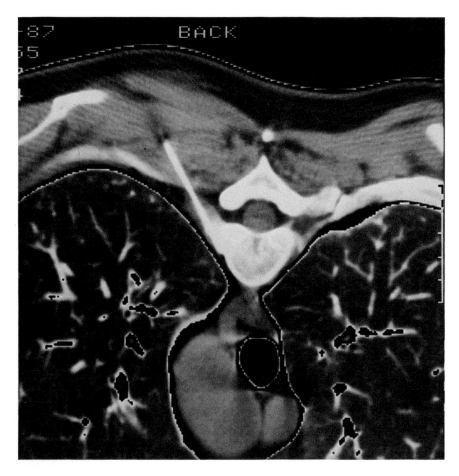

Fig. 4.5.

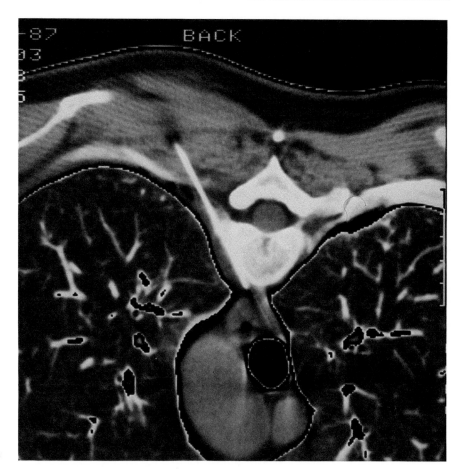

Fig. 4.6

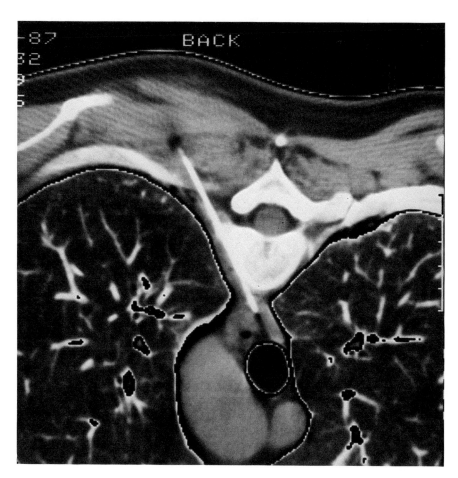

Fig. 4.7

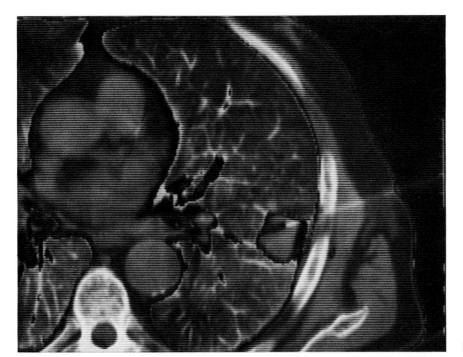

Figs. 4.8. and **4.9.**
Rounded mass in the periphery of the left lung. CT guided FNA from a lateral approach revealed bronchial carcinoma.

Fig. 4.8

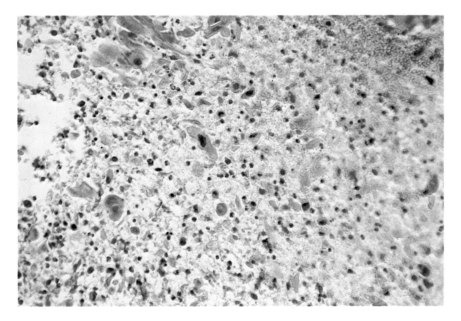

Fig. 4.9

Table 4.4. Origin of pulmonary metastases in 91 (14.1%) of the 644 patients.

Renal cell carcinoma	23.0%
Breast carcinoma	18.7%
Colorectal carcinoma	12.1%
Thyroid carcinoma	8.8%
Urothelial carcinoma	6.6%
Liposarcoma	6.6%
Osteosarcoma	5.5%
Non-Hodgkin lymphoma	4.4%
Hodgkin's lymphoma	3.3%
Chondrosarcoma	2.2%
Plasmocytoma	2.2%
Thyroid sarcoma	2.2%
Ovarian carcinoma	2.2%
Carcinoma of the vulva	2.2%

With fine-needle biopsy of metastatic masses one can check whether a further dedifferentiation has taken place or if the metastasis histologically corresponds to the primary tumor. An example is a female patient with a resected uterine carcinoma. In this patient the biopsy of an intrapulmonary mass showed metastatic spread of a breast carcinoma. As a result appropriate therapy could be initiated.

Punctured benign lesions could not be differentiated radiologically from malignant processes. The majority of lesions presented an intrapulmonary mass without calcification. The punctured pleuromas were located at typical locations in the lung 10 segments [10]. Tuberculosis and abscess-forming pneumonias were also frequently diagnosed by fine-needle biopsy (Table 4.5.).

Figs. 4.10. and **4.11.**
A mass is identified in the right lung with extension into the mediastinum. FNA was performed from a posterior approach with the patient in the prone position. Histology revealed a bronchial carcinoma.

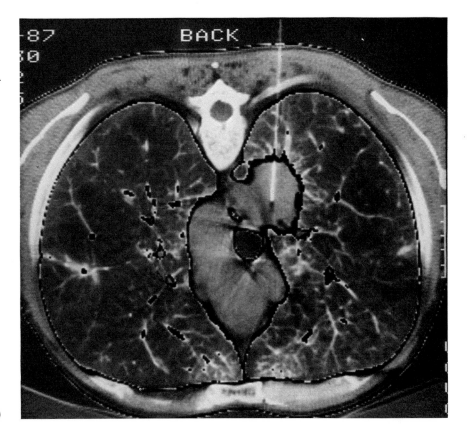

Fig. 4.10

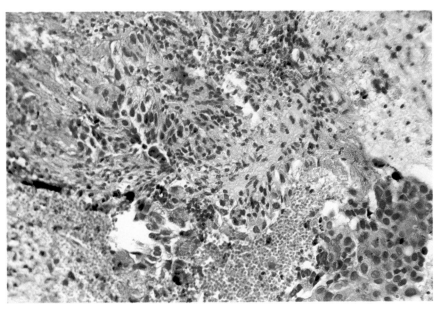

Fig. 4.11

Table 4.5. Benign alterations in 95 (14.8%) of the 644 patients.

Tuberculosis	32.6%
Pneumonia with abscess	31.6%
Non-specific pneumonia	12.6%
Sarcoidosis	8.4%
Fibrosis	6.3%
Pleuroma	5.3%
Adenochondroma	2.1%
Chronic bronchitis	1.1%

Complications

The complication rate depends on additional pulmonary diseases such as emphysemas or fibrosis and the location of the lesion. In peripheral changes with contact with the pleura, side-effects are unlikely. Contrary to the authors' initial thoughts, neither puncture of the central regions of the lung nor the mediastinum increased the risk of complication (Table 4.10.). Puncture of small, basal and centrally located masses may be more time-consuming due to their greater respiratory movement. In these cases the needle tip, if not sufficiently flexible, may damage the lung parenchyma and lead to a pneumothorax. There is a lower incidence of complications if the needle tip rests for several minutes within a solid focus before performing the biopsy. The frequency of complications also depends on the type of biopsy needle used (Table 4.6.).

Table 4.6. Frequency and type of complication.

	n	%
Pneumothorax, total	48	7.5
needing treatment	4	0.6
Shoulder pain	10	1.6
Hemoptysis	9	1.4
Cutaneous emphysema	1	0.2
Total number of patients with one or more complication	54	8.5

Pneumothorax

The most frequent complication after fine-needle biopsy of the lung is the occurrence of a partial pneumothorax. 48 pneumothoraces occurred which is equivalent to 7.5% of the patients.
In only four cases (0.6%) was therapy necessary to treat the pneumothorax. These patients had a chest tube in place. In the other patients the partial pneumothorax was spontaneously absorbed in a few days. A drain is only required when the patient shows dyspnea or if a tensin pneumothorax has occurred. In protracted courses of smaller pneumothorax a complete absorption was proven without therapy.

Hemoptysis

In eight patients a minimal hemoptysis occurred shortly after puncture, which stopped after a few minutes. In one patient with a metastatic renal cell carcinoma and pronounced emphysema, a massive endobronchial bleeding occurred with a reflex resulting cardiovascular arrest during puncture of a basal and central-located metastasis with a cutting-biopsy needle.

Pain

Ten patients experienced ipsilateral shoulder pain approximately 4-8 hours after puncture. In each case, this was due to a small pneumothorax.

Cutaneous Emphysema

One patient with a pneumothorax developed subcutaneous emphysema at the area of the puncture 24 after the procedure. This patient had a chest tube in place because of the pneumothorax.

Comparison of Frequency and Type of Complications by CT- and Fluoroscopy-Guided Puncture

The authors did not find any significant difference in frequency and type of complication in CT- and fluoroscopic-guided punctures using this technique (Table 4.7.).

Table 4.7. Frequency and type of complications when using a CT- or fluoroscopy-guided puncture.

	n = 338 CT-guided puncture		n = 306 fluoroscopy-guided puncture	
	n =	%	n =	%
Pneumothorax, total	28	8.2	20	6.5
needing therapy	0	0	4	1.3
Hemoptysis	3	0.9	6	2.0
Shoulder pain	5	1.5	5	1.6
Cutaneous emphysema	0	0	1	0.72
Total 55 patients	30	8.9	25	8.2

Complications and Age of Patients

The average age of patients who experienced complications was 68.33 years, higher than the age of the other patients (average 60.87 years). The difference between the two groups is statistically significant.

Complications and Size of the Punctured Mass

The average diameter of the mass in patients who suffered complications was 1.46 cm. In the other patients the average diameter measured 2.09 cm. This difference is statistically significant (Table 4.8.).

Table 4.8. Complications versus age of patients and size of tumor.

	Complication	No complication
Age* (years)	68.33	60.87
Size of tumor* (cm)	1.46	2.09

*$p < 0.005$

Location of the Punctured Alterations versus Complications

In tumors with pleural contact no complication was observed after puncture. Complications occurred most frequently after biopsies of the middle lobe (23.9%). A contributing factor for this high complication rate was the puncture point, which was always anteriorly located when puncturing the middle lobe (Tables 4.9. and 4.10.).

Table 4.9. Complications in the relationship with the puncture site.

	Complications n	%
Puncture posterior (n = 483)	27	5.6
lateral (n = 52)	6	11.5
anterior (n = 109)	22	20.2

Table 4.10. Complications versus location of the mass.

	n	% of total punctures
Puncture indeterminated* (n = 78)	5	6.4
Upper lobe (n = 226)	20	7.5
Lower lobe (n = 201)	17	8.5
Middle lobe (n = 46)	11	23.9
Mediastinum (n = 93)	2	2.2
Total	55	8.5

* No specific lobe could be identified

Complications versus Type of Puncture Needles Used

Until 1983, lung punctures were performed with simple puncture needles, 70–90 mm in length and 0.9 mm in diameter or with a Chiba-needle. In 152 procedures using this type of needle, six complications occurred including three pneumothorax. 44 punctures were then performed with a cutting-biopsy needle. Complications occurred in 26 cases. Punctures were performed with newly developed biopsy needles 448 times: in 22 cases a partial pneumothorax occurred (Table 4.11.).

Biopsy Needle

The reason for the development of a new biopsy needle was because of an interest in

Table 4.11. Complications versus biopsy needle used.

	Simple cannula	Cut-biopsy needle [7]	Sei-bel-biopsy needle
Patients with complications	6	26	23
Percentage of patients	3.9	59	5.1
Pneumothorax	3	23	22
Hemoptysis	3	3	3
Pain	3	5	2
Cutaneous emphysema	0	1	0
Drainage after pneumothorax	0	2	2
Total number of punctures	152	44	448

obtaining suitable cylinders for histological examination without increasing the complication rate (Table 4.11.). Thus, a new lung-biopsy needle was developed. The needle can cut tissue cylinders due to a special interior and exterior design. The use of a mandrin prevents the needle from becoming congested with tissue from the thoracic wall, it can also close very tightly so that air embolism is almost impossible even when the needle remains within a vessel for a long period of time. The slanted cut of the needle tip allows repeated puncture of the mass after withdrawing the mandrin without tearing the surrounding lung parenchyma. The repeated puncture of the lesion at different peripheral locations is more accurate because the risk of obtaining only necrotic or unspecific material is reduced. In addition, extremely precise punctures with CT-guidance are possible by using the 1 cm graduated scale on the needle (Fig. 4.12.).

Discussion

Any mass in the lung has to be considered as malignant until proven to the contrary. Because, on the one hand, an early diagnosis of lung tumors by laboratory diagnosis is not possible and, on the other, an X-ray morphology cannot exclude a malignant process, a biopsy diagnosis is desirable even in the case of a smaller lesion. Sputum cytology and bronchoscopy normally fail in cases of small peripheral masses. Furthermore, sputum diagnoses are not sufficiently reliable. Hüttemann found after specific bronchial secretion examination, a cytologically positive result in only 35% of lesions of less than 3 cm diameter [3].

After bronchoscopy, frequently only non-specific tissue can be identified in the examined material, especially when the bronchus has been displaced by inflammatory mucous swellings.

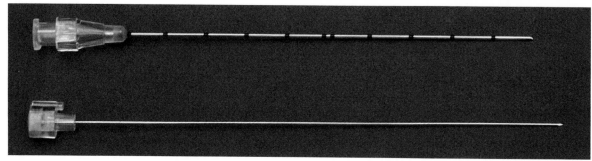

Fig. 4.12. The fine needle developed by the Muelheimer Krankenhaus Institut is well-suited to precise punctures because of the calibrated scale. The special double-cut makes it possible to obtain tissue for histologic evaluation with the minimum of trauma of the surrounding structures. During the biopsy procedure, multiple fan-shaped punctures with aspirations are performed with the needle. The stylet is removed just before the aspiration of the tumor to prevent the needle from clogging with normal tissue.

With a histologic diagnosis of 92%, the percutaneous fine-needle biopsy represents a safe low-risk method for clarification of peripheral as well as central pulmonary masses. A peribronchial specimen can be obtained as well as endobronchial specimen. Furthermore, as opposed to bronchoscopy, it is also possible in post-stenotic infiltrates to diagnose the infectious agent. By examining infiltrates caused by radiation a demonstration of the infectious agent can be made with the fine-needle biopsy (FNB) [8]. Anaerobic bacilli are frequently found using this technique.

FNB considerably shortens the time taken to perform a diagnosis and the length of stay in hospital. We also conducted the procedure in out-patients. They could leave hospital after a stay of approximately 2–3 hours provided that they return the next day for a follow-up examination. After the histologic diagnosis these patients were, if necessary, admitted for further study.

X-ray morphologic criteria and follow-up films can only lead to an approximation of the origin of an intrapulmonary mass. Although calcifications within a mass and a lack of growth point towards benignity, one example revealed after puncturing a calcified focus in the upper lobe, which had not increased in size for years, a squamous cell carcinoma within a tuberculoma. This patient was followed up for pulmonary tuberculosis for several years. The age and history of inhalation of contaminants of a patient can aid the diagnosis of the malignancy of a pulmonary mass. Young patients rarely have a malignant process, but the youngest patient in our examinations with a small cell bronchial carcinoma was only 16 years old.

The time needed for a diagnosis can be shortened because of the minimal risk from FNB. Thus FNB can be used in an increasing number of cases to clarify the presence of intrapulmon-ary masses. In an optimal case with a central tumor in the left hilus, the diagnosis of a small cell bronchial carcinoma was made the same afternoon after performing a FNB and therapy could be initiated the same day.

FNB makes early diagnosis of primary lung tumors in a pre-clinical stage possible. In small stage I bronchial carcinomas (by TNM-classification) after resection, 5-year survival rates of 40-60% can be obtained. In patients with an extensive tumor, where a curative resection is not possible, a diagnostic thoracotomy is unnecessary. After histologic diagnosis with FNB, radiation therapy or chemotherapy can be initiated.

Sinner found in more than 5300 fine-needle punctures of the lung that more than 50% of the patients had a benign process [9, 11]. These results often lead to "overtreatment" to perform primarily (without histologic clarification) surgical intervention in every patient with a pulmonary mass. Similar results are also shown by Toomes et al. in surgically treated patients at the Thorax Clinic in Rohrbach [12].

Secondary tumors of lung rarely require surgical treatment. Many surgeons also abstain from resection in small cell bronchial carcinoma. In more than 40% of our patients with FNB, surgical treatment was unnecessary, and diagnostic thoracotomy could be eliminated.

The appearance of intrapulmonary masses after diagnosis of a malignant growth is frequently equated with metastatic spread. In many cases this results in the discontinuation of further therapy. However, frequently it is a secondary tumor which can be treated for a cure after diagnosis with FNB (Fig. 4.13.).

With the development of a new biospy needle, which can also be used in the abdomen and mediastinum, we were able to reduce the complication rate to approximately 5%. The advantage of this needle is the possibility to extract

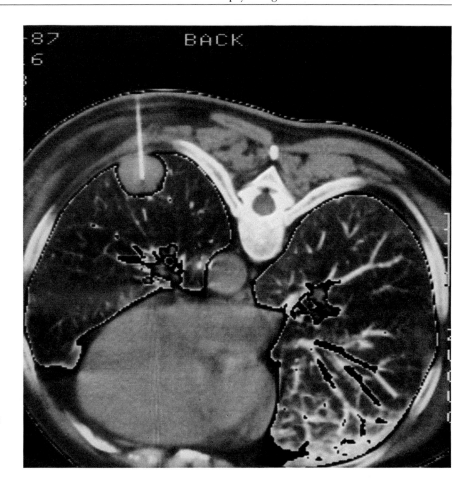

Fig. 4.13. Peripheral mass in the left lower lobe close to pleura. Histologic diagnosis: oat-cell carcinoma.

suitable cylinders of lung tissue for histologic examination. With only one puncture it is possible to obtain tissue from different regions of a mass without increasing the risk of complication.

Small peripheral masses that move with breathing are ideal targets to puncture under fluoroguidance (Figs. 4.14. and 4.15.). CT makes an exact mediastinal, hilar, and pleural puncture possible due to the high tissue differentiation (Figs. 4.16.–4.23.). With Angio-CT vessels in hilus can be differentiated from the tumor. Even the most difficult localities can be reached by CT. A biopsy under CT guidance is also possible in patients with right heart insufficiency using Angio-CT. The 3-D documentation of the needle tip is an additional advantage of CT-puncture.

Summary

The results for FNB of the lung show the following.
1. In 92% of cases histologically usable tissue was obtained that allowed differentiation between benign and malignant processes.
2. The biopsy reduces the time for diagnosis.
3. FNB makes an early diagnosis in the preclinical stage of bronchial carcinomas possible.
4. Differentiation between primary and secondary tumors is possible.
5. Optimum planning of therapy can occur.
6. Follow-up therapy is possible in tumor treatment.
7. Minor complications arise in approximately 5% of cases with the use of the new biopsy needles. This is valid for peripheral location of the punctured mass as well as central location.

The percutaneous FNB under CT guidance and fluoroscopy is today the most safe and precise technique for the biopsy classification of intrapulmonary, pleural, or mediastinal masses. The high histologic efficacy with minor side-effects makes extensive use of this method possible. In difficult cases we also use combination methods with CT and flurosocopy. In this way we utilize the advantages of both methods to reduce further the complication rate and produce a higher efficacy (see Chapter CT- and fluoroscopy-guided percutaneous nucleotomy).

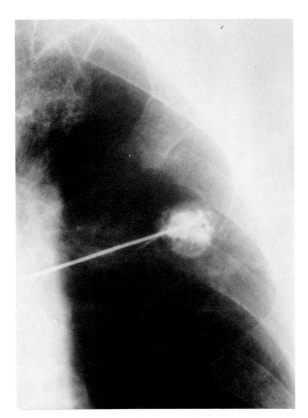 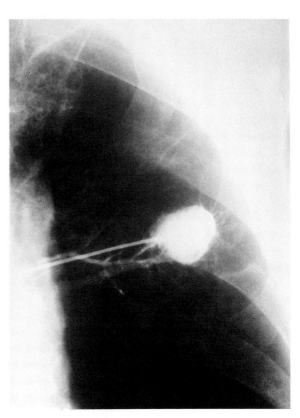

Figs. 4.14. and **4.15.** A solitary focal mass located in the left upper lobe. Blood was aspirated during the puncture. Contrast medium was then injected for a direct angiogram in order to exclude a vascular deformity. The supplying artery and vein to this mass are well defined. Histologic diagnosis: renal cell carcinoma metastasis. Following this study a 2.5 cm renal cell carcinoma was identified in the left kidney. Following nephrectomy and resection of the lung mass, the patient has remained free from cancer for the last six years.

Instruments and medications	
Needle	10-15 cm 20-G needle DTMB 20-15.0 S1 (Cook)
Local anesthetic	10-15 ml Mepivacaine 1%

References

1. Dahlgren S.E., Nordenström B.: Transthoracic-needle biopsy. Year Book Med. Publ., Chicago 1966.
2. Denck H.: Die Chirurgie des Bronchuskarzinoms. Therapiewoche 29 (1979) 8758–8772
3. Hüttemann U.: Die diagnostischen Verfahren bei den unterschiedlichen Erscheinungsformen des Bronchuskarzinoms. Onkologie 1 (1978) 66–69.
4. Leyden O.O.: Über infektiöse Pneumonie. Dtsch. med. Wschr. 9 (1883) 52
5. Menetrier P.: Cancer primitive du poumon. Bull. Soc. anat. Paris 11 (1886) 643
6. Nordenström B., Sinner W.N.: Needle biopsy of pulmonary lesions. Fortschr. Röntgenstr. 129 (1979) 414
7. Otto R.Ch.: Sonographische Feinnadelpunktion: Indikation und Ergebnisse. Dtsch. Ärztebl. 81 (1984) 3573
8. Seibel R.M., Wendt B.K.: Immunglobuline zur Prophylaxe der Strahlenpneumonitis nach großvolumiger Bestrahlung beim Bronchialkarzinom. Onkologie 9 (1986) 43–47
9. Sinner W.N.: Wert und Bedeutung der perkutanen transthorakalen Nadelbiopsie für die Diagnose intrathorakaler Krankheitsprozesse. Fortschr. Röntgenstr. 123 (1975) 197–202
10. Sinner W.N.: Pleuroma – a cancer mimicking atelectatic pseudotumor of the lung. Fortschr. Röntgenstr. 133 (1980) 578
11. Sinner W.N.: Fine needle biopsy of solitary pulmonary metastasis, Europ. J. Radiol. 4 (1984) 9
12. Toomes H., Delphendal A., Manke H.-G., Vogt-Moykopf I.: Der solitäre Lungenrundherd. Differentialdiagnose und Beurteilung. Dtsch. Ärztebl. (1981) 1717–1722

Figs. 4.16. and **4.17.**
This patient has a lymphoma in the upper mediastinum which is relatively difficult to reach. A biopsy from the anterior is not possible because of the anatomy. From a posterior approach the mass can be punctured by advancing the needle near the hilar vessels. Histologic diagnosis: Hodgkin's disease rich in lymphocytes.

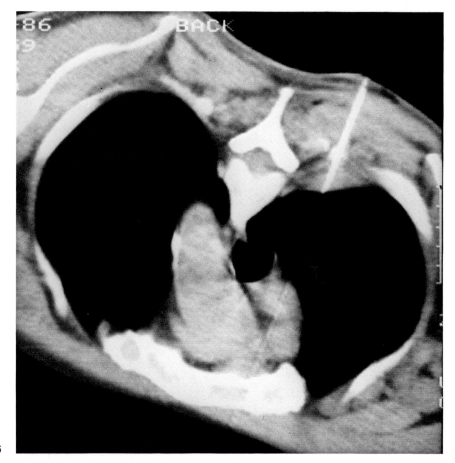

Fig. 4.16

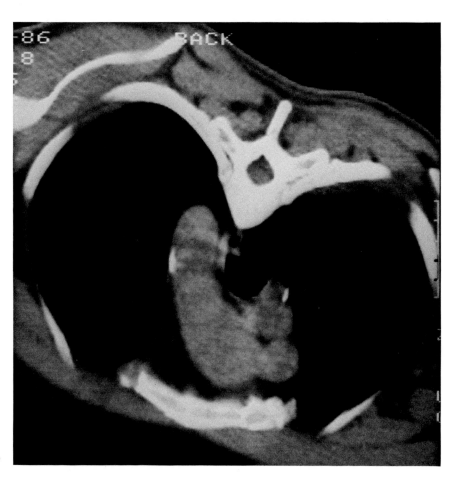

Fig. 4.17

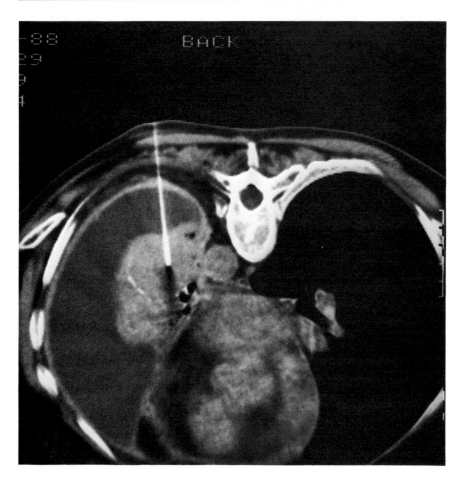

Fig. 4.18. Female patient after mastectomy for breast carcinoma. No tumorous cells were identified in the pleura effusion after multiple punctures. The CT-guided fine-needle biopsy of the left hilum showed the presence of breast cancer cells.

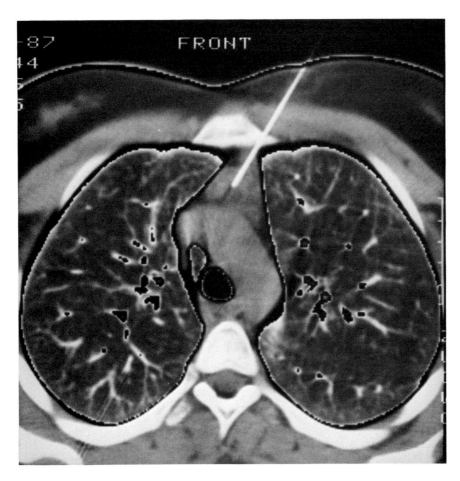

Fig. 4.19

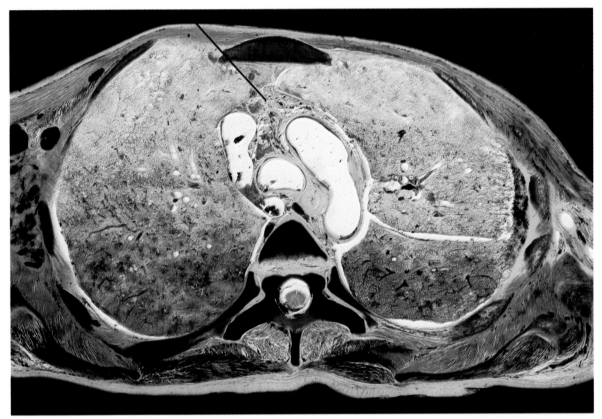

Figs. 4.19.–4.21. These figures demonstrate how the anterior mediastinum can be punctured without injuring the lung. The anatomic cut shows the difficulty in biopsing the anterior upper mediastinum in the vicinity of the great vessels (Fig. 4.20.). The CT puncture is made through the sternocostal joint (Fig. 4.19.). Histologic diagnosis: benign thymoma.

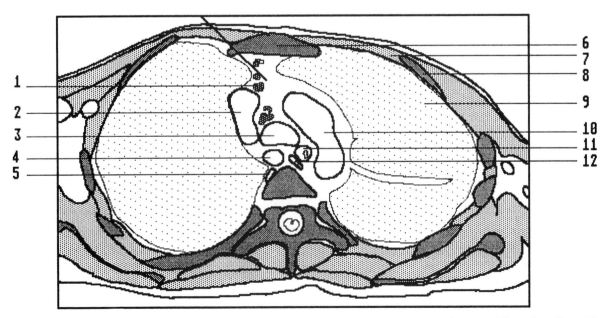

Figs. 4.20. and **4.21.** Simulated biopsy of an anterior upper mediastinum lesion. Anatomic cut and illustration. It would be impossible in this anatomic cut to biopsy the mediastinum from the left without injuring the lung, therefore the puncture is simulated from the right. *1* Lymph node; *2* superior vena cava; *3* trachea; *4* azygos vein; *5* intercostal vein; *6* sternum; *7* pectoralis major muscle; *8* rib; *9* lung; *10* aortic arch; *11* esophagus; *12* accessory hemiazygos vein.

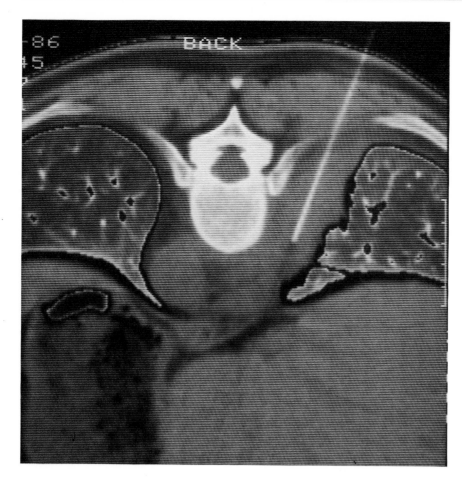

Fig. 4.22. Patient with intercostal neuralgia. A pleura mesothelioma is demonstrated with extension into the posterior mediastinum. Puncture from posterolateral.

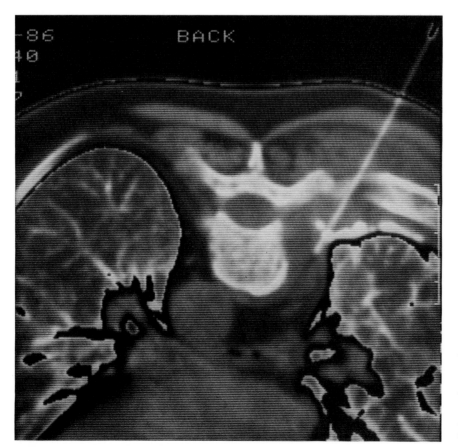

Fig. 4.23. Patient with intercostal neuralgia. A paravertebral mass can be seen with evidence of an erosion of the lateral vertebral body. Furthermore, calcified pleura is identified. Histological tuberculosis.

Chapter 5
CT-Guided Liver Biopsy

B. Kramann

Indications

The radiologic differential diagnosis of focal liver lesions is subject to considerable uncertainty. This uncertainty is the cause of the increasing interest in CT-guided punctures. The CT-guided technique is safer than US-guided biopsy, especially in small and/or deep-seated lesions. Furthermore, the ability to avoid high-risk biopsy routes and to collect material from the non-necrotic tumor margins is greater with the CT-guided technique than with sonography. Two main advantages of the CT-guided biopsy are better control of the needle tip and improved documentation of the needle position. Indications for CT-guided liver biopsy are any focal lesions where a suspicion of malignancy cannot be excluded and where obtaining the diagnosis can be followed by therapy.

Contraindications

A significant coagulopathy is a contraindication to this technique. The danger of puncturing a hemangioma is not a contraindication, since it has been clearly demonstrated in the literature that there is only a minimal risk of such a puncture. Earlier reports estimated a high risk of hemangioma puncture, but more recent articles have shown a much lower risk of hemorrhage [4]. Prior to the puncture of any cystic lesion, echinococcosis must be excluded serologically. However, one must be careful since the echinococcosis complement fixation test can have false negative results.

Examination Technique

The access route to a liver lesion is determined by the topography. Normally, the shortest distance is preferred (Fig. 5.3.). However, in cases where a hemangioma is in the differential diagnosis, a longer intraparenchymatous puncture tract should be selected. This longer tract can self-tamponade after a hemorrhagic puncture [3]. The longer puncture tract is especially helpful for lesions located close to the liver surface (Figs. 5.1. and 5.2.). In cases of subphrenic masses, a transpleural access is technically easier to perform than a puncture directed medial and superior, which avoids the pleural space. If a pleurocentesis cannot be circumvented with maximum inspiration, then it is recommended to perform the puncture at maximum expiration or with the patient in the lateral position (Fig. 5.4.), because under these conditions the pleural recesses will contain little or no lung tissue [3].

The selection of puncture needles depends on tumor size as well as on the puncture route. There have been numerous reports comparing cutting biopsy versus fine-needle aspiration biopsy. Andriole et al. [1] experimentally examined different biopsy needles with calibers between 14 and 22 gauge. They found that the amount of material obtained was 15 times greater with the utilization of a 14-G needle than with a thin caliber 22-G needle. Histologic assessment of the tissue specimen was possible from a caliber of 20-G and larger. Furthermore, artifacts caused by the puncture technique were less frequently observed in tissue specimens obtained with large caliber needles. These experimentally obtained results were also verified by clinical examinations [2, 6]. Pagani reports a sensitivity of 84% with the utilization of 14-G and 18-G needles [7]. The high success rates from biopsies with large diameter cannulas by comparison with needles with a small lumen have also been reported by other authors [2, 6]. Additionally, the specificity with the use of a cutting biopsy is higher when compared with a fine-needle aspiration biopsy, because histochemical examinations can also be conducted. Lüning et al. [5] pointed out that a large number of aspirates per biopsy is needed, therefore, he recommended that biopsy material be obtained at least four different times.

The possibilities of incorrect cytologic diagnosis are well-known. Apart from the quality of the material and its preparation, difficulties can arise from the differentiation of pseudoatypical changes caused by inflammation from genuine

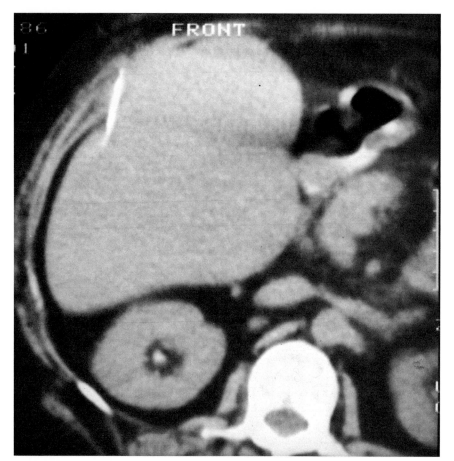

Figs. 5.1. and **5.2.** 58-year old female patient with cirrhosis of the liver, acute icterus and a bilirubin of 15 mg%. A liver biopsy was ordered to determine the cause of her icterus. The patient had a reduced pro-thrombin value of 50%. In these cases, a CT-guided fine-needle biopsy can be performed with only a minor danger of bleeding. The needle was placed from the anterior approach deep into the parenchyma along the periphery of the liver. With this technique the large intrahepatic vessels are not punctured. Histo-logic diagnosis – chronic progressive cirrhosis of the liver.

Fig. 5.1

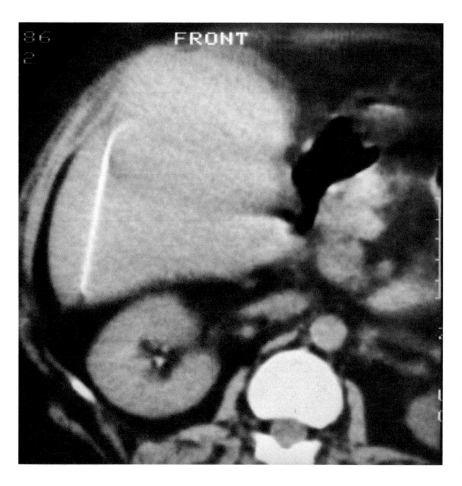

Fig. 5.2

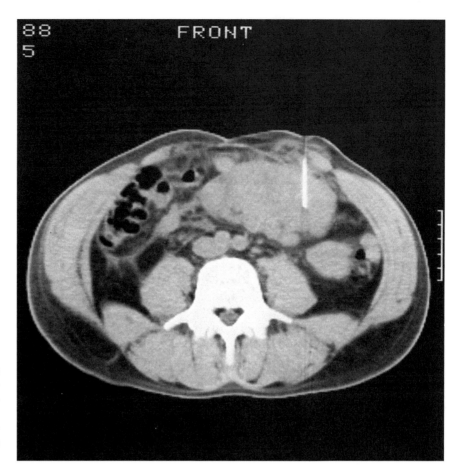

Fig. 5.3. Extensive metastasis to the left lobe of the liver. Evidence of mesenteric and peritoneal metastases are also present. Histologic diagnosis – metastasis to the liver from a colorectal carcinoma.

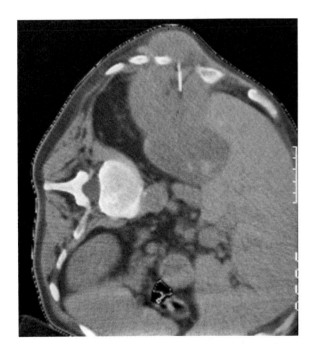

Fig. 5.4. With the patient lying on the left side, a puncture is performed of an extensive mass, originating in the right liver lobe, which has extended through the thoracic wall. Histologic diagnosis – malignant histiocytic lymphoma. The patient was treated with intratumoral therapy with MRI-guidance (see Chapter 23, Figs. 23.30.–23.31.).

atypical cells, which is always difficult and can sometimes be impossible.

The value of a cutting biopsy is often greater than that of FNA, especially in cases of benign processes. CT-guided fine-needle punctures with needles smaller than 20-G should preferably be performed only in the neighborhood of high risk structures, such as the vicinity of the porta of the liver or within the subphrenic region. Otherwise, it is recommended to use a 20-G needle, DTMB 20–15 SIN (Cook, Inc.) as, even with this small caliber, a cutting biopsy is still possible (Figs. 4.5. and 4.6.). Furthermore, another advantage of the 20-G needle is that the needle can be inserted in a fan-like fashion into different tumor areas as with the puncture for aspiration biopsy.

Complications

Complications are rare with the CT-guided liver biopsy. Martino et al. [6] report two cases of hemorrhage and one case of hematoma. The authors describe a complication rate of 0.9% with the fine-needle biopsy and 1.4% with the cutting biopsy. Furthermore, it is remarkable that even in punctures of hemangiomas with

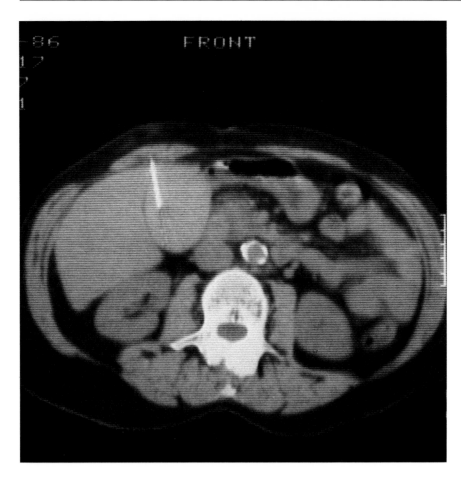

Fig. 5.5. Homogeneous thickening of the gall-bladder wall. CT-guided biopsy of the gall-bladder wall was performed from an anterior approach. Histologic diagnosis – gall-bladder carcinoma.

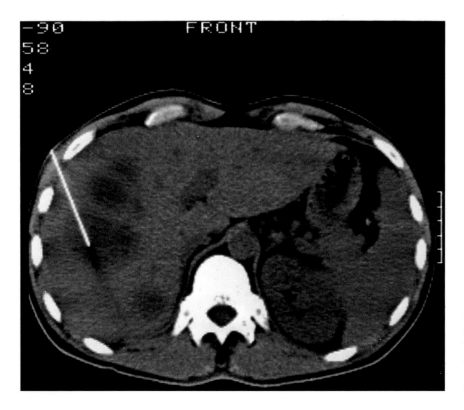

Fig. 5.6. Four large hypodense masses in the right lobe of the liver. CT-guided fine-needle biopsy from an anterolateral intercostal approach. Histologic diagnosis – abscess of amoeba.

cutting biopsy cannulas there were no reports of severe bleeding.

References

1. Andriole J.G., Haaga J.R., Adams R.B., Nunez C.: Biopsy needle chracteristics assessed in laboratory. Radiology 148 (1983) 659
2. Feuerbach S.: Perkutane Biopsie. In: Clausen C., Felix R. (Hrsg.) Quo vadis CT: Berlin, Heidelberg, New York 1988, 284
3. Haaga J.R., LiPuma J.P., Bryan P.J., Balsara V.S., Cohen A.M.: Clinical comparsion of small- and large-caliber cutting needles for biopsy. Radiology 146 (1983) 665
4. Klose K.Ch., Günther R.W.: CT-gesteuerte Punktionen. In: Günther R.W., Thelen M. (Hrsg.) Interventionelle Radiologie, Stuttgart 1988, 459
5. Lackner M., Landwehr P., Schlolaut K.-H., Feyrabend Th.: CT-gesteuerte Punktionen. In: Friedmann G., Steinbrich W., Angioplastie, Embolisation, Punktion, Drainagen. Interventionelle Methoden der Radiologie. Konstanz 1989, 147
6. Lüning M., Schmidt B., Hoppe E.: CT-gestützte Feinnadelbiopsien bei Leberraumforderungen. Ein Vergleich der Ergebnisse einer Arbeitsgruppe von zwei Zeiträumen. Röntgenpraxis 42 (1989) 1974
7. Martino C.T., Haaga J.R., Bryan P.J., LiPuma J.P., El Yousef S.J., Alfodo R.J.: CT-guided liver biopsies: Eight years' experience. Radiology 152 (1984) 755
8. Pagani J.: Biopsy of focal hepatic lesions. Comparison of 18 and 22 gauge needles. Radiology 147 (1983) 673

Chapter 6
Pancreas

D.H.W. Grönemeyer, R.M.M. Seibel

Figs. 6.1. and **6.2.**
Anatomic cut and illustration of the abdomen at the level of the pancreas.
1 Pancreas; *2* splenic artery; *3* inferior vena cava; *4* adrenal gland; *5* latissimus dorsi muscle; *6* liver; *7* kidney; *8* diaphragm; *9* back musculature.

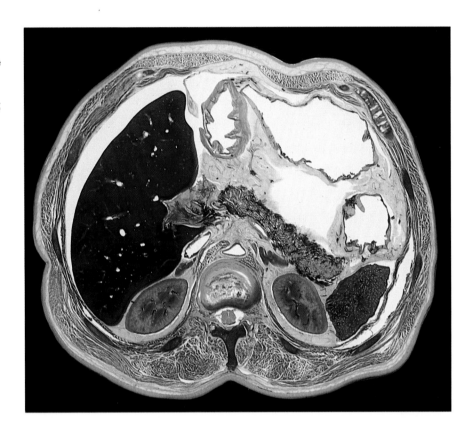

Fig. 6.1

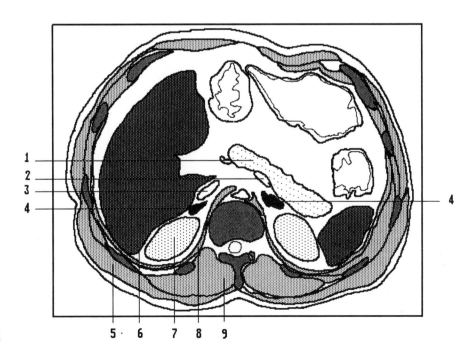

Fig. 6.2

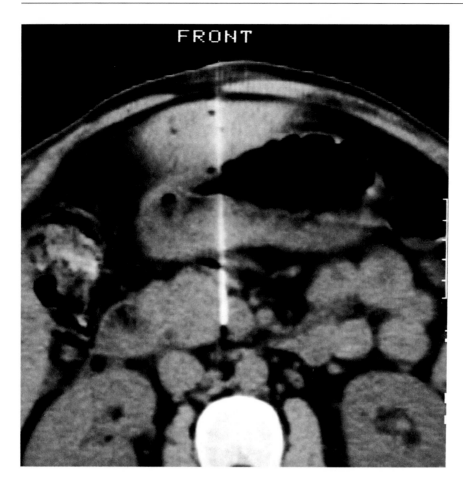

Fig. 6.3. Angio CT shows a hyperdense mass in the region of the uncinate process, measuring 1.5 cm in diameter. The CT-guided fine-needle biopsy was performed through the left lobe of the liver and the stomach. The needle tip is positioned within the tumor. Histologic diagnosis – pancreatic carcinoma.

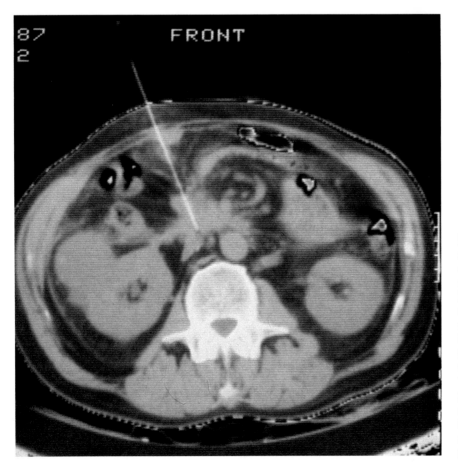

Fig. 6.4. 45-year old man, status post-Whipple's operation two years earlier for carcinoma of pancreas head. CT was suspicious of a local recurrence with compression and infiltration in the mesentery. A metastasis of the right kidney was also suspected. The CT-guided biopsy was planned at an angle to avoid puncturing the intestine. Histologic diagnosis – recurrent pancreatic carcinoma.

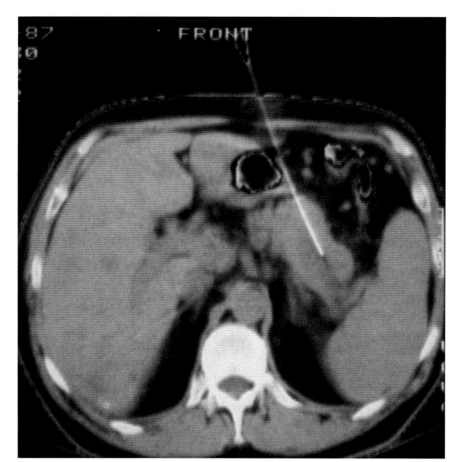

Fig. 6.5. Inhomogeneous enlargement of the pancreatic tail. The CT-guided fine-needle biopsy was performed perigastrically without endangering the splenic vessels. Histologic diagnosis – pancreatic carcinoma.

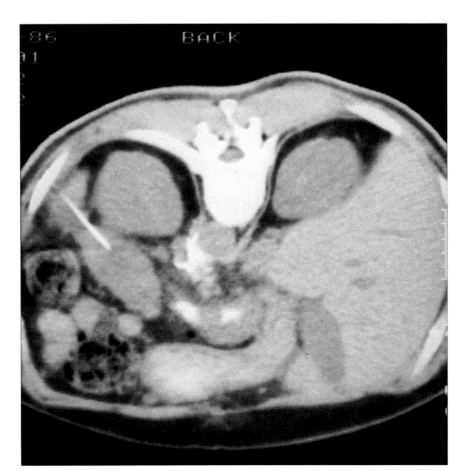

Fig. 6.6. Inhomogeneous enlargement of the pancreatic tail. A puncture was performed from a posterolateral approach in the prone position. The needle biopsy was carried out in the tail of the pancreas below the spleen. Histologic diagnosis – pancreatic carcinoma.

Chapter 7
Adrenal Gland

D.H.W. Grönemeyer, R.M.M. Seibel

Figs. 7.1. and **7.2.** *1* Back musculature; *2* diaphragm; *3* kidney; *4* liver; *5* latissimus dorsi muscle; *6* adrenal gland; *7* inferior vena cava; *8* splenic artery; *9* pancreas.

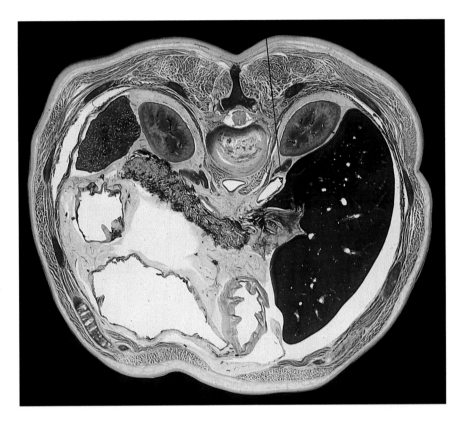

Fig. 7.1. Anatomic cut at the level of the adrenal glands with a simulated puncture of the right adrenal gland. The position of the kidney and the vena cava can make this puncture difficult. Also, the posteroinferior recess of the pleura can extend deep into this region. Therefore, in these cases a caudocranial approach is normally selected for puncture to avoid the risk of a pneumothòrax (3-D puncture).

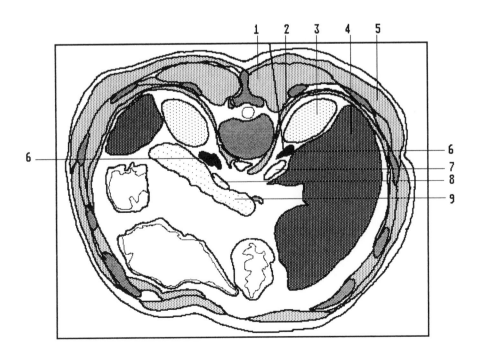

Fig. 7.2. Drawing of the anatomic dissection.

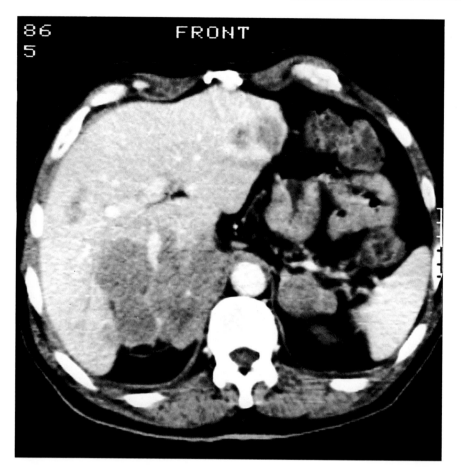

Figs. 7.3. and **7.4.** 68-year old patient who had a malignant melanoma removed 6 years earlier. An abdominal ultrasound showed evidence of multiple liver and right adrenal gland metastases. Angio-CT demonstrates an anterolateral displacement of a compressed vena cava.

Fig. 7.3

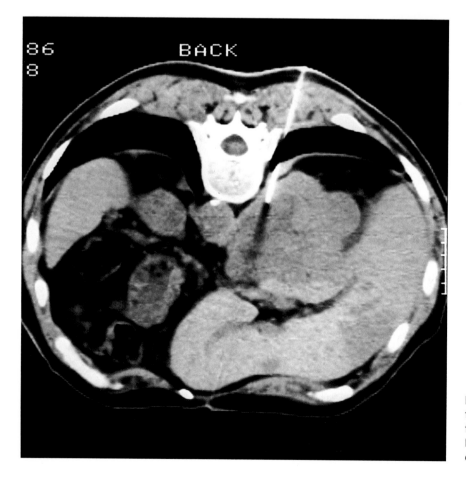

Fig. 7.4. CT-guided puncture from posterior through the inferior pleural recess. Histologic diagnosis – small cell carcinoma of the lung.

Figs. 7.5.–7.8. 71-year old patient with a peripheral lung mass. CT shows a mass in the left adrenal gland, suspicious of a metastasis. The right adrenal gland is moderately enlarged and arteriosclerosis is identified in the abdominal aorta. A puncture of the left adrenal gland was performed with a special dual-needle technique. The first needle is a 22-G, which is placed next to the kidney (Figs. 7.5. and 7.6.) to avoid any injury to the kidney. This puncture is performed in expiration and below the inferior pleural recess. Then a second needle is introduced with the tip tilted medially. This second puncture is performed with a 20-G needle (Fig. 7.7.). In this scan, the tip of the needle is within the tumor. Histologic diagnosis – small cell lung carcinoma metastasis.

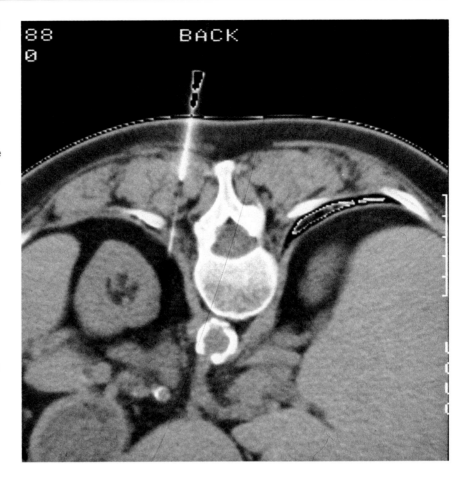

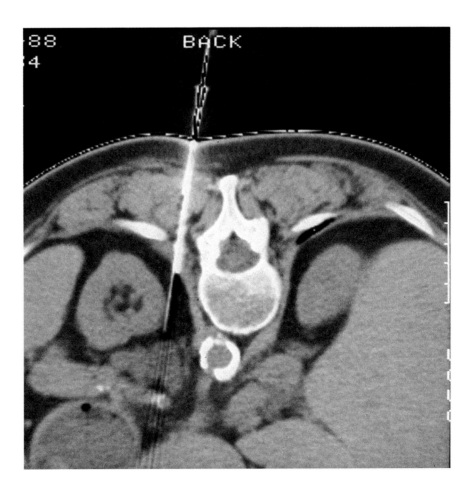

Fig. 7.6

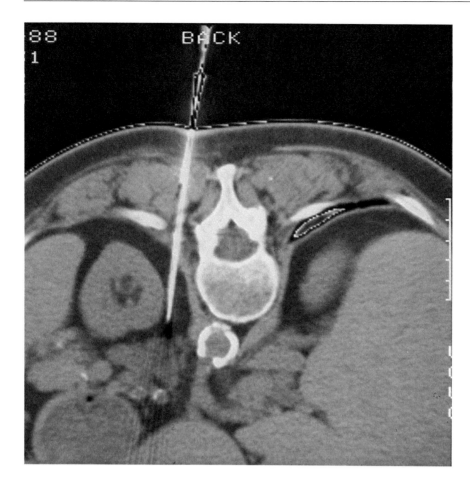

Fig. 7.7

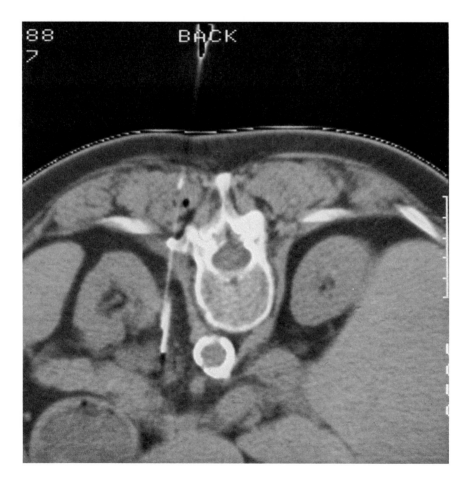

Fig. 7.8

Figs. 7.9.–7.12. In this case a steep caudo-cranial tilt to the needle is used in this puncture. The cutaneous puncture point (Fig. 7.9.) is located below the inferior pleural recess. The needle's cranial course is documented step by step (Figs. 7.10.–7.12.). The needle tip rests at the edge of the mass (Fig. 7.12.). In this case a dual-needle technique was selected, thereby fixing the tissue in this subdiaphragmatic route (Fig. 7.12.).

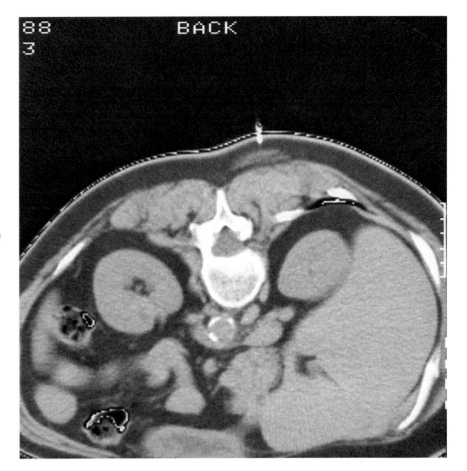

Fig. 7.9

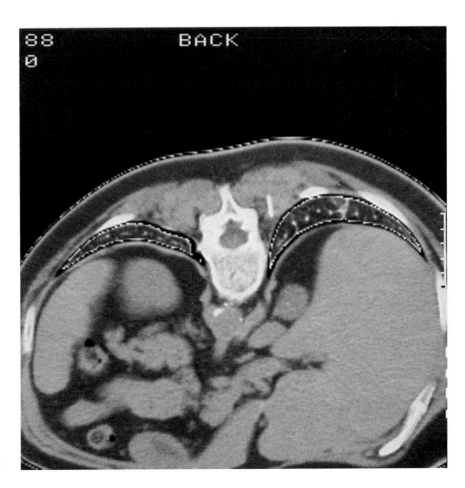

Fig. 7.10

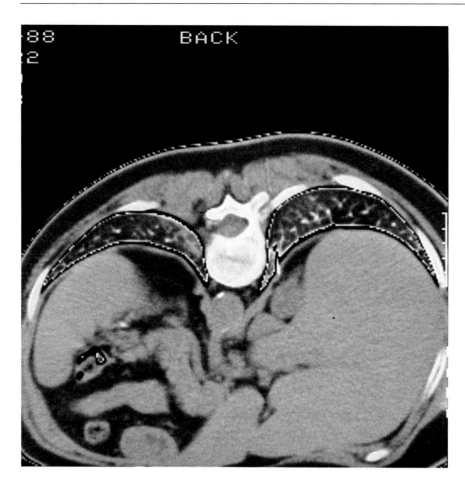

Fig. 7.11

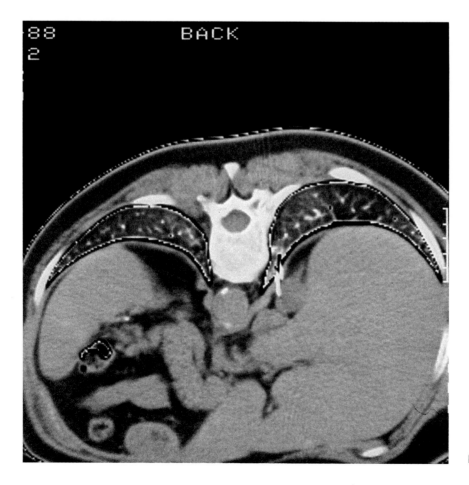

Fig. 7.12

Figs. 7.13. and **7.14.** A difficult puncture immediately medial to the left kidney. In this case the puncture needle must be advanced past the transverse process of the thoracic vertebrale superiorly to the left renal artery into the adrenal mass.

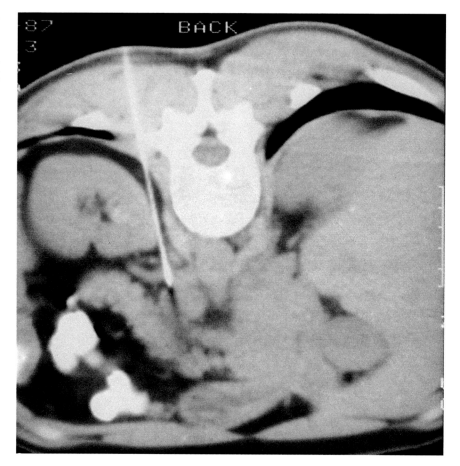

Fig. 7.13

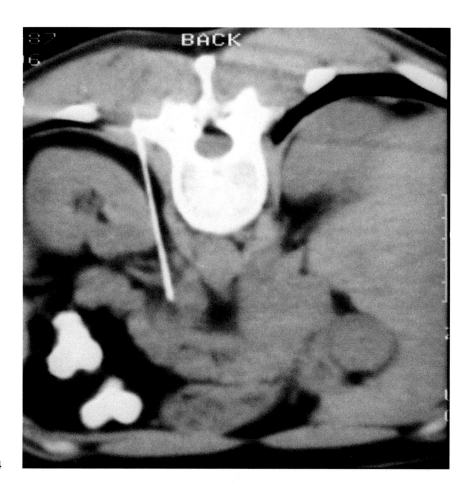

Fig. 7.14

Figs. 7.15. and **7.16.**
Puncture of the right adrenal gland with a 20-G fine needle from a posterior approach. The margins of the tumor were punctured due to the possibility of necrois in the center (Fig. 7.15.). Histologic diagnosis – small cell carcinoma of the lung.

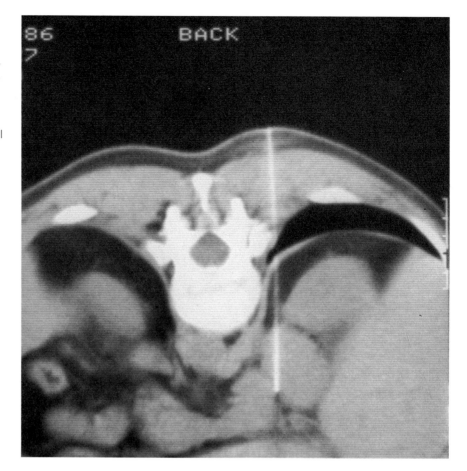

Fig. 7.15

Fig. 7.16

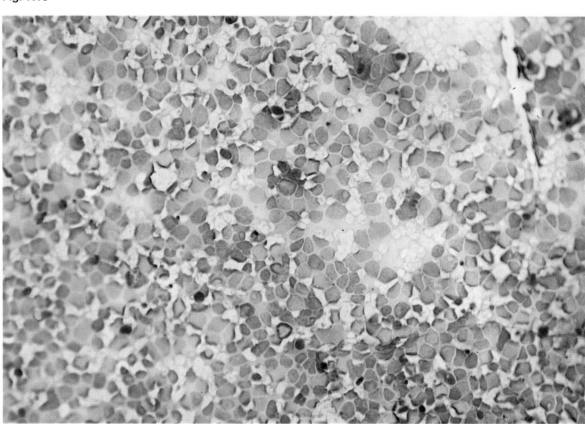

Chapter 8
Kidney

D.H.W. Grönemeyer, R.M.M. Seibel

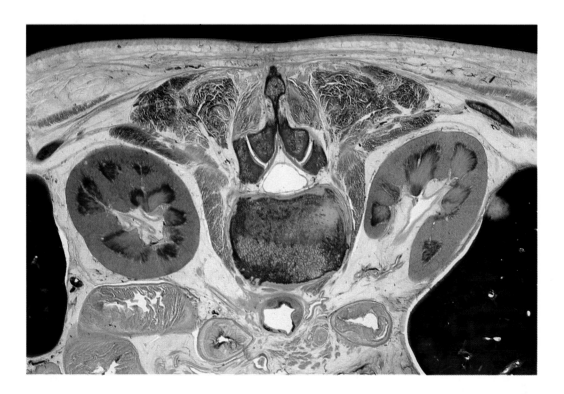

Fig. 8.1

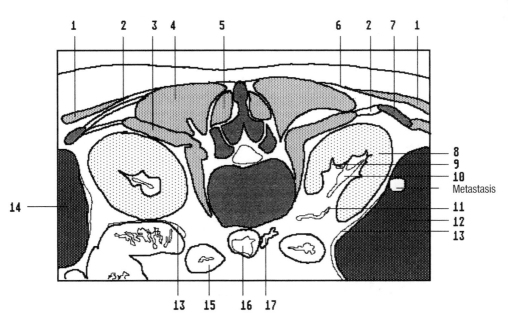

Fig. 8.2

Figs. 8.1. and **8.2.** Anatomic cut and illustration at the level of the renal pelvis. The anatomic cut demonstrates a subcapsular metastasis in the liver. *1* Latissimus dorsi m.; *2* thoracolumbar fascia; *3* diaphragm; *4* iliocostal m.; *5* spinal muscles; *6* thoracolumbar fascia; *7* rib; *8* kidney; *9* renal papilla; *10* renal pelvis; *11* ureter; *12* liver; *13* peritoneum; *14* spleen; *15* intestine; *16* aorta; *17* inferior vena cava.

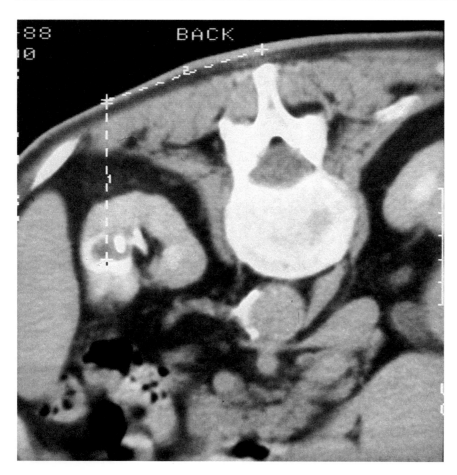

Fig. 8.3. Renal biopsy planning-CT. The left kidney is shown after contrast-medium infusion. A half-moon shaped area of contrast enhancement around a hyperdense space-occupying mass in the region of a lateral group of calyces is shown (1.8 cm in diameter).

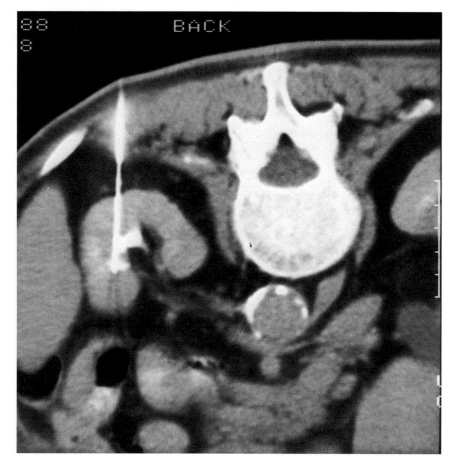

Fig. 8.4. Renal biopsy. Puncture was performed in the prone position through the back musculature (lateral segment) lateral to the major psoas m. through anterior portions of the diaphragm. The tip of the needle is in the anterior portion of the half-moon shaped contrast-medium area. The contrast medium was tapped and a tissue specimen was obtained. Diagnosis – renal tuberculoma with an area of caseation. Further review of the CT shows the renal artery and renal vein in their entire course. The kidney outline shows a wave-like configuration and has fine peripheral stranding of the perirenal fat. These findings point towards inflammatory sequelae.

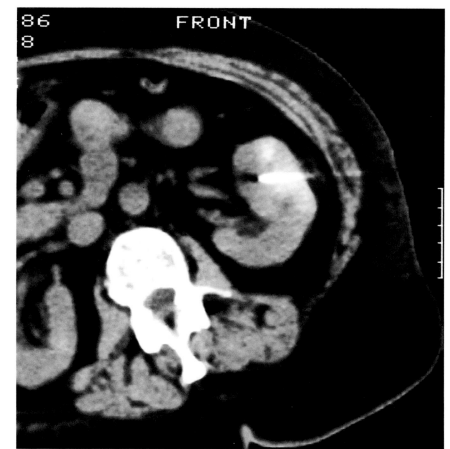

Fig. 8.5. Sonographic suspicion of a mass in the left kidney. Renal biopsy was carried out in the area of the thickened lateral parenchyma. The puncture was performed in the supine position through the following muscles (sequence from lateral to medial): External oblique m.; internal oblique m.; transverse m. The position of the needle tip is documented by the medial hyperdense (black) metal artifact ahead of the tip. Result of biopsy – kidney variation with normal parenchyma.

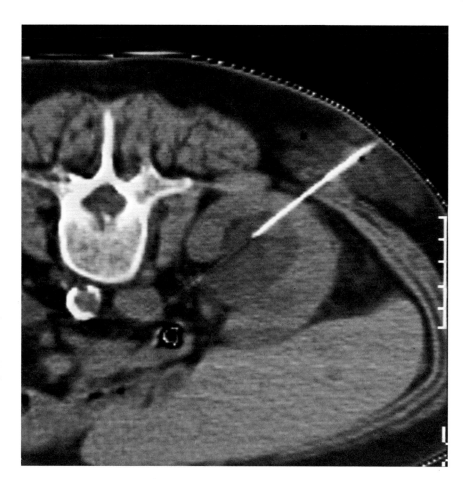

Fig. 8.6. CT-guided biopsy of the renal pelvis from right posterolateral approach. This female patient had a pyogenic pyelonephritis with a surrounded membrane. As a follow-up to the biopsy a percutaneous nephrostomy was placed for abscess drainage.

Chapter 9
Pelvis

D.H.W. Grönemeyer, R.M.M. Seibel

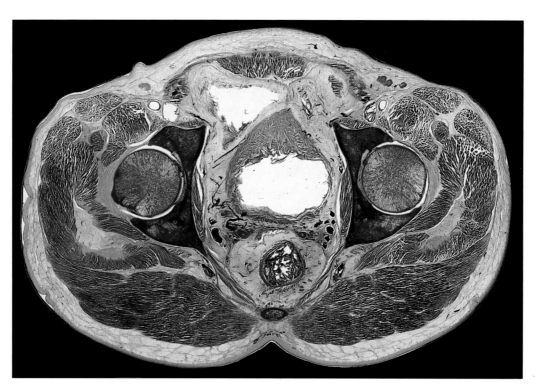

Fig. 9.1

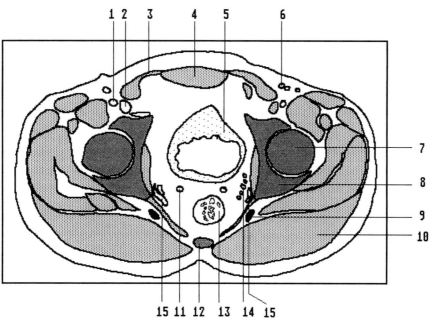

Fig. 9.2

Figs. 9.1. and **9.2.** Anatomy of pelvis at level of the femoral head. Anatomic cut and illustration. *1* Femoral artery; *2* femoral vein; *3* internal oblique m.; *4* rectus abdominis m.; *5* bladder; *6* lymph node; *7* head of the femur; *8* ischium; *9* inferior gluteal vein and sciatic nerve; *10* gluteus maximus m.; *11* ureter; *12* coccyx; *13* rectum; *14* internal iliac artery and vein; *15* sacral plexus.

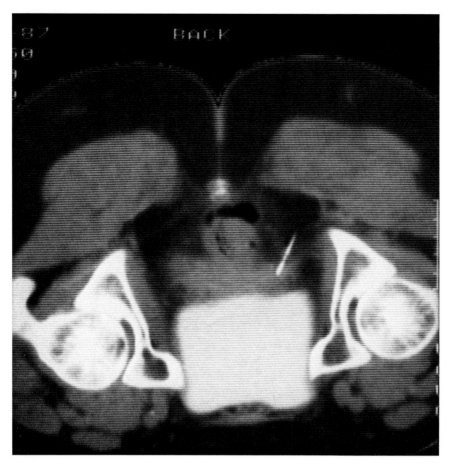

Fig. 9.3. CT of a male pelvis at the level of the hip joints. A retrovesical mass with infiltration into the anterior wall of rectum is identified. CT-guided biopsy was performed from a posterolateral approach through the gluteal muscles. In this scan the needle tip is in the retrovesical mass. Histologic diagnosis – carcinoma of the prostate.

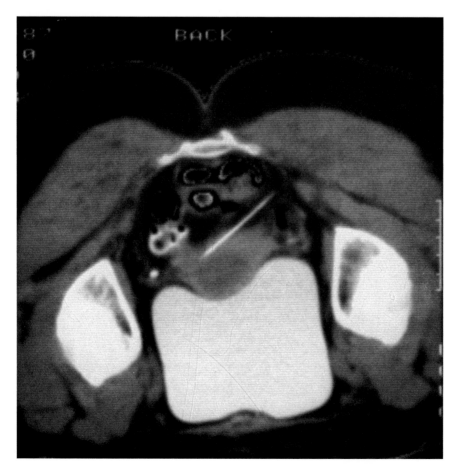

Fig. 9.4. 62-year old female patient with a hysterectomy for carcinoma of the cervix 4 years ago. CT demonstates a partially cystic, partially solid retrovesical mass at the level of the vaginal stump. CT-guided biopsy was performed from a posterolateral approach. Histologic diagnosis – recurrence of cervical carcinoma.

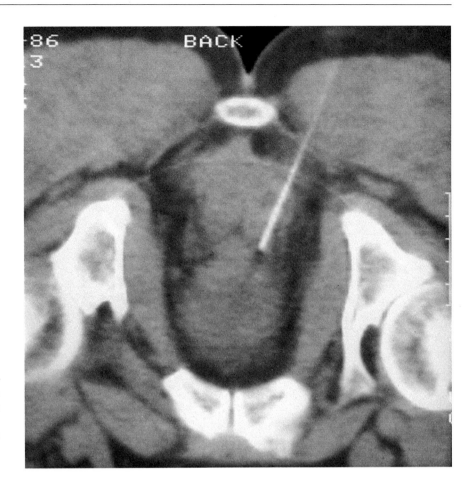

Fig. 9.5. 49-year old patient one year after resection of the rectum. The patient had normal tumor markers, CEA and no pain symptoms. Follow-up CT shows a precoccygeal mass. Histologic diagnosis – recurrent rectal carcinoma.

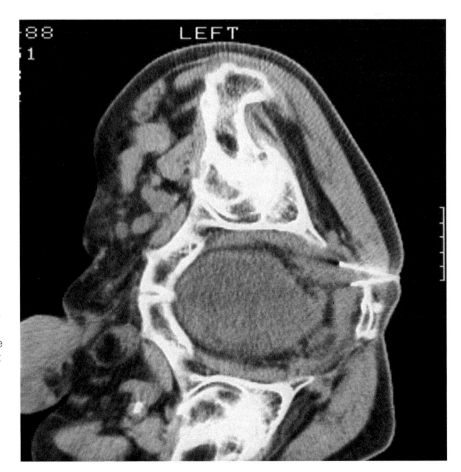

Fig. 9.6. 64-year old patient, status post resection of the rectum for carcinoma. Follow-up CT shows a strong suspicion of extensive recurrence in the region of the pelvic wall. CT-guided biopsy was performed with the patient lying on the right side. Tissue was obtained from different areas of the tumor during the same session using two different needles. The sciatic nerve is located just lateral to the tumor. Histologic diagnosis – recurrent rectal carcinoma.

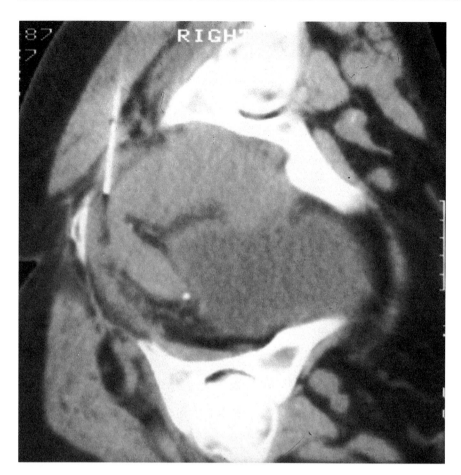

Fig. 9.7. CT shows an extensive tumor located predominantly in the right and posterior pelvic wall. CT-guided biopsy was performed from a lateral approach with the patient lying on the left side. The needle tip is precoccygeal. Histologic diagnosis – extensive recurrent carcinoma of the cervix.

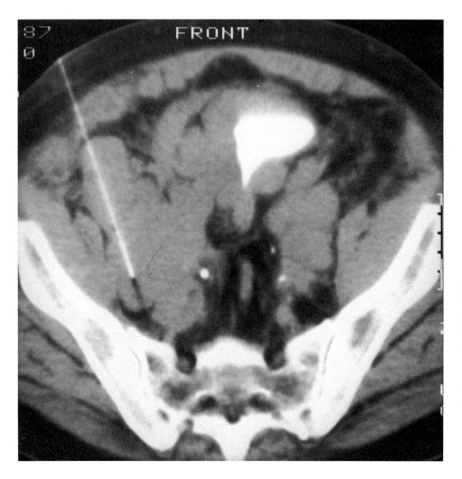

Fig. 9.8. 61-year old patient with thrombosis of the pelvic veins. The CT shows the cause to be an extensive tumor alongside the right iliac vessels. Additionally, this tumor had infiltrated the bladder wall. CT-guided fine-needle biopsy was performed from an anterior approach. Histologic diagnosis – myxoid liposarcoma.

Chapter 10
Retroperitoneum

D.H.W. Grönemeyer, R.M.M. Seibel

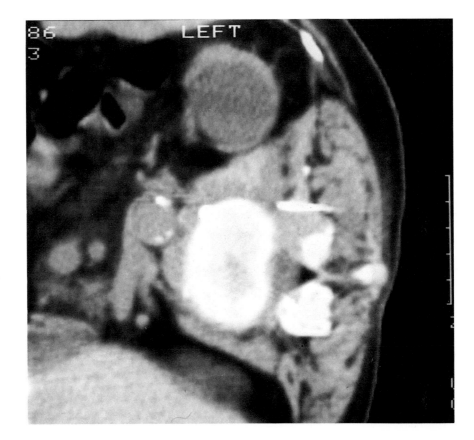

Fig. 10.1. Tumor destruction of the left vertebral arch by an osteolytic metastasis extending to the left psoas muscle. CT-guided biopsy was performed from a posterior approach with the patient lying on the right side. Histologic diagnosis – malignant histiocytoma.

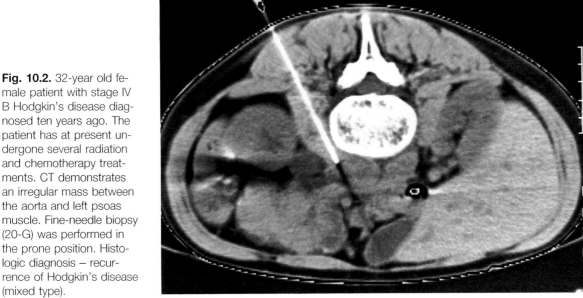

Fig. 10.2. 32-year old female patient with stage IV B Hodgkin's disease diagnosed ten years ago. The patient has at present undergone several radiation and chemotherapy treatments. CT demonstrates an irregular mass between the aorta and left psoas muscle. Fine-needle biopsy (20-G) was performed in the prone position. Histologic diagnosis – recurrence of Hodgkin's disease (mixed type).

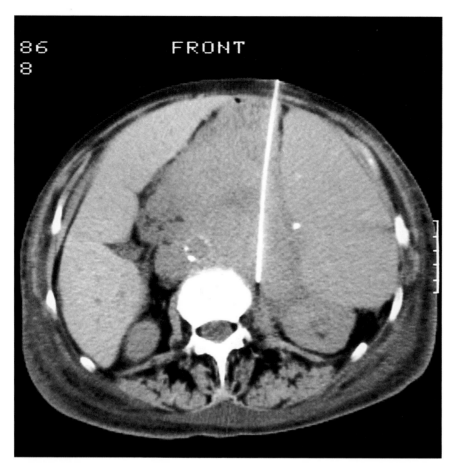

Fig. 10.3. 72-year old female with extensive tumor that has displaced the aorta to the right. The vena cava is compressed by this tumor. The mass extends to the hilus of the liver, to the splenic hilum and anteriorly to the peritoneum of the anterior abdominal wall. Hepatosplenomegaly is also identified. A CT-guided biopsy with a 20-G fine-needle was performed from an anterior approach. Histologic diagnosis – centrocytic-centroblastic malignant lymphoma.

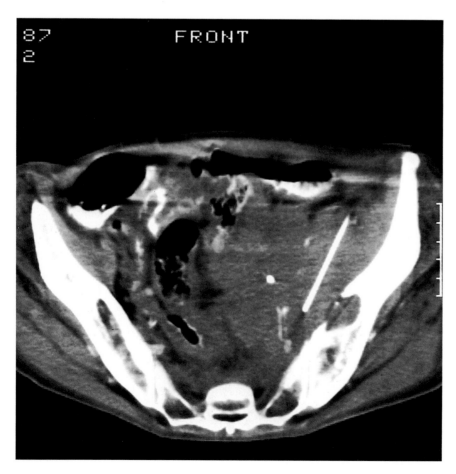

Fig. 10.4. CT demonstrates extensive retroperitoneal tumor in the left pelvis with thrombosis of the femoral and iliac veins and also destruction of the left ilium. The tumor has displaced the large and the small intestine. Histologic diagnosis – fibrosarcoma.

Figs. 10.5. and **10.6.** 26-year old patient with a 4 cm mass located in front of the vena cava. CT-guided fine-needle biopsy was performed from a posterolateral approach. The needle was advanced into the tumor past a loop of small intestine, just below the right kidney pole and beside the ureter.

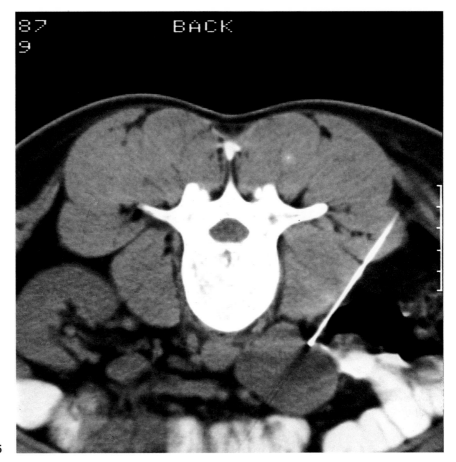

Fig. 10.5

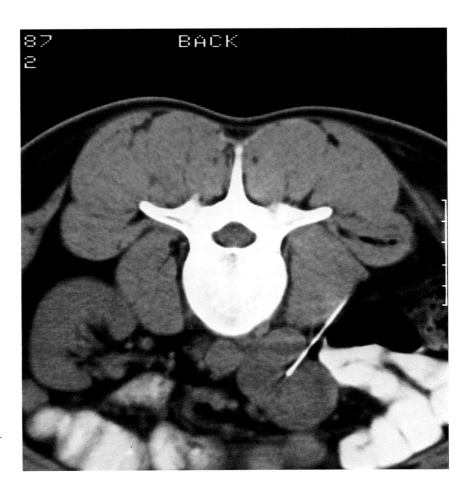

Fig. 10.6. The needle was advanced into the mass past the vena cava. Now the vena cava can be separated from the mass by this needle. Histologic diagnosis – neurofibroma (unusual location).

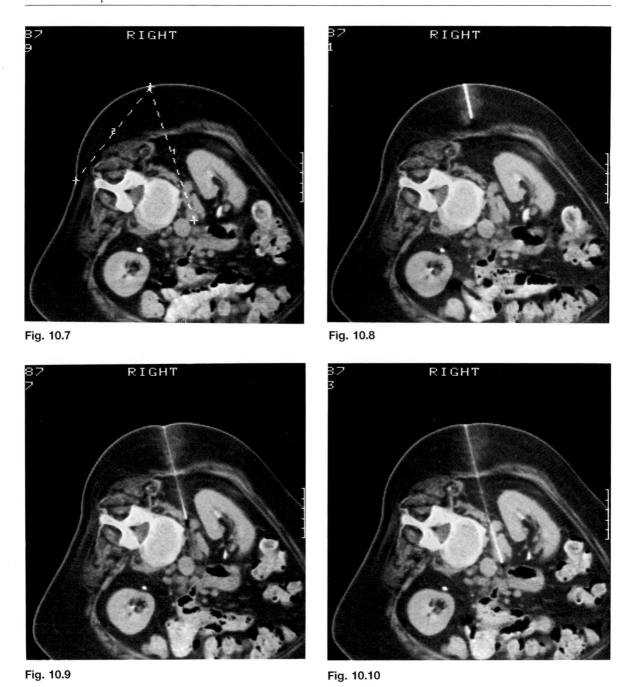

Fig. 10.7

Fig. 10.8

Fig. 10.9

Fig. 10.10

Figs. 10.7.–10.10. Technical approach for a retroperitoneal lymph node biopsy. Behind the vena cava three lymph nodes are identified, which are displacing the cava anteriorly. A puncture was performed with the patient in an oblique position. After the planning-CT (Fig. 10.7.), a guiding needle was advanced in the plane of the mass and at the correct puncture angle (Fig. 10.8.). The distribution of local anesthetic could be recognized by the increase in density surrounding the needle tip (Fig. 10.8.). A biopsy of all three nodes on the same pass was performed using an interventional needle (Fig. 10.9.). The distance between the needle and the vena cava was only 1 mm. The result of the puncture was a non-specific inflammatory process.

Chapter 11
Skeleton

D.H.W. Grönemeyer, R.M.M. Seibel

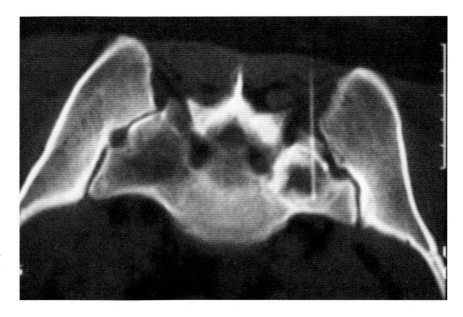

Fig. 11.1. 2 cm large osteolytic mass in the right lateral sacrum with associated sclerosis. CT-guided fine-needle biopsy was performed with a 20-G needle. Histologic diagnosis – benign bone cyst.

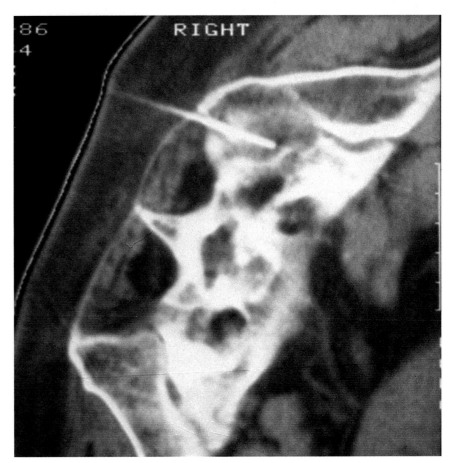

Fig. 11.2. Irregulary bony lesion of the right sacro-iliac joint. CT-guided biopsy was performed with a 20-G fine needle. Histologic diagnosis – alteration of the sacro-iliac joint with no indication of malignancy.

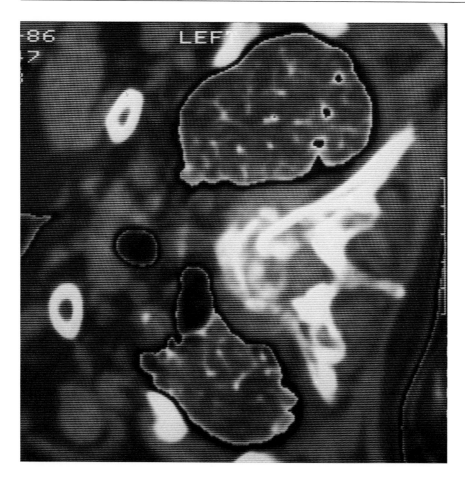

Fig. 11.3. (soft tissue window) and **Fig. 11.4.** (bone window). Osteolytic destruction of the T5 vertebra resulting in the patient being completely paraplegic at this level. CT shows expansion of the paravertebral space by the tumor. Additionally, a pathologic fracture of the T5 vertebral body and extension of the tumor into the spinal canal are visualized on CT.

Fig. 11.3

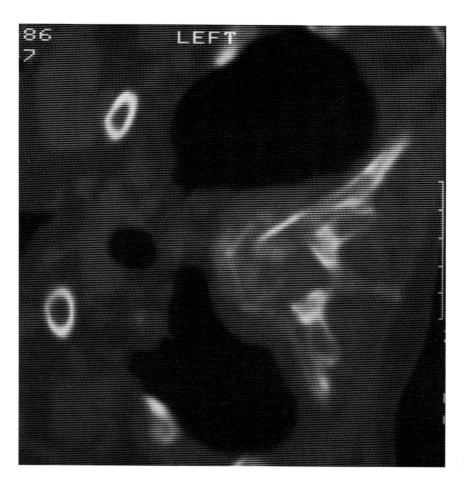

Fig. 11.4

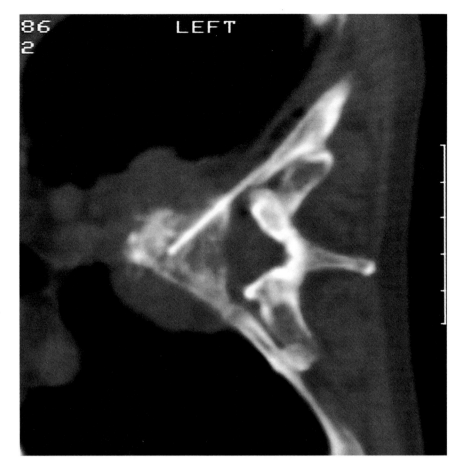

Fig. 11.5. CT-guided biopsy from a posterolateral approach (same patient as in Figs. 11.3. and 11.4.). The needle was introduced into the vertebral body alongside the rib. The bulk of the tumor is located in the left paravertebral space and has directly infiltrated the thoracic vertebral body. Histologic diagnosis – squamous cell carcinoma of the lung.

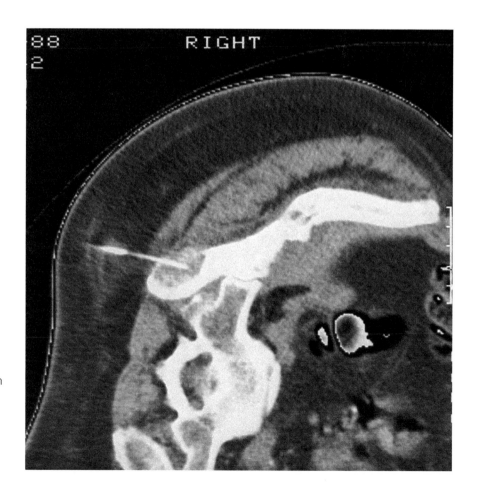

Fig. 11.6. Osteolytic lesion of the right ilium. CT-guided fine-needle biopsy with a 20-G needle was performed. Histologic diagnosis – breast cancer metastasis.

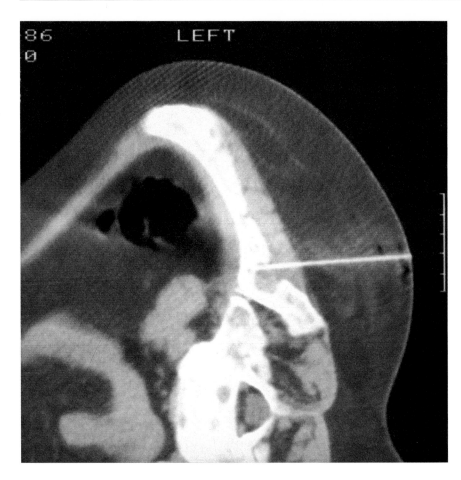

Fig. 11.7. CT-scan demonstrates several osteolytic metastases of the ilium and also small osteolytic lesions of the sacrum. With the patient in the right lateral position a puncture was performed from a posterior approach. Histologic diagnosis – signet ring cell carcinoma.

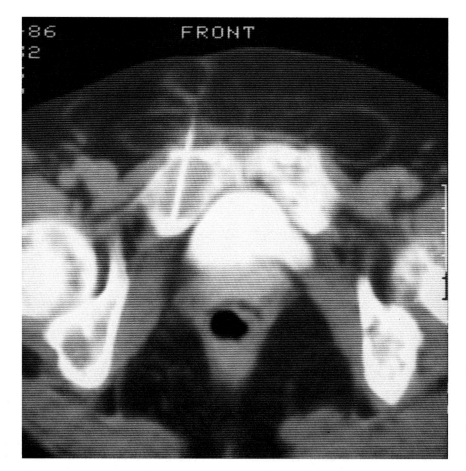

Fig. 11.8. Osteolytic metastatic lesion of the right pubic bone. The CT-guided biopsy was performed from an anterior approach. Histologic diagnosis – breast cancer metastasis.

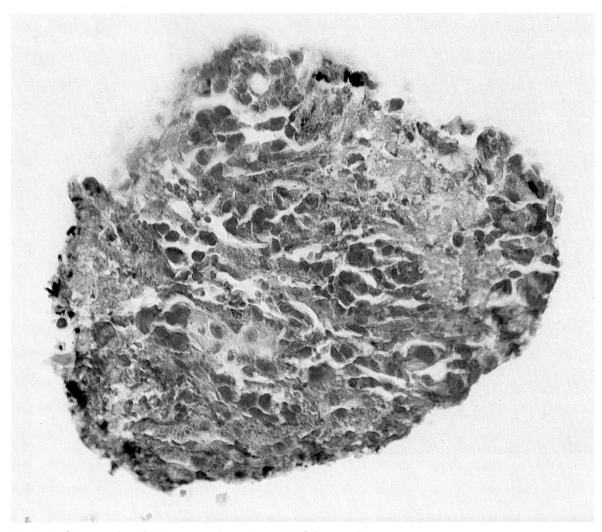

Fig. 11.9. Cross-section of a biopsy specimen from a 20-G fine needle.

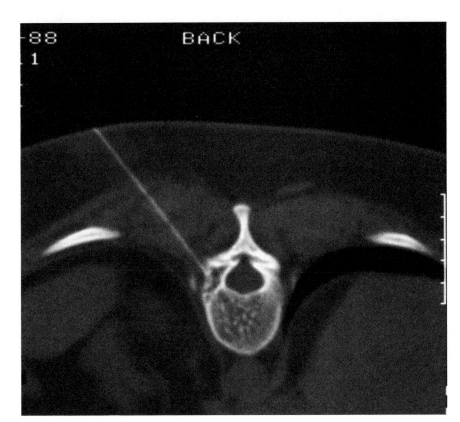

Fig. 11.10. Osteolytic lesion of the left T11 vertebral arch. Four years earlier this woman had a mastectomy for breast cancer. The CT-guided biopsy was performed from a posterolateral approach with a 20-G fine needle. Histologic diagnosis – breast cancer metastasis.

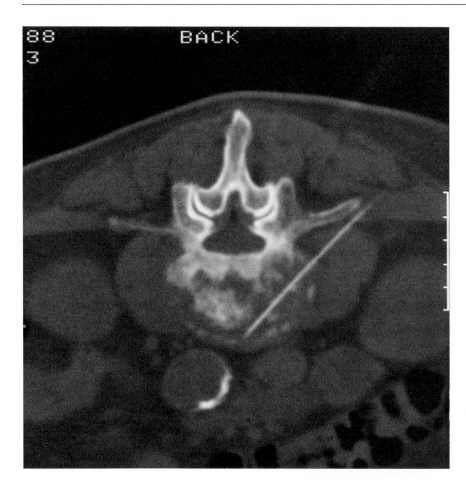

Fig. 11.11. Osteolytic lesion of the L4 vertebral body with extension to L5. A CT-guided biopsy was performed from the posterolateral approach. Histologic diagnosis – breast cancer metastasis.

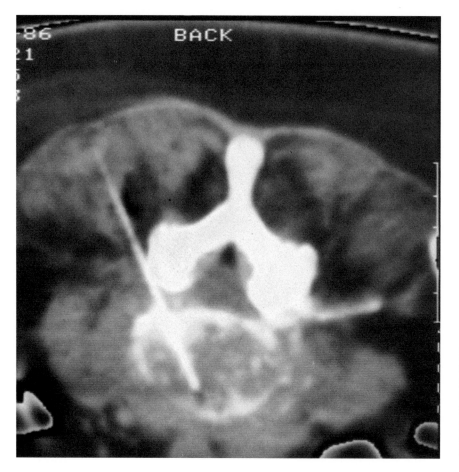

Fig. 11.12. Osteolytic destruction of the L4 vertebral body with extension into L5. CT-guided fine needle biopsy demonstrates non-specific spondylitis and diskitis with microbiologic evidence of staphylococci.

Therapeutic Procedures

Chapter 12
Autonomic Nervous System (ANS)

D.H.W. Grönemeyer, R.M.M. Seibel, W.H. Arnold

History

In 1664, the British anatomist Thomas Willis named and described the sympathetic trunk of the "autonomic nervous system" (Schiffter). However, for a long time after this, it was still called the "intercostal nerve". Then, 150 years before Horner, in 1727, Pourfour de Petit identified during his investigation of the neck region of the "intercostal nerve" the syndrome, that is today called the Horner syndrome. In 1789, Günther described the N. intercostalis s. sympathicus magnus and its connections to the gastro-intestinal tract, heart etc.

The term "negative" (autonomic) nervous system was first used in 1801 by Bichat and then in 1807 by Reil. They differentiated between autonomic functions, which are involuntary and subconsciously regulated, and animal functions, which are consciously controlled. In 1816, Dupuy investigated the regulation of sweat glands by the nervous system. The first anatomic preparation of nerve fibers in the vicinity of sweat glands was performed in 1859 by Koellicker and Tomsa. In 1844, Claude Bernard was able to reproduce a Horner syndrome and mydriasis after stimulation of the cervical sympathetic trunk. After this, in 1851, he obtained a mydriasis, a Dalrymple's sign, and sweating after stimulation of the cervical sympathetic trunk. In 1852, Budge found the ciliospinal center. The Zurich ophthalmologist Horner described in an 1869 paper a form of ptosis, a syndrome later bearing his name (consisting of ptosis, miosis, enophthalmos, and anhydrosis, all on the same side of the face). With this finding he was able to prove that innervation of the sweat glands is through the sympathetic nervous system. In 1873, Nikati described a classification of sympathetic trunk injuries. In 1875, Friedrich Goltz was able, by stimulating the sciatic nerve of a cat, to induce outbreaks of sweating. He also researched vegetative stimulation at the spinal cord and its significance in rectal and urogenital function.

The neuronal mechanisms of the vasomotor system were first described in 1851 by Claude Bernard and then in 1852 by Brown-Séquard. Research by Henlé from 1855 to 1871 and Koel-

licker in 1896 confirmed the sympathetic cross-linkage of arteries by their anatomic-histologic findings. Already in 1812, Le Gallois had discovered a center for respiratory control in the medulla oblongata. In 1871, Owsjannikow instigated further research with his multiple cuttings of this center which he called "life node". In 1874, Hitzig obtained mydriasis and miosis by stimulation experiments on the occipital cortex of dogs. In 1845, the Weber brothers were for the first time able to slow down the heart rate by vagus nerve stimulation. In 1866, the De Cyon brothers increased the heart rate by stimulating the sympathetic trunk.

Another major advancement in the understanding of ANS was detection of the autonomic nerve plexi and their effect on the gastro-intestinal wall by Meissner (1857) and Auerbach (1862). The submucosal plexus was named after Meissner and the myenteric plexus after Auerbach.

Intensive neurologic research by Gaskell from 1885 to 1916 led to his postulation of an involuntary nervous system consisting of a stimulating and supressing segment. He recognized the connection of this system with the central nervous system. He then subdivided the involuntary system into three segments: 1 Bulbo-parasympathetic; 2 thoracolumbar-sympathetic and 3 sacral-parasympathetic.

In 1905, Langley subdivided the autonomic nervous system into only two parts, the sympathetic and parasympathetic compartment.

After this, research into the area of central-autonomic regulations pursued by Pawlow/Keidel and Hess/Karplus from 1909 until 1918. Other outstanding clinical practitioners who added to the research into the ANS are Head, Förster, Guttmann, L.R. Müller, Romberg and in more recent times Hansen, Schliack, Monnier, Umbach, Johnson, Spalding and Schiffter.

Organization of the Autonomic Nervous System

The autonomic nervous system is a complexly connected system which automically regulates

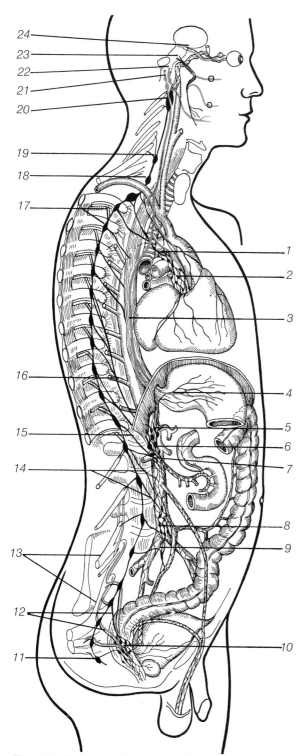

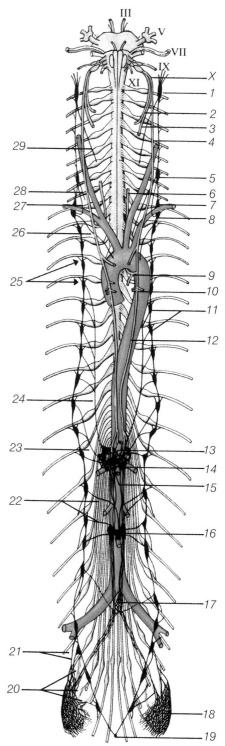

Fig. 12.1. Synopsis of the construction of the autonomic nerve system (modified after Krieg), (B). Blue = parasympathetic system; black = sympathetic system; cited after Rohen J.W., Funktionelle Anatomie des Nervensystems, F.K. Schattauer Verlag, Stuttgart, New York, 1985, 286, Fig. 168).

1 Pulmonary plexus; *2* cardiac plexus; *3* vagus nerve; *4* gastric plexus; *5* celiac plexus; *6* aorticorenal ganglion; *7* superior mesenteric ganglion; *8* inferior mesenteric ganglion; *9* superior hypogastric plexus; *10* inferior hypogastric plexus; *11* coccygeal ganglion; *12* pelvic splanchnic nerves; *13* lumbosacral plexus; *14* lumbar splanchnic nerves; *15* lesser splanchnic nerve; *16* greater splanchnic nerve; *17* sympathetic trunk; *18* inferior cervical ganglion; *19* middle cervical ganglion; *20* superior Cranial ganglion; *21* cranial nerve X; *22* cranial nerve IX; *23* cranial nerve VII; *24* cranial nerve III.

Fig. 12.2. Anatomy of the autonomic nervous system in relation to the spinal metamere region of the spinal cord (simplified after Mattuschka) (B). Black = sympathetic system; yellow = parasympathetic system; red = aorta (cited after Rohen J.W.: Funktionelle Anatomie des Nervensystems, F.K. Schattauer Verlag, Stuttgart, 1985, 286, Fig. 170).

III Cervical nerve III; V cervical nerve V; VII cervical nerve VII; X cervical nerve X; XI cervical nerve XI; *1* superior cervical ganglion; *2* superior laryngeal nerve; *3* superior cervical cardiac nerve; *4* vagus nerve; *5* middle cervical ganglion; *6* recurrent laryngeal nerve; *7* inferior cervical ganglion; *8* thoracic ganglion 1; *9* recurrent laryngeal nerve with inferior cardiac nerve; *10* pulmonary branches; *11* sympathetic trunk; *12* vagus nerve; *13* celiac plexus; *14* aorticorenal ganglion; *15* mesenteric ganglion; *16* inferior mesenteric ganglion; *17* superior hypogastric plexus; *18* inferior hypogastric plexus; *19* coccygeal ganglion; *20* pelvic splanchnic nerves; *21* sacral splanchnic nerves; *22* lumbar splanchnic nerves; *23* lesser splanchnic nerve; *24* greater splanchnic nerve; *25* white and grey communicating branches; *26* inferior cervical cardiac nerve; *27* subclavian loop; *28* middle cervical cardiac nerve; *29* superior cervical cardiac nerve.

organ functions and adjusts these functions to an organism's needs. Through numerous connections with the sensory, motor, and limbic apparatus, the autonomous nervous system influences the voluntary (animal) nervous system (Figs. 12.1. and 12.2.).

Functionally and anatomically, there are three organizational levels that can be differentiated in the ANS. The highest level is the dienkephalon and reticular formation which control and regulate the functions of the target organ systems. The medial level is subdivided into a sympathetic and a parasympathetic system. These systems are closely linked and antagonistic in their effect on the target organs. Both systems use acetylcholine as transmitting substance at the preganglionic synapse. However, in the peripheral intramural ANS, the sympathetic and parasympathetic system are distinguished by their different transmitting substances. The postganglionic parasympathetic neuron is cholinergic, whereas the postganglionic sympathetic neuron is adrenergic. The peripheral intramural system is under the control of central-autonomic feed-back mechanism, but can act autonomously within limits.

Unfortunately, the important role of the autonomic nervous system is often not taken into consideration in research, teaching, and every-day medical practice, as it should be. The significance of autonomic functional disorders, the involvement of the sympathetic and parasympathetic systems in pathologic changes, and diseases of these systems are often ignored, even though the autonomic nervous system is extensively involved in all body reactions and diseases. This is especially true for acute and chronic pain. Many doctors are often overwhelmed by the numerous autonomic symptoms which they observe daily. These autonomic reactions can range from tension headache and constipation all the way to the collapse of vital organ function. Often only symptoms of organic disorders are noticed, and the neurologic-systemic connections are missed.

It would be beyond the scope of this book to describe in detail the autonomic system and its connections. The references at the end of this chapter are for readers interested in a more detailed review. For practical reasons the authors have limited themselves predominantly to a discussion of the sympathetic nervous system near the spine. This is because the therapeutic methods described in this book occur mainly in this area.

Organization of the Sympathetic Nervous System

The pericaryons (cell bodies) of the preganglionic sympathetic fibers are located in the thoracal and lumbar segments of the spinal cord (intermediolateral nucleus). In this area, the sympathetic trunk has a rigorous segmental structure, that is one segment consists of one dermatome, myotome, enterotome, angiotome, sclerotome, etc. Similarly segmentally structured are the sensory, motor, and autonomic innervation for a segment.

The preganglionic sympathetic fibers exit from the spinal cord via the anterior root, along with the efferent fibers of the peripheral nerve. After leaving the anterior root, they are called white communicating branches (medullated nerve fibers) and extend to the paired sympathetic trunk (truncus sympathicus) on both sides of the vertebral bodies. The sympathetic trunk extends from the base of the skull to the coccyx. On each side of the trunk, there are approximately 22 sympathetic trunk ganglia which are interconnected by interganglionic branches. In the neck region, there are three large ganglia, the superior, middle and inferior (stellate ganglion or cervicothoracicum) cervical ganglion. In the thoraco-lumbar region, the sympathetic trunk is in a rigorous metamere structure. Caudally, there exist four lumbar and four sacral pairs of ganglia and a single rudimentary coccygeal ganglion.

A part of the preganglionic sympathetic fibers synapses at the sympathetic trunk ganglion to form the postganglionic neurone. From there the postganglionic fibers rejoin the spinal segmental nerve as thinly myelinated gray communicating branches. Then, they accompany the sensory peripheral nerves to the segmental dermatome. Thus, the postganglionic fibers follow the skin dermatomes. In this way, the skin (including the sweat glands, vessels, and erector muscles of the hairs) over the entire body surface area has sympatethic innervation.

A part of the preganglionic fibers traverses – either ascending or descending – the interganglionic branches without forming synapses through several sympathetic trunk ganglia. They then synapse with the postganglionic neuron either above or below these segmental ganglia. A preganglionic ganglion can divide into up to ten nerve fibers and supply up to eight postganglionic neurons. This means that the experimental or therapeutic stimulation of a single preganglionic neuron can affect up to eight dermatomes, angiotomes etc, whereas the stimulation of a postganglionic neuron will affect only one segment. On the other hand, interruptions of a single preganglionic nerve fiber will not result in symptoms, because of the overlap of postganglionic innervation. Another group of the preganglionic sympathetic neurons passes through the sympathetic trunk ganglion without synapsing and leaves the ganglia as the splanchnic nerves. The splanchnic nerves extend to the unpaired prevertebral ganglion and to the intramural plexus. There, they synapse and form the post-ganglionic neurons. Located in the region of the ganglia there are always autonomic plexi. These plexi are predominantly in the region of the lung hilus, heart and large vessels (cardiac, pulmonary, celiac plexus etc.). All preganglionic neurons for the thoracic organs originate between C8 and T5. Furthermore, all fibers for the abdominal and pelvic organs originate between T5 and L2. The postganglionic fibers of the abdominal and pelvic cavities begin from plexi and do not travel with the segmental nerves, but with the vessels to the intramural plexi as periadventitial reticulum.

The segmental autonomic reflex arches have been extensively explored and have great clinical significance. All sensory afferent impulses (including those from all organs) extend to the posterior root of the spinal cord over the dendrites of the spinal ganglionic cells and their axons. From there, they pass via the posterior white columns and Gowers's tract to the brain. At segmental cord level, the visceral-sensory afferent impulses (i.e. visceralgia) reach the synapses of the sympathetic neurons at the columna lateralis via the so-called D-cells of the spinal ganglion and their axons. The reflex arch will be closed when sensory stimulations from internal organs (e.g. for contraction of the bladder) lead to the reflex response (viscero-visceral reflex). In this reflex arch, sensory afferent impulses from the skin (A-cells of the spinal ganglion) and motor efferent impulses to the striated musculature are also interlinked via collaterals and interneurons to the spinal cord. Pain stimuli from an enterotome (e.g. from the large intestine) lead to spasm of the associated striated musculature of the abdominal wall (rigid abdomen) in the myotome (viscero-motor reflex). The reflex can also cause hyperesthesia with painful sensations in the associated dermatome – with or without a vascular reaction, sweat gland activation, or pilo-erection: viscero-cutaneous reflex. Within the dermatomes and also overlapping them, there are maximum zones which are linked to certain organs and react strongly to stimulation (Head's zones). In the reverse direction, physical-therapeutic treatment can affect the cutaneo-visceral reflex. The effect of most different types of physical therapy can be explained by this reflex, such as water therapy, massage, or electric stimulation methods. Spasms, pain, and functional disorders in the segment can respond in a favorable manner

to these treatments (see Chapter Electro Stimulation).

Organization of the Parasympathetic Nervous System

Contrary to the sympathetic system, the origins of the preganglionic nerve fibers of the parasympathetic nervous system (PNS) are in well-defined brain-stem nuclei and in the so-called sacral-autonomic center in the intermediolateral nucleus of the lateral horn in the spinal cord region of S1-S3.

The preganglionic fibers of the PNS for the head traverse with the cranial nerves (oculomotor nerve, facial nerve [intermediary nerve] and glossopharyngeal nerve) to the corresponding ganglia, where they synapse to form the postganglionic fibers. From there, they mainly traverse with the branches of the trigeminal nerve to their target organs. The internal organs of the thorax and abdominal cavity are supplied by the vagus nerve with parasympathetic nerve fibers. The ganglia of the parasympathetic trunk are located near these organs, mostly in intramural plexi. The vagus nerve innervation of the internal organs extends all the way to the left colon flexure, the so-called Cannon-Böhm point (border line between the innervation of the vagus nerve and the sacral parasympathetic system, between the medial and left third of the colon transversum). Distal to the Cannon-Böhm point, the intestinal segments and genital organs have parasympathetic innervation from the sacral autonomic center. The preganglionic fibers leave the spinal along with the spinal nerves and traverse to the intramural ganglia where they synapse with the postganglionic fibers.

Pain Conduction and Referred Pain

Besides the sensory somatic fibers, a considerable part of the autonomic system is involved in the pain process. This is especially true for all angiodynias, i.e. all types of primary or secondary pain from pathologic blood vessels or pain caused by compression of vessels. This is also valid for intestinal pain.

Knowledge of the somatic-segmental nerves and the origin of the sympathetic fibers, which are responsible for the autonomic supply of organs and vessels, is important. This knowledge is necessary in order to understand the blocking interaction of somatic nerves and the corresponding part of the sympathetic trunk. Table 12.1. contrasts the segmental somatic and sympathetic innervation, and demonstrates an appropriate clinical approach. It must be stated

Table 12.1

Organ	Pain projection	Pain conduction via segmental nerves	Origin of preganglionic fibers
meninges	scalp	sens. nucleus of cervical n. V. – (1st branch), IX, X, XII	T1–T2 (3)
eyes	orbital cavity and frontal area	sens. nucleus of cervical n. V. – (1st branch)	T1–T3 (4)
lacrimal glands	orbital cavity	nucl. of the solitary tract n. VII and IX	T1, T2
parotid gland	region of the parotid gland	nucl. of the solitary tract n. V. via VII and IX	T1, T2
submandibular gland	region of the submandibular gland	nucl. of the solitary tract ling. n. via n. VII and ganglion geniculi	T1, T2
larynx	larynx, anterior cervical region	sup. laryngeal n.	T2–T7
trachea, bronchi, lung parenchyma	sternal region insensitive to pain	T2–T7 insensitive	T2–T7 T2–T7
parietal pleura in the region of:			
shoulder	shoulder	C3–C5	
supraclavicular	supraclavicular (brachial plexus)	C8–T1	
intercostal	intercostal nerves of the affected region	T1–T12	
heart	left precordium	T1–T4 (5) (left) arm	T1–T4 (5)
thoracic aorta	upper half of the thorax and neck	T1–T5 (6)	T1–T5
abdominal aorta	lower half of the thorax	T6–T12	T6–L2
esophagus upper half lower half	medial part of the sternum (horizontal)	T5–T8	T2–T5 T5–T8
stomach	epigastric area, interscapular region	T(6), T8(9)	T(5)6–T10(11)
liver and gall bladder	right hypochondrium	T(5)6–T8(9) + phrenic n.	T6–T11 right
pancreas	epigastric area, midline of the back at T10 and TII	T(5)6–T10(11) + vagus n., cellac ganglion	T5–T11
spleen	left hypochondrium	T6–T8	T6–T8
small intestine: duodenum jejunum and ileum cecum and ascending colon	epigastric area and navel suprapubic	T(5)6–T7(8)* T9–11 T9–T11	T6–T11 T8–T11 right
appendix	right lower quadrant	T10–T11 (-L1)	T8–T11 right
descending colon and sigmoid colon	deep in pelvis anus	L1 and L2 S2–S4	T11–T12 L1–L4 left
suprarenal gland	none	none	T6–L2 unilateral
kidney	lower paravertebral area and groin	T10–L2	T10–L1(2)
ureter	lower pravertebral area and groin	T11–L2	T11–L1(2) unilateral

* Oral part on the right, the other part on the left and vagus nerve

Table 12.1. (Cont.)

Organ	Pain projection	Pain conduction via segmental nerves	Origin of preganglionic fibers
bladder			
fundus	suprapubic	T11–L1	L1–L2
testes	testes	T10	T10–L1
prostate	perineum and back	T10, T11, and S2–S4	T10–L1
ovaries and fallopian tubes	both lower abdominal quadrantts	T10	T6–L2
uterus	perineum	T10–L1 S2–S4	T6–L2
female genitalia	perineum	S2–S4	L1–L2
blood vessels, sweat glands, hair follicles, etc at:			
upper extremity	skin area	C5–T1	T2–T8(9)
trunk	skin area	T1–T12	T1–T12
lower extremity	skin area	L4–S3	T10–L3

that different authors have reported different associations between organs and referred spinal segments (especially in the sympathetic nervous system).

In Table 12.1. those segments are listed on which most authors agree. The present authors have found the best results by treating the middle of the listed segmental nerves. Furthermore, it should be borne in mind during treatment that after injection, the medication (e.g. ethanol, local anesthetic) will spread into neighboring caudal and cranial segments.

References

1. Auerbach L.: Fernere vorläufige Mitteilung über den Nervenapparat des Darmes. Virchows Arch. path. Anat. 30 (1864) 457–460
2. Bichat M.F.X.: Anatomie générale appliquée á la physiologie et á la medicine. 2. Vols. Paris 1801
3. Bernard C.: Lecons sur la Physiologie et la Pathologie du Système Nerveux. Vol. 11, Paris 1858
4. Gaskell H.W.: The involuntary nervous system. London 1916
5. Günther D.E.: Kurzer Entwurf der anatomischen Nervenlehre. Düsseldorf 1789
6. Head H.: Die Sensibilitätsstörungen der Haut bei Viszeralerkrankungen. Berlin 1898
7. Hess W.R.: Zwischenhirn. Basel 1954
8. Hitzig E.: Untersuchungen über das Gehirn. Zbl. med. Wiss. (1874) 548
9. Horner F.: Über eine Form von Ptosis. Klin. Mbl. Augenheilk. 7 (1869) 193–198
10. Jenkner F.L.: Nervenblockade auf pharmakologischen und auf elektrischem Weg. Wien, New York 1983
11. Karplus J.P.: Physiologie der vegetativen Zentren. In: Bumke W., Foerster O. (Hrsg.): Handbuch der Neurologie. Bd. 2 1937, 402–475
12. Kölliker R.A. von: Handbuch der Gewebelehre des Menschen. Leipzig 1896
13. Langley J.N.: The autonomic nervous system. 1. Cambridge 1921
14. Meissner G.: Über die Nerven der Darmwand. Z. rat. Med. 8 (1857) 364–366
15. Monnier M.: Physiologie des vegetativen Nervensystems. Stuttgart 1963
16. Müller I.R.: Die Lebensnerven Berlin 1857
17. Owsjannikow P.H.: Die tonischen und reflektorischen Zentren der Gefäßnerven. Ber. Verh. Sächs, Ges. Wiss. Leipzig. Math. Phys. Cl. 23 (1871) 135–147
18. Pawlow J.P.: Sämtliche Werke Bd. 1–6. Berlin (DDR) 1954
19. Pourfour de Petit F.: Mémoire dans la quel il est démonstré que les nerves intercostaux fournissent des rameaux que portent des esprits dans le yeux. Hist. Acad. roy. Sci., Paris 1727
20. Rohen J.W.: Funktionelle Anatomie des Nervensystems. New York 1985
21. Romberg M.H.: Lehrbuch der Nervenkrankheiten des Menschen. Berlin 1985
22. Schiffter R.: Neurologie des vegetativen Systems. Berlin, Heidelberg, New York, Tokyo 1985

Further Reading

Brücke F.: Zur Physiologie der vegetativen Innervation der Haut. Acta neuroveg. 18 (1958) 203

Mislin H.: Zur vergleichenden Anatomie und Physiologie des vegetativen Nervensystems. In: Monnier M. (Hrsg.), Physiologie des vegetativen Nervensystems. Stuttgart 1963

Moruzzi G., Magoun H.W.: Brain stem reticular formation and activation of the EEG. Elektroenceph. Clin. Neurophysiol. (Can.) 1 (1949) 455

Chapter 13
Local Anesthetics in Interventional Radiology

D. Reinking, A.M. Schmidt, D.H.W. Grönemeyer, R.M.M. Seibel

Introduction

Local anesthetics produce a reversible blockade of the conduction of nerve impulses. These drugs are used for local, reversible blockade of peripheral nerves. Cocaine, a naturally occurring alkaloid, was the first local anesthetic discovered, and was used as early as 1884. Today, many synthetic local anesthetics are used, and lidocaine is often thought of as the standard by which other local anesthetics are judged.

Mechanism of Action

Transmission in a nerve cell is affected by an action potential which spreads along the cell membrane. The action potential results from a rapid depolarization of the cell membrane. The depolarization arises from the sudden change in permeability for cations, allowing sodium ions to quickly flow to the intracellular space. Local anesthetics prevent depolarization of the nerve cell by impeding this rapid inflow of sodium. This results in an unexcitable nerve fiber.

Although the blockade of pain fibers is the goal of local anesthetic use, other nerve fibers, including the sympathetic and motor fibers, as well as fibers transmitting pressure and touch, are also affected to varying degrees.

Multiple factors influence how the nerve fiber is affected by the local anesthetic. Myelinated and unmyelinated fibers are affected differently. Myelin acts as an insulator that limits access of the local anesthetic to the nerve membrane, except at the nodes. Since much of the local anesthetic is absorbed by the myelin, a higher concentration of local anesthetic is needed to block myelinated nerve fibers, compared to unmyelinated fibers. Also, since nerve impulses can skip over one or two blocked nodes, at least 5 or 6 mm of nerve must be bathed in anesthetic solution to achieve a total blockade of a myelinated fiber. Another factor is the size of the nerve. In general, nerve fibers of thinner diameter are more readily blocked than thicker fibers. Due to these differences, a differential nerve block can be produced. For example, when anesthetizing a peripheral nerve, pain may be completely obtunded (a Delta, the smallest of the A fibers, and C fibers, which are unmyelinated, are blocked) while the motor function and touch (alpha and beta fibers, the largest of the A fibers) are unaffected. Clinically, since the large, harder to block fibers convey touch and pressure, many patients will continue to feel touch and pressure, and some of these patients may complain that the local "isn't working".

The typical local anesthetic molecule consists of a tertiary amine (hydrophillic portion) and an unsaturated aromatic ring, usually a benzene ring (lipophillic portion). These two portions are linked together by an intermediate chain, which may be either an ester (–CO–) or an amide (–CNH–) bond. Thus, by this bond, the local anesthetics can be described as either an ester-type or amide-type local anesthetics. The ester and amide local anesthetics differ in several characteristics.

Alterations in the substitutions in the area of either the tertiary amine or aromatic ring affect the hydrophilic/lipophilic nature of the local anesthetic molecule and its subsequent characteristics. For example the more lipophillic molecules can more easily pass into membranes and are more potent and of longer duration than the more hydrophillic drugs. Local anesthetics are weak bases that exist in a chemical equilibrium between the basic, uncharged (lipid soluble) form (B) and the charged cationic form (BH+). The drug's pKa is the pH at which the concentration of the uncharged local anesthetic base is equal to the concentration of the charged cation. Since only the uncharged, lipid soluble form can diffuse through nerve cell membranes, factors affecting the pH also alter the effectiveness of the drug. This dependance on pH explains why local anesthetics are less effective in infected tissue, with its more acidic pH causing more of the local anesthetic to exist in the charged, cationic form. Local anesthetic potency is greatly influenced by its lipid solubility, while duration of action of local anesthetics is influenced by protein binding.

Local Anesthetics

Local anesthetic drugs are either of the ester type or the amide type. The amide local anesthetics undergo metabolism in the liver and are subsequently excreted in the urine, whereas the ester local anesthetics undergo rapid hydrolysis by esterases located principally in the plasma. Para-aminobenzoic acid is a metabolic byproduct of the ester type local anesthetics, and has been implicated in the development of allergic reactions. Due to their slower and more complex metabolism of the amide type local anesthetics, cumulative drug effects and systemic toxicity are more likely to occur with this class of drug.

The amide type local anesthetics include lidocaine (Xylocaine), mepivicaine (Carbocaine), etidocaine, bupivicaine (Marcaine), and prilocaine. The ester type include procaine (Novocaine), Chlorprocaine (Nesacaine), tetracaine and cocaine. Local anesthetics are frequently used for 1) topical anesthesia, 2) local infiltration, or 3) conduction anesthesia or major nerve block.

Amides

Lidocaine is an ideal agent for most block procedures when a rapid onset is desired. It is useful for infiltration, nerve block and topical anesthesia of mucous membranes. Effective infiltration anesthesia can be produced with 0.5 or 1% solutions and onset of anesthesia is almost immediate. The 1% solution has a duration of approximately 120 minutes or 240 minutes with epinephrine. The recommended safe dose is 200–400 mg if a solution without epinephrine is used; if epinephrine has been added the recommended safe dose is 500 mg. Lidocaine is cleared rapidly from the body, primarily due to rapid extraction by the liver. The serum half-life of lidocaine is approximately 1.6 hours. Impaired liver function, or decreased blood flow to the liver, such as seen in low cardiac output states, will delay lidocaine clearance.

Mepivicaine is not effective topically, but is otherwise similar to lidocaine in potency and toxicity. The concentrations used for infiltration, nerve block and epidural anesthesia are the same as for lidocaine. The safe dosage is 400 mg or 500 mg with epinephrine.

Bupivicaine is used for infiltration, peripheral nerve block, and epidural anesthesia. It is approximately four times as potent as lidocaine, and appears to be more toxic than lidocaine. Commonly used solutions are 0.25% and 0.5%, with and without epinephrine. During infiltration anesthesia, onset is rapid, and the duration is approximately 200 minutes, 400 minutes with epinephrine. The safe dose is 150 mg, with epinephrine 200 mg. For peripheral nerve block, 0.5% solution is usually preferred, and the onset is slow, approximately 10 to 20 minutes. After nerve block, duration of anesthesia is quite variable and can continue up to 24 hours.

Esters

Cocaine is used for topical anesthesia and is commonly used in 1% to 10% solutions. The 1% solution is adequate for corneal anesthesia while 4% solution is adequate for anesthesia of the mucous membranes of the oro- and nasopharynx. Unlike other local anesthetics, cocaine has its own vasoconstrictive properties. This is thought to be due to its prevention of reuptake of catecholamines at the nerve endings. 150 to 200 mgs is regarded as a safe dose. The CNS effects of cocaine vary from mild euphoria and mental alertness seen at moderate blood levels, to excitement, seizures and coma seen at very high levels. Tachycardia and hypertension are seen at low to moderate doses, and high doses are followed by myocardial depression which may become rapidly fatal.

Procaine (Novocaine) has very poor spreading properties, and is not effective topically. Effective concentrations for infiltration and nerve block are similar to lidocaine but it has a longer onset and shorter duration.

Epidural block with procaine frequently results in missed segments. The safe dose is 500 mg, or 750 mg with epinephrine.

Chlorprocaine (Nesacaine) is not effective topically. It has a rapid onset and very low toxicity due to its very rapid hydrolysis in the blood. Chlorprocaine's main disadvantage is its short duration. For infiltration anesthesia or peripheral nerve block, a 1% solution has a duration of 45 to 60 minutes, or 70 to 80 minutes with epinephrine. Safe dose is 600 mg, 800 mg with epinephrine.

Tetracaine (Pontocaine) is approximately four to six times as potent as lidocaine, but also much more toxic. It is frequently used for spinal anesthesia and can also be used for topical anesthesia.

Epinephrine, usually in a concentration of 1:200,000, is frequently used with local anesthetics to delay absorption, leading to increased duration and decreased systemic toxicity. Higher concentrations of epinephrine do not produce a correspondingly increased vasoconstriction. A total dose of 200 micrograms of epinephrine should not be exceeded and the patient with hypertension or arrhythmias may warrant a reduction in this total dose. Epinephrine containing solutions are generally not recommended for use on appendages, due to the possibility that the vasoconstriction from the epinephrine could result in ischemia to the appendage.

Adverse Reactions to Local Anesthetics

Immediate adverse reactions to local anesthetics can be 1) allergic reactions, 2) systemic toxicity due to a high plasma concentration of the drug or of the added vasoconstrictor, or 3) physiologic reaction from the nerve block itself.

Allergic Reactions

Allergic reactions to local anesthetics are uncommon. Although many patients state that they have had "allergic reactions" to local anesthetics, careful questioning will often reveal that the patient may have actually suffered 1) a vasovagal reaction, with bradycardia, faintness, or even loss of consciousness, 2) toxicity from high serum levels following rapid absorption or intravascular injection, or 3) systemic effects (palpitations, hypertension) from the epinephrine used in dental preparations. Most reports of allergic reactions to local anesthetics have been after the use of ester type local anesthetics (procaine, tetracaine) which produce metabolites related to para-aminobenzoic acid. Amide type local anesthetics (lidocaine, mepivicaine, bupivicaine) are not metabolized to para-aminobenzoic acid and are much less likely to produce an allergic reaction. True allergic reactions, when they occur, will be accompanied by symptoms of histamine release, such as urticaria, pruritus, edema, erythema, hypotension, dyspnea and wheezing. Treatment of allergic reactions includes airway maintenance, oxygenation, support of the blood pressure with fluids, positioning and vasopressors, administration of antihistamines, epinephrine, and possibly corticosteroids. Aminophylline may be needed for the accompanying bronchospasm. Edema may also occur in the airway, precipitating obstruction. While true allergic reactions to local anesthetics are very rare, systemic toxicity due to overdose, intravascular injection or rapid absorption of local anesthetics is much more common.

Systemic Toxicity due to High Serum Levels of Local Anesthetics

Central Nervous System Effects

CNS effects are frequently seen in a toxic reaction to local anesthetic, as the local anesthetic passes easily into the CNS. Signs and symptoms include tinnitus, circumoral numbness, drowsiness, restlessness, muscular twitching, slurred speech, and visual and auditory disturbances. As the serum levels continue to increase, generalized seizure activity may be seen, and the reaction may progress to CNS depression and coma.

Cardiovascular Effects

The cardiovascular toxicity of local anesthetics is generally seen at higher serum levels of local anesthetics than are needed to produce the CNS toxicity. Hypotension can result from both relaxation of arteriolar vascular smooth muscle and direct myocardial depression caused by toxic levels. Local anesthetics are believed to block the sodium channels in myocardial cells, as occurs during conduction blockade in the peripheral nerves. At low concentrations, this can be a useful effect, treating arrythmias. At higher concentrations many channels can also become blocked, depressing automaticity and conduction. This can be seen on the ECG as an increased PR interval and QRS duration, and sinus bradycardia.

Although in general, the cardiovascular system appears to be more resistant than the CNS to toxic effects of local anesthetics, bupivicaine is relatively more cardiotoxic than the less potent, less lipid soluble anesthetics such as lidocaine.

Treatment of local anesthetic toxicity is supportive. Airway maintenance, oxygenation, and support of the circulation with fluids, positioning and vasopressors should be carried out. If marked CNS excitation or seizure activity is present, this can be treated with small doses of diazepam or a barbiturate. Adequate oxygenation is particularly important during seizure activity, as seizures increase the oxygen consumption of the brain. A neuromuscular blocking agent such as succinylcholine may be used to control the muscular activity and may be needed to allow the physician to gain control of the airway and adequately ventilate the patient; it will not, however, alter the seizure activity seen on the EEG.

Prevention of local anesthetic toxicity by use of the smallest effective dose of drug, repeated aspiration to prevent direct intravascular injection, and recognition of early signs of toxicity by continuous verbal contact with the patient is optimal. If any signs or symptoms suggestive of systemic toxicity with a local anesthetic appear, the physician should discontinue the injection and proceed with supportive care as needed. Premedication with a drug that raises the seizure threshold such as diazepam can increase the CNS toxic threshold but does not alter the cardiovascular toxic threshold.

References

Auberger H.G., Niese H.C.: Praktische Lokalanaesthesie. Stuttgart 1982

Covino B.G., Scott D.B.: Epidurale Anaesthesie und Analgesie. Weinheim 1988

Noisser H.G., Osswald M.W.: Schmerzbehandlung in Klinik und Praxis. Z. Allg. Med. 57:1981

Schmidt R.F., Thews G.: Physiologie des Menschen. Heidelberg 1980

Suggested Reading

Stoelting R.K.: Pharmacology and Physiology in Anesthetic Practice. Lippincott Philadelphia 1987

Cousins M.J., Bridenbaugh P.O.: Neural Blockade in Clinical anesthesia and Management of Pain. Lippincott, 1980

Miller R.D.: Anesthesia. Churchill Livingston 1986

Treatment of Spinal Column Diseases

Chapter 14
The Vertebral Column

W.H. Arnold

Bony elements

The 24 vertebrae of the vertebral column form a chain-like structure, which in adults takes on a double s-shape, because of the upright human posture (cervical lordosis, thoracic kyphosis, lumbar lordosis, sacral kyphosis). Due to the upright posture, the weight of the head is entirely supported by the vertebral column. Because of this posture, there is a reduction in neck musculature and nuchal ligament in comparison with four-footed animals. Human vertebrae are exposed to increasing stress with increasing distance from the head. Due to this stress, the shape of the vertebrae, the positioning of the vertebral joints, and the axis of motion, change from the cranio to caudal direction.

The diameter of the vertebral bodies increases from the head to the pelvis (Figs. 14.1. and 14.2.). Furthermore, the cancellous bone in the vertebral body occupies a larger part of the total volume than the compact bony substance. For this reason, the porous portion of each vertebral body increases from the cervical spine to the lumbar spine. The spongy trabaculae are tractionally arranged depending on the stress to which the vertebral body is exposed to (Figs. 14.3. and 14.4.). Therefore, a collapse of the vertebral body occurs more often in the lumbar region than in the thoracic or cervical region.

The gap between two vertebral bodies is occu-

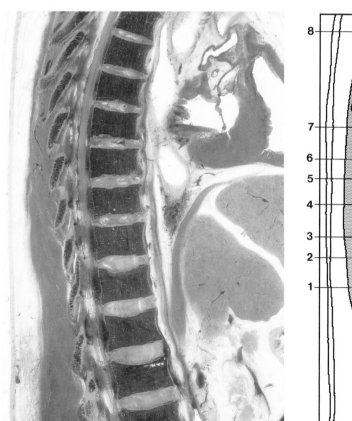
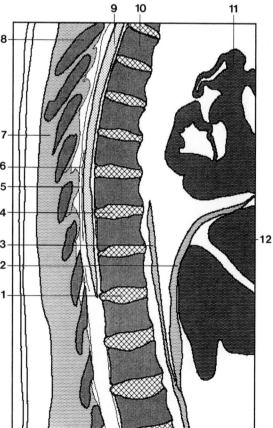

Figs. 14.1. and **14.2.** (Anatomy and drawing) *1* Intervertebral disc; *2* diaphragm; *3* prevertebral musculature; *4* intervertebral disc; *5* epidural space; *6* posterior spinal artery and vein; *7* back musculature; *8* spinous process; *9* spinal cord; *10* vertebral body; *11* heart; *12* liver.

pied by the intervertebral disc (see below). The vertebral arches are attached dorsally to the vertebral body and together form the vertebral canal.

From each vertebral arch rise the paired transverse processes and the spinous process. These processes serve as origin and insertion points for the perivertebral back musculature. In the region of the thoracic spine, the spinous processes are relatively long and directed caudally, so that they overlap and cover the vertebral canal. Normally, the spinous processes can be palpated from the 6th cervical vertebral body down and serve as important landmarks for localization of internal organs.

Besides the spinous and transverse processes, from each vertebral arch rise four joint processes which guide the movement between the vertebral bodies and also limit the vertebral motion in certain directions. There are also a variety of costal processes in different parts of the vertebral column. In the cervical spine, the paired costal processes are only rudimentary and merged with the transverse process. Only in the cervical spine, between these processes, an opening remains – the transverse foramen. In the transverse foramina the vertebral artery

transverses from the 6th cervical vertebra to the brain through the foramen magnum.

In the thoracic spine the 12 rib pairs are fully developed and articulate with the vertebral bodies and transverse processes. In the lumbar vertebra, the costal processes arise directly from the vertebral arches as rudimentary processes, and the actual transverse process becomes a small mamiliary process. The obvious transverse bony element of the lumbar spine in the plain film, which is often called „transverse process", is a rudimentary rib. Finally, in the region of the sacrum all bony structures are fused by synostosis.

The Ligaments of the Vertebral Column

The vertebral bodies are attached and stabilized over their entire length by rigid ligaments that run ventrally and dorsally (anterior and posterior longitudinal ligament [Figs. 14.5. and 14.6.]). They greatly limit the range of motion between each individual vertebra. The anterior longitudinal ligament is firmly attached to the vertebral bodies, but not to the annulus fibrosis.

In contrast, the posterior longitudinal ligament is tightly attached to the intervertebral disc, but

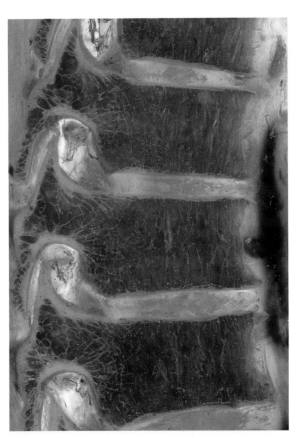
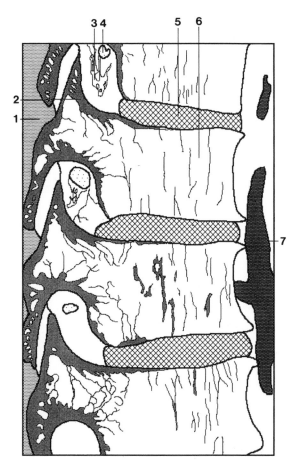

Figs. 14.3. and **14.4.** (anatomy and drawing) *1* Back musculature; *2* cortical bone of the vertebral arch; *3* venous plexus; *4* spinal ganglion; *5* vertebral disc; *6* spongy trabecular substance of the vertebral body; *7* azygos vein with a lumbar branch.

not to the midposterior surface of the vertebral bodies. Therefore, the anterior longitudinal ligament connects the vertebral bodies with each other and the posterior longitudinal ligament connects the intervertebral discs. To understand the function of the vertebral column, it is important to note that the tensions on these two ligaments are maintained by the volume of the intervertebral disks, which push the vertebral bodies apart. Therefore, a loss in volume of a single segment leads to a generalized loss of tension, especially in the posterior longitudinal ligament. This quickly results in destabiliziation of the vertebral column at several levels.

The vertebral arches are connected by the ligamenta flava. These arches are under strong longitudinal tension with stretches the spine backwards. Therefore, the ligamenta flava work against the tendency of the body to tip forward. This function is also supported by the perivertebral musculature. Between the spinous processes is the interspinal or supraspinal ligament. The function of the interspinal ligament is to stabilize the flexion motion of the vertebral column. With flexion of the vertebral column, the spinous processes separate from each other because they are posterior to the transverse axis of the vertebral body.ʼ

The Intervertebral Disc and its Relationship to the Mobility of the Vertebral Column

The form and function of the vertebral column are primarily determined by the intervertebral discs. The height of the intervertebral discs increases in the cranial to caudal direction and their form adapts to the curvature of the spine (Figs. 14.1.–14.6.). In the region of the cervical and lumbar lordosis, the intervertebral discs are wedge-shaped. The tip of the wedge is directed dorsally, contrary to the thoracic discs which are uniform in thickness.

The intervertebral discs contain a gelatinous center (the nucleus pulposus) which is surrounded by fibrocartilage material (the annulus fibrosis) (Figs. 14.5. and 14.6.). The fibers of the annulus fibrosis are coil-shaped and interconnected with the collagenous fibers of the lower and upper end plates of the vertebral bodies. In this way, the vertebral bodies are connected by synchondrosis (Figs. 14.3. and 14.4.). In the region of the cervical spine, the annulus fibrosis can often have a gap which can almost separate the disc in two halves (uncovertebral joint), but does not function as a joint (see Chapter Pathophysiology).

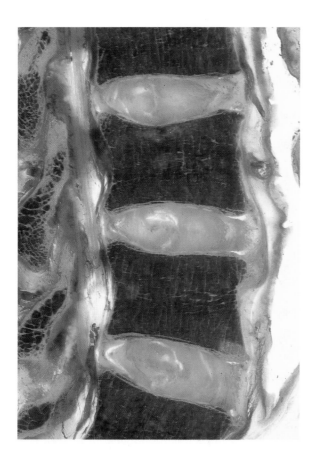
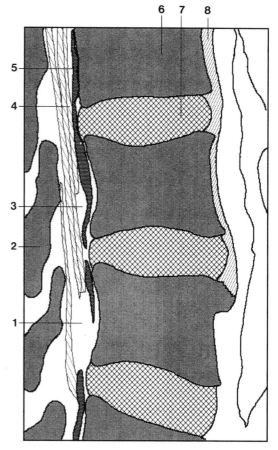

Figs. 14.5. and **14.6.** (Anatomy and drawing) *1* Intervertebral foramen, *2* spinous process; *3* intervertebral foramen; *4* nerve root; *5* venous plexus: *6* vertebral body; *7* intervertebral disc; *8* anterior longitudinal ligament.

The nucleus pulposus itself has few fibers and is of a liquid consistency. It serves as a cushion for pressure equalization in the annulus fibrosis, accommodates in shape to the movements of the spine, and allows for adjustment in height of the intervertebral disc. Water is pushed out of the nucleus pulposus and through the cartilaginous tissue of the annulus fibrosis, due to the weight of the body. This physiologic loss of disc height occurs during the course of the day in the upright position.

The mobility between individual vertebrae is different in each region of the spine. In general, the range of motion between any two vertebrae is relatively small. The total range of motion is a summation of the single movements between the vertebrae.

The greatest range of motion is found in the cervical spine. Here the facet articular surfaces are nearly flat and are tilted downward in anteroposterior direction approximately 45°. From cranial to caudal, the joint surfaces align more and more toward the coronal plain. In the lumbar spine, the facets are additionally tilted in the sagittal axis. Finally, in the sacrum all elements are fused and no movement is possible. Therefore, the range of motion is decreased from cranial to caudal by the changes of joint positioning. Thus, in the lumbar spine, only bending and stretching are possible. In conclusion, because of the shape of the facet joints, the cervical spine has the greatest mobility, whereas in the caudal region the function is primarily static.

The Vertebral Canal

The vertebral canal contains the spinal cord, the cauda equina, the arteries and veins, and the pia, arachnoid, and dura (Figs. 14.1. and 14.2.). In the adult, the spinal cord ends at the lumbar 1–2 level. The cord continues in the vertebral canal as the cauda equina, which contains the nerve roots of the lumbosacral plexus.

The dural sac extends from the foramen magnum to the second sacral vertebra, where it is firmly attached by the filum terminale which extends to the first coccygeal vertebra. Between the dura mater and the periosteum of the vertebrae is the expansive epidural space which contains fat and the vertebral venous plexus. This fat, as well as the extensive vertebral venous plexus in the epidural space, serves as a cushioned space for the movements of the spine (Figs. 14.1. and 14.2.).

The arachnoid membrane is attached to the dura mater inside the dural sac and encloses the subarachnoid space, which contains the cerebrospinal fluid (CSF). The spinal cord, the anterior spinal artery, and the paired posterior spinal arteries that supply the spinal cord are all enclosed by the pia mater. All spinal nerves originate in the spinal cord by their anterior and posterior root and exit the spinal canal through the intervertebral foramen at each segment. The intervertebral foramen is bordered cranially by the inferior margin of the pedicle, anteriorly by the vertebral body, posteriorly by the articular processes and caudally by the superior margin of the pedicle of the next lower vertebra. Also, in the intervertebral foramen lies the spinal ganglion which is surrounded by dura mater (Figs. 14.2. and 14.3., Figs. 14.7. and 14.8.).

Vessels and Nerves

A. Arteries and Veins

The arteries that supply the cervical cord arise from the vertebral artery and the deep cervical artery. In the thoracic and lumbar spine, the arterial supply originates from segmental arteries off the aorta (Figs. 12.7. and 12.8.). Each dorsal branch has a branch that traverses the intervertebral foramen to the spinal canal (spinal ramus). The dorsal branches also supply the perivertebral musculature as well as the vertebral arches. The vein flow follows similar tracks.

B. Nerves

Each spinal segmental nerve, after leaving the intervertebral foramen, separates into four branches: 1 meningial branch; 2 communicating branches; 3 posterior branch; 4 anterior branch. The meningial branch is a sensory nerve and twice during its course it traverses through the intervertebral foramen. It innervates the meninges, the inner lining of the vertebral canal, and the anterior portion of the intervertebral joint capsule (facet joint).

The communicating branches are autonomic nerve fibers that end in the sympathetic trunk. Through the gray communicating branches the spinal nerve receives the postganglionic autonomic nerves that innervate the peripheral vessels and the skin (Head's zones).

The dorsal branch is a mixed nerve that innervates the perivertebral musculature, the posterior trunk, and the posterior portion of the facet capsule. Changes in the spinal canal (see segmental movements) may cause an increase in involuntary tension of the perivertebral musculature via the dorsal branch of the spinal nerve.

The ventral branch is the longest branch of the spinal segmental nerve. It extends to the anterior lateral trunk and segmentally innervates the

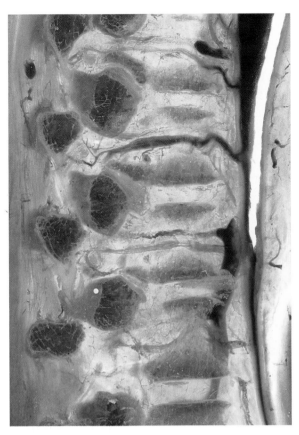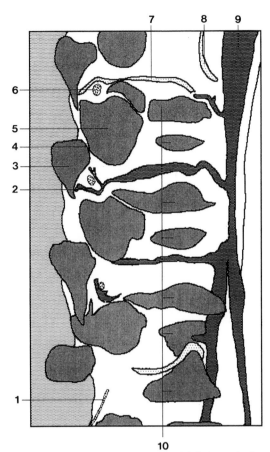

Figs. 14.7. and **14.8.** (Anatomy and drawing) *1* Exiting spinal segmental nerves; *2* intervertebral vein; *3* inferior articular process; *4* facet joint; *5* superior articular process; *6* spinal ganglion; *7* and *8* intercostal artery; *9* azygos vein; *10* partial volume of the vertebral bodies.

skin and underlying musculature. In the region of the extremities, these ventral branches form multiple plexi.

The Motion Segment

The term "motion segment" was coined by Junghanns in 1951. It encompasses all elements that are involved in the movement between two vertebrae. The bony structure of this motion segment is composed of the two vertebrae and the connecting intervertebral disc. Also, the intervertebral foramen with its accompanying nerve pathways, the ligamentous apparatus, the perivertebral musculature and the joints of the vertebrae make up the "motion segment".

The motion segment is a functional unit and, when affected, tends to be totally involved in the pathological processes. It is difficult to understand the total picture of intervertebral disc diseases without fully understanding the anatomy of the complex "motion segment".

Degenerative changes in the intervertebral disk primarily lead to a laxity of the motion segment. If a protrusion or a disc prolapse occurs, the nerve routes and vessels in the intervertebral foramen can be compressed. The consequences can be ischemia to the affected area, edematous changes, painful tension of the back musculature, paresthesias, pareses, and autonomic disturbances. Furthermore, involuntary tension of the back musculature can lead to further narrowing of the affected intervertebral foramen of the motion segment. In this way, the process becomes a self-perpetuating vicious circle. Finally, irreversible damage to the nerve root may occur.

Further Reading

1. Benninghoff A., Goerttler K.: Lehrbuch der Anatomie des Menschen. Band 1, München 1978
2. Junghans H.: Die funktionelle Pathologie der Zwischenwirbelscheiben als Grundlage für klinische Betrachtungen. Arch. Klin. Chir. 267 (1951) 393–417
3. Rohen J.W.: Funktionelle Anatomie des Menschen. Stuttgart 1984
4. Rohen J.W.: Topographische Anatomie. Stuttgart 1984
5. Rohen J.W.: Anatomie des Menschen. Photographischer Atlas, Stuttgart 1988
6. Schiebler T.H., Schmidt W. (Hrsg.): Anatomie. Berlin 1987

Chapter 15
Pathophysiology of Diseases of the Vertebral Body/Intervertebral Disc Functional Unit

A.M. Schmidt, D.H.W. Grönemeyer, R.M.M. Seibel

The intervertebral discs have an immense influence on the mobility of the vertebral column. The vertebral disc consists of obliquely arranged connective tissue fibers (the fibrous ring or anulus fibrosus) and a gelatinous central portion (the nucleus pulposus). The anatomic structure of the intervertebral disc has already been described in detail in the previous chapter. The collagen of the nucleus pulposus initially consists mostly of glycosamin-glycanes which are replaced, as one ages, by dermatansulfate. Also due to the high portion of glycosamin-glycanes, the nucleus pulposus is able to bind water. Additionally these proteoglycanes are important for the nutritive exchange. The nucleus of the disc acts as a buffer between the vertebral bodies due to its great water binding capacity [1]. Where there is an eccentric strain on the disc, it will give way to the weak side. In cases where the resistance of the anulus fibrosus is reduced, the nucleus gives way in the direction of the weakest point. If this point is in the cartilage of the upper or lower plate of the vertebral body, a disc herniation (Schmorl's node) will result [8]. This point physiologically is within the area of the notochord (chorda dorsalis). If the nucleus either partially or completely perforates the fibrous ring, a disc prolapse will result.

Compression and decompression of the disc during movement and rest causes a kind of pumping action. This leads to a shifting of fluid within the area of the disc. This mechanism can be observed by the circadian decrease in height of the the intervertebral space caused by continuous pressure on the disc. This fluid exchange is important for understanding the nutritive and mechanical physiology and pathophysiology of the disc. Due to the continuous variation of pressure, a fluid movement in the direction of the disc takes place through the fine perforated cartilage of the vertebral body plates. In this way nutrient supply to the disc is ensured.

With a progressive degeneration of the nucleus pulposus the disc becomes more and more rigid. This decreases the diffusion of nutrient and then leads to a vicious circle by which inadequate nutrition adds to progressive degeneration. A consequent decrease in disc height leads to stability loss at that segment. If the back musculature then compensates, a discopathy can follow.

Sensory innervation is in the outer areas of the anulus fibrosus (see chapter 14 – The vertebral column) [5].

Microfractures after strain or due to degenerative processes at the outer area of the fibrous ring may also cause acute pain. The intervertebral disc is provided with blood vessels up to the interior layers of the anulus. However, the nucleus is free of vessels. Already at infancy the blood vessels have receded. This triggers the aging process in the form of a progressive dehydration. The dehydration of the intervertebral disc can be seen at MRI with T2-weighted images as an increasingly hypointense area within the region of the nucleus. With dehydration the nucleus loses its gelatinous consistency and shrinks. Due to this shrinking process of the nucleus, the disc will lose its buffer function. With the pressure load on the dehydrated anulus, radial tears can occur. This condition is also called "Dérangement interne" [3]. Following this, nuclear material can more easily invade the anulus ring, overstretch the fibrous ring and ligamentous system. If this material bulges into the spinal canal, it is called protrusion. If it penetrates through the fibrous ring, it is called disc prolapse. This mechanism is most distinct at the region of lordosis, due to the mechanical load strain here [1]. The protrusion or prolapse can cause a compression of the intraspinal venous plexus with a corresponding dilation of these vessels. The subsequent delevioration in perfusion of the segmental nerves leads to an increased development of perineural granular tissue with local inflammatory reaction [2]. Thereby, a degenerative process of the nerve is initiated, which leads to well-known painful conditions. The discopathy can lead to a painful perineural fibrosis, caused by venous compression and obstruction with insufficient fibrinolytic activation as well as through fibrin deposition.

The factors which are responsible for the insufficient fibrinolytic activation are unknown [2]. Periradicular fibrosis is well observed at CT as well as at MRI, as a thickened nerve root. The cartilage plates which separate the intervertebral space from the vertebral bodies, can also show tears due to chronic stress. Through these lesions blood vessels can invade into the anulus. The subsequent metaplastic processes can lead to calcifications and gaseous inclusions (nitrogen) in the disc region. In the radiologic literature, this is considered a sign of advanced detoriation. The detection of gaseous inclusions within the disc tissue is called vacuum phenomena [6]. Due to the decrease in the intervertebral space, reactive periosteal bone neoformation can develop [7]. In cases with associated enchondral ossification of the prolapsed disc, there may also exist a continuous connection between vertebral body and exostosis.

Some fibers of the anulus radiate into the anterior longitudinal ligament. In cases of nuclear degeneration and preserved anulus, there is increased stress at the periostium of the ventral and lateral vertebral body [1]. Stimulation sufficient to prompt new bone formation can result. Consequently, the spondylosis deformans that develops is not an independent illness, but rather more a reactive change.

If the nucleus and the anulus are both degenerated, there is an increased pressure load on the neighboring vertebral body plates. This leads to a subcartilaginous hyperostosis. These alterations are summarized under the term osteochondrosis vertebralis, which often follows an increased stress on the vertebral column. This causes hypertrophy of the facet joints. The intervertebral foramina are narrowed and a nerve root compression may occur. These types of degenerative vertebral joint changes are called spondylarthrosis deformans.

In cases of primarily osseous narrowing intervertebral foramen, a minor disc protrusion can lead to additional root damage. Clinically this type of damage demonstrates radicular signs and symptoms.

With an increasing loss of cartilage within the region of the facet joints, instability and partial dislocation of these joints may occur. This acts as a stimulus for a subsequent hypertrophy of the yellow ligaments as well as hypertrophy of the vertebral arches. These changes will lead to a narrow spinal canal which clinically presents as a painful cauda-syndrome or spinal claudication.

The vertebral canal is anteriorly limited by the posterior longitudinal ligament (PLL). This is considerably wider at the retrodiscal section than at the retrovertebral section. Therefore it has a rhombus-like appearance. The PLL is affixed to the middle section of the disc leaving a large part of the disc without ligamental reinforcement on the lateral portion. As a result, discs prolapse more frequently to mediolateral than to medial [3].

A median prolapse at L5/S1 level is located most often between the S1 roots, so that radicular signs and symptoms are frequently absent. The mediolateral prolapses lead to a nerve root compression with the pathophysiologic changes described above. In most cases these prolapses show monoradicular signs and symptoms. If the prolapse is far lateral, then the nerve root from the upper segment can also be damaged.

References

1. Doerr W.: Organpathologie. Stuttgart 1974
2. Baumgartner H.: 2. Europäischer Kongreß der International Back Pain Society, Mai 88, Montreux/Schweiz, Der Schmerz 3 (1989) 46–49
3. Gerlach J.: Grundriß der Neurochirurgie. Darmstadt 1981
4. Grote W.: Neurochirurgie. Stuttgart 1975
5. Lange M.: Lehrbuch der Orthopädie und Traumatologie. 2. Band, II, Stuttgart 1965
6. Piepgras U.: Neuroradiologie. Stuttgart 1977
7. Remmele W. (Hrsg.): Pathologie. Heidelberg 1984
8. Sandritter W., Beneke G.: Allgemeine Pathologie, Stuttgart 1974

Chapter 16
New Methods of Treatment of Spinal Column Diseases Using Interventional Radiological Techniques

R.M.M. Seibel, D.H.W. Grönemeyer, Th. Grumme

Introduction

Degeneration of the spinal column is a common disease. In the Federal Republic of Germany (FRG), treatment of back pain is the primary pain therapy next to headaches. Based on Federal Association of Pharmaceutical Industries data for 1983/84, the overall sale of analgesics and rheumatoid medications in 1982 amounted to 781.8 million Deutschmarks (approximately US$ 400 million), an increase of 130% compared with 1971 [76]. An estimated 30–40% of this amount is spent on treatment of back pain. In 1983 the frequency of back pain in the female population was 62–81% and for males 68-70% [4]. 52–60% of these cases were connected with their work [4]. Furthermore, only 50% of the patients suffering from back pain for more than 6 months ever returned to work. Moreover, the cost of early payment of social security benefits for these cases is enormous and is far above the cost of treatment.

Additionally, 60% of all applications for disability benefits and a major part of all applications for extended care centers [40] are due to recurrent and unresponsive cases of back pain.

Statistics from the General Health Insurance show that in 1981 700,000 cases of back pain were reported and resulted in a loss of 13 million days of work for this group [76]. The curative and rehabilitation measures for chronic back pain, especially for treatment of low-back pain (LBP), are a heavy burden on the health and social budget.

The reported rate of success of intervertebral disc operations differs widely in the literature [3, 29, 34]. Operative results are different depending on the technique used and experience of the surgeon [33, 46, 69, 70]. Ebeling et al. found that, after 495 operations, 39% showed excellent, 31% good, and 19% satisfactory results [13].

Oppel et al. [49] reported that, after major surgery such as multiple disc operation or hemilaminectomy, the results were less favorable than after less invasive surgery. Simular results were also reported by Mattmann [38, 39]. Schepelmann et al. [53] reported delayed wound healing after extensive operations compared with less invasive surgeries.

The average complication rate from conventional operative techniques is between 5.1 and 6.5%, but there are reports of complication rates between 8% and 15.8%. These complications include discitis, impairment of wound healing, mortality and neurological deficits etc. Literature data available at present indicates that an average of 7.4% of the patients need a second back operation with 4.5% of the cases having residual material [18, 31, 39, 40, 42, 46, 49, 52, 53, 60, 65, 67, 71, 72].

Great Britain spends 240 million DM per year (4.28 DM per capita) and the United States spends 2.4 billion DM (11.80 DM per capita) per year just for treatment of LBP [28]. Unfortunately, no comprehensive epidemiological data are available for the FRG at present. Therefore, it is a great medical and economic challenge to find an effective treatment of back pain which would result in a full recovery of function. Besides surgery and conservative treatment, interventional radiology is finding its niche. Interventional radiology has shown promising results from new techniques that can offer an accurate, minimally invasive procedure for the relief of back pain.

Because of the many causes of back pain, an exact diagnosis is often difficult. This diagnosis requires an extensive history and often accurate general medical and neurologic evaluations. It can be very difficult to distinguish between root pain caused by a disc lesion or by an osseous compression at the neuroforamen etc., and facet pain (pseudoradicular pain within the area of the facet joints). Therefore, neurological studies must be compared carefully with the radiologic examinations.

Neurological Examination

Nerve lesions can lead to pain that projects into the somatome of the affected nerve fibers. In cases with typical pain and hyperesthesia at the appropriate dermatome, the neurologic diagnosis can be easy. In most cases, however, the entire nerve is not affected but only parts of the dorsal or ventral ramus. The varying nerve irritations and nerve deficits can cause a symptom complex which can take different forms depending on the involvement of individual touch, motor, sympathetic or pain fibers (Table 16.1.). Often, radicular pain, pseudo-radicular pain, and even tumor pain are present simultaneously. Also, even totally peripheral pain may originate in the spinal column. The afferent symptoms of a damaged spinal level can be distributed over several segments and consequently can produce different pain syndromes, as demonstrated in the example of lesions at the L4–5 vertebral level (Table 16.2.).

Table 16.1. Back pain terminology.

Lumbago	acute or sub-acute pain in the lumbar region of the back
Lumbalgia	chronic pain in the lumbar region of the back
Sciatica	nerve pain in the leg (sciatic nerve - supply area: L2-S2)
Lumbosciatica	back pain with pain extending to the legs

Table 16.2. Innervation region and damage level in the area of L4 level (after Auberger [1]).

1. Skin over L4 vertebral body	T 11 and T 12 nerves
2. Subcutaneous tissue, superficial muscles	L1 and L2 nerves
3. Longitudinal ligaments, parts of dura	L2 and L3 nerves
4. Facet joints	L3 to L5 nerves
5. Deep paravertebral muscles, part of vertebral arch, deep parts of interspinous ligament	L4 nerve

A thorough neurological examination, possible diagnostic blocks, and/or diagnostic electro-stimulation test (for post-discectomy syndrome) can often make the correct diagnosis and therefore the proper treatment possible.

It is routine procedure at the author's institute that a detailed pain history and documentation of motor activity are recorded, the flexibility of the spine (rotation, bending forward, backward, and to the side) is tested, and the Trendelenburg sign is carefully checked (for possible paresis of the gluteal musculature – L5 syndrome). The status of the biceps, triceps tendon and the radial reflexes of the arm are also examined. In the leg, the Achilles tendon reflex and the quadriceps tendon reflex are checked. Furthermore,

the fanning of toes and the finger-floor distance are evaluated. Then the small Schober (range of flexion in the lumbar spine), Ott, Lasègue signs (normal, reversed, crossed) and the Bragard sign (dorsiflexion of the foot by straight leg) are checked, and the ileosacral joints are examined. This is followed by the documentation of any area of abnormal touch and pain sensation. For diffuse pain involving the buttock or thigh and extending to the knee, it is necessary to examine the movement of the hip and knee joint. The level of the two hip joints must be evaluated. The joints of the lower extremities are also examined for pain after loading and pressure. Finally, the pulses in each extremity are checked.

Radiological Diagnosis

Before each treatment, anteroposterior (A-P) and lateral X-rays are obtained of the affected regions in the cervical, thoracic or lumbar area and, if necessary, functional radiograms. These X-rays are to confirm or rule out inflammation, degenerative disorders, tumors, osteoporosis, or spondylolisthesis.

Since a disc prolapse cannot be diagnosed on the plain film, after 4 weeks of unsuccessful conservative treatment or in the presence of neurological deficits, a CT scan and possibly an MRI should be performed. Experience in Germany shows that both CT and MRI are not used as frequently as they could be. CT and MRI are of great value in the evaluation of the disc in relation to the nerves and to the spinal cord. The indications for myelography have decreased, since it can reliably be replaced by non-invasive methods such as CT and MRI. In difficult cases, doubtful diagnosis, or negative CT and MRI scans (approximately 12% of all cases) a myelo-CT or a conventional myelography may be needed. The frequently used argument of lower cost for myelography can be refuted by pointing out the follow-up cost and the relatively frequent side-effect of a CSF-loss syndrome with violent headaches.

An advantage of MRI, besides the high morphologic differentiation, is the multiplanar capabilities which allow imaging in any plane without the use of ionizing radiation. However, osseous structures can be more clearly delineated using CT. If the CT scan is unclear, an MRI examination is indicated (Beyer [3]) such as in the case of a post-discectomy syndrome. This syndrome may be caused by the pathophysiological processes listed in Table 16.3., which can often be differentiated by MRI.

Furthermore, MRI is the method of choice for the evaluation of post-operative complications,

Table 16.3. Causes of a postdiscotomy or postnucleotomy syndrome.

– prolapse at another level
– new protrusion prolapse
– intra- or extradural scar
– intra- or extradural sequester
– incomplete removal at first surgery
– overlooked sequester
– inadequate indication for surgery
– inadequate surgical technique
– segmental spine column instability as consequence of surgery
– nerve root lesion
– instability of spine
– spondylolisthesis
– root cysts
– spurious (pseudo) meningocele
– bony spinal stenosis
– varicose veins
– facet syndrome
– spondylitis
– discitis
– iliosacral joint changes
– hip-joint diseases
– diseases of the tendons
– other diseases (i.e. Pyruvate-calcinosis, tumors, etc.)

i.e. for an early diagnosis of iatrogenic, traumatic or post-operative inflammatory spinal column change or alterations at the cauda equina and/or individual nerve roots. MRI can often reliably evaluate patients post-operatively, i.e. in a partial disc resection or in a fat implant. MRI should be used as a matter of routine in these cases and also after percutaneous nucleotomy (Figs. 16.1. and 16.2.).

Differential Diagnosis of Back Pain

For each case of back pain, one is inclined to attribute the symptoms to a disc lesion. In order to avoid an erroneous diagnosis, detailed knowledge of the multiple etiology of back pain is mandatory. The differential diagnosis includes degenerative, inflammatory processes, tumor changes, myotenositis and vessel alterations (i.e. thrombosis, angioma or Mondor's disease). Also, organic diseases of the liver, pancreas and stomach as well as alterations of the aorta and the vena cava can provoke back pain. Another frequent cause of pain in the spinal column is pain referred by changes in the urogenital region. A comprehensive differential diagnosis for back pain is shown in Tables 16.4. and 16.5. and Fig. 16.3.

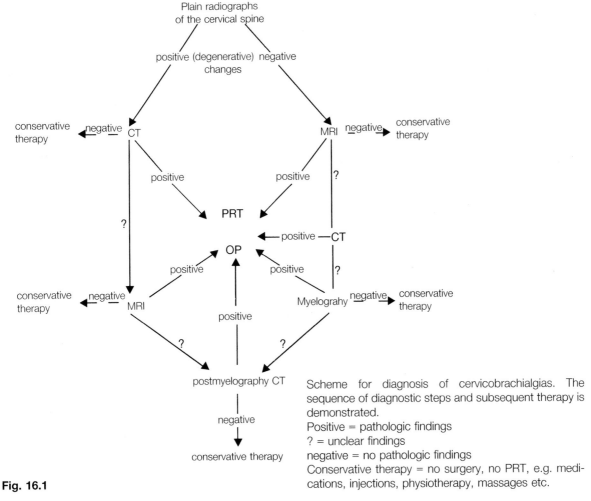

Scheme for diagnosis of cervicobrachialgias. The sequence of diagnostic steps and subsequent therapy is demonstrated.
Positive = pathologic findings
? = unclear findings
negative = no pathologic findings
Conservative therapy = no surgery, no PRT, e.g. medications, injections, physiotherapy, massages etc.

Fig. 16.1

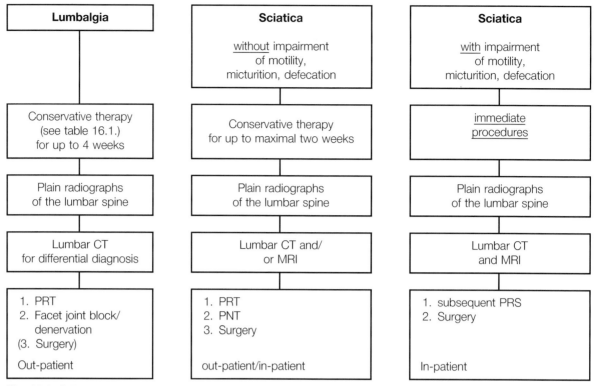

Lumbalgia	**Sciatica**	**Sciatica**
	without impairment of motility, micturition, defecation	with impairment of motility, micturition, defecation
Conservative therapy (see table 16.1.) for up to 4 weeks	Conservative therapy for up to maximal two weeks	immediate procedures
Plain radiographs of the lumbar spine	Plain radiographs of the lumbar spine	Plain radiographs of the lumbar spine
Lumbar CT for differential diagnosis	Lumbar CT and/ or MRI	Lumbar CT and MRI
1. PRT 2. Facet joint block/ denervation (3. Surgery) Out-patient	1. PRT 2. PNT 3. Surgery out-patient/in-patient	1. subsequent PRS 2. Surgery In-patient

Fig. 16.2. Scheme for diagnosis and therapy in patients with suspicion of discopathy.

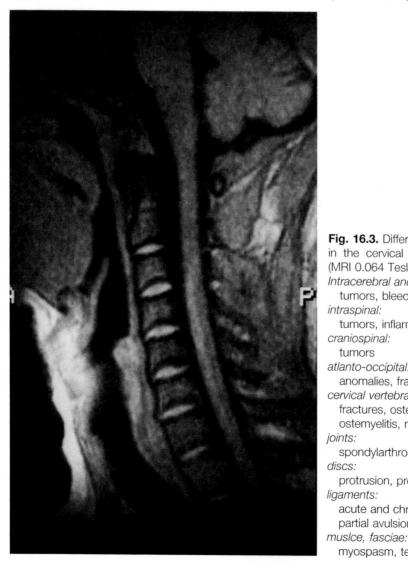

Fig. 16.3. Differential diagnosis of pathologic causes in the cervical spine region by cervicobrachialgias (MRI 0.064 Tesla)

Intracerebral and intracerebellar:
    tumors, bleeding, inflammation
intraspinal:
    tumors, inflammation, syrinx
craniospinal:
    tumors
atlanto-occipital:
    anomalies, fractures, inflammation
cervical vertebra:
    fractures, osteochondrosis, osteoporosis, ostemyelitis, metastases
joints:
    spondylarthrosis, inflammation
discs:
    protrusion, prolapse, discitis, abscess
ligaments:
    acute and chronic alteration after whiplash, partial avulsion, laxity, inflammation
muslce, fasciae:
    myospasm, tendomyosis

Table 16.4. Differential diagnosis for back pain of thoracic and lumbar spine.

Area of lesion	Cause	Symptoms/Pain localization
Heart	1 Angina pectoris 2 Infarct	Circular in the back Radiating into left arm
Thorax	1 Mesothelioma 2 Bronchial carcinoma 3 Emphysema 4 Pleurisy, acute lobar pneumonia	One or both sides, i.e. behind shoulder Back/shoulder pain Feeling of pressure in chest and back Shoulder pain
Vessels	1 Aneurysm 2 Venous: Thrombosis, i.e. superficial thoracic veins	Severe, intermittent back pain Feeling of tension, hyperesthesia, pressing pain at the lateral thoracic wall (Mondor syndrome)
Gall Bladder	Stones, tumor	Shoulder pain
Pancreas	Pancreatitis, tumor, pseudo-cysts	Circular into back
Kidney	1 Obstruction 2 Inflammation 3 Tumor 4 Trauma	Pain projection into lumbar region and groin
Bladder	Tumor	Pain in the lumbar region

Genitals	1 Tumor (uterus, prostate)
	2 Alterations in position:
	   – retroflexion of uterus
	   – descensus, prolapse
	3 Inflammation
	   – prostatitis, vesiculitis sem.
	4 Endometriosis
	5 Premenstrual syndrome
		Pain in the lumbar region and perineum possible

Intestine	Tumor	Radiating into buttocks and/or perineum
Spinal cord	1 Myelitis 2 Spinal angio-dysgenesis 3 Myelomalacia 4 Tumor	Belt-type symptom, neurologic deficits Belt-type symptom, neurologic deficits Segmental pain, syringomyelic dissociation, neurologic deficits Belt-type symptom, radicular pain, neurologic deficits

Spinal root	1 Herpes zoster
	2 Compression by
	   – Disc
	   – Tumor
	   – Scar
	   – Bone alterations
		Skin anthema on one side, severe, partly burning, radicular pain
		Radicular or diffuse pain, neurologic deficits, possible perspiration disorders

Peripheral nerve	– Scar tissue – Tumor – Inflammation	Peripheral functional deficits
Muscle	1 Myotenositis 2 Myositis	Local pressure pain
Spreading pain	Diseases of various organs	Irritation of the Head's zones, dermatome pain
Local processes	1 Tietze's syndrome 2 Friedrich's syndrome 3 Cyriax syndrome	Rib cartilage swelling with parasternal spontaneous pressure and motion pain Pain, swelling, redness, demineralization at the sternoclavicular joint Abnormal mobility of inferior rib, paroxysmal pain at the costal arch, hyperesthesia in segment T9-depending on movement.

Table 16.5. Differential syndrome by lumbosciatica.

1 Radicular pain	4 Anteromedial mononeuropathic pain (L1-L4)
2 Arthrogenic pain	– iliohypogastric nerve
– facet syndrome	– ilioinguinal nerve
– iliosacral syndrome	– genitofemoral nerve
– knee-hip joint alterations	– lateral cutaneous nerve of the thigh
3 Plexus pain	– femoral nerve and saphenous nerve
– lumbar plexus	– obturator nerve
– lumbosacral plexus	5 Posterolateral mononeuropathic pain (L5-S4)
– plexus pudendus nervosus	– gluteal nerve
– coccygeal plexus	– sciatic nerve
	– tibial nerve

A. Facet Therapy

Often pain in the lumbar region can be treated by facet denervation. These facet joints are sensorily innervated from the adjacent segments. Serious arthritic changes can cause facet pain which can be alleviated by CT-guided denervation.

In 1971 Rees [51] introduced a method of multiple bilateral percutaneous lumbar facet denervation with a scalpel. This method was modified by Shealy [56, 57], who separated the nerves with an electrocoagulation probe to avoid large hematomas, which Rees experienced in 20% of cases. Since that time, the method has been called "Facet Rhizotomy" or "Facet Denervation".

During further development of this treatment, the procedure was performed with fluorscopy-guided injections of corticosteroids or a local anesthetic. The use of a physiologic solution to provoke pain as well as facet denervation with 96% ethanol have also been attempted.

Facet Pain Syndrome

The typical symptom of a facet syndrome is diffuse back pain which increases with motion. This pain can radiate to the pelvic girdle and the inguinal region, to the buttocks and/or into the thighs. Occasionally, the pain can reach below the knee. The facet pain is not confined to any segmental borders ("pseudoradicular pain") and can occur in addition to a radicular pain. Furthermore, the hypertrophic changes of the facet joints can also produce radicular pain symptoms by bony spondylarthrosis compression of the neuroforamina.

The facet joint capsulae are well innervated with pain fibers. Pain in this area can be caused by vertical displacement of the joint facets, improper straining, as well as reactive muscular tension and poor posture. Also, changes in these joints can be from misalignment from a postdiscectomy syndrome. After disc surgery, the facet joints have to cushion an increasing pressure load due to the lack of elasticity of the surrounding ligaments and discs. This increased pressure, which is transmitted to the facet joints, can lead to arthrosis which can be very painful (Fig. 16.4.). The facet pain is often described as sharp, burning and penetrating. In the cervical spine this pain is mostly superficial. In the lumbar vertebrae the facet pain is described as deep.

Cervical Vertebrae

Cervical facet pain can radiate into the arms and can be caused by movement. This can involve muscle tension type pain with curtailment of mobility ("Twisted Neck", "Stiff Neck"). Normally the pain caused at the C3 and C4 level radiates diffusely into the neck region, whereas the pain originating at the C5 and C6 level is described as radiating into the shoulder or arm. Following this, there is often associated progressive muscular tension. The pain can possibly be elicited by axial compression or movement in the direction of tension.

Thoracic Vertebrae

Thoracic facet pain is described as a sharp pain shooting into the chest wall occurring with motion, which then disappears quickly. Later

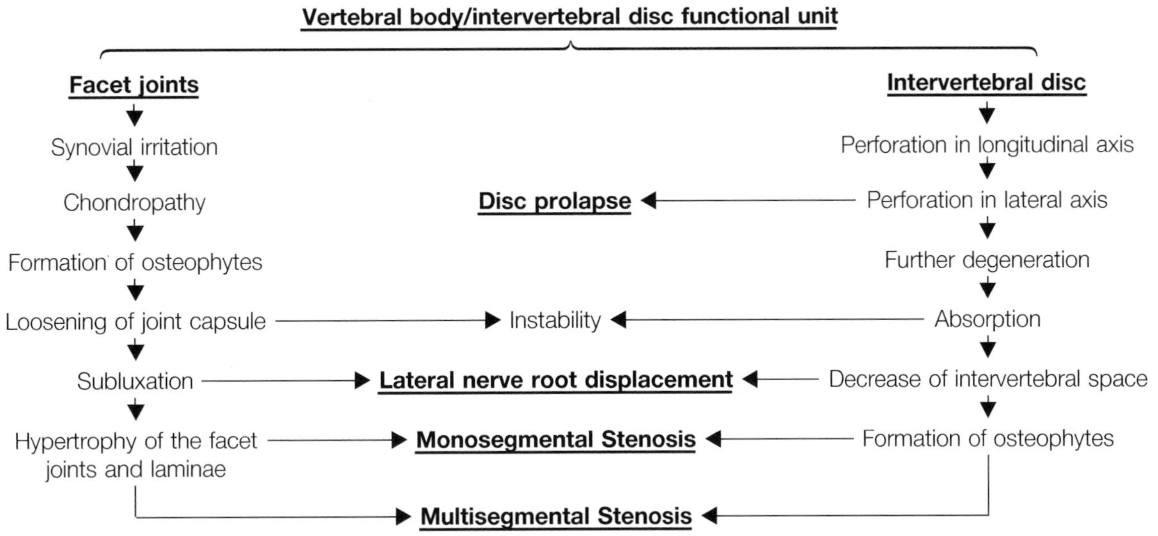

Vertebral body/intervertebral disc functional unit

Facet joints		Intervertebral disc
↓		↓
Synovial irritation		Perforation in longitudinal axis
↓		↓
Chondropathy	**Disc prolapse** ←	Perforation in lateral axis
↓		↓
Formation of osteophytes		Further degeneration
↓		↓
Loosening of joint capsule ——→	Instability ←	—— Absorption
↓		↓
Subluxation ——→	**Lateral nerve root displacement** ←	—— Decrease of intervertebral space
↓		↓
Hypertrophy of the facet ——→ joints and laminae	**Monosegmental Stenosis** ←	—— Formation of osteophytes
└——→	**Multisegmental Stenosis** ←	——┘

Fig. 16.4. Demonstration of the complex changes in the vertebral body/intervertebral disc functional unit. The pathologic alterations are schematically shown.

this pain is overlapped by pain from muscular tension. It can often be reduced by rest. Furthermore, patients sometimes complain of a feeling of chest tightness or constriction. Finally, this thoracic facet pain can also be provoked by rotation or extension of the back.

Lumbar Vertebrae

Changes of the lower lumbar facet can cause pain which can radiate into the sacral illiac joint, into the region of the iliac roll, back of upper thigh, to the ischium and sometimes also into the lower leg. The upper facets can cause pain in the iliac crest, lumbosacral angle and inguinal area [1, 8, 54].

Anatomy

The facet joints are supplied by the fibers of the medial branch of the dorsal ramus of the spinal nerve (Figs. 16.5. and 16.6.). Just behind the spinal ganglion, the dorsal ramus divides into a medial and lateral branch. The skin and paraspinal musculature are supplied by the lateral branch. The medial branch supplies both the facet joint capsulae at the same level as the nerve and also the facet joint just below this

level. Consequently, the joint capsulae are bisegmentally innervated. This medial branch crosses the lower facet joint process. Furthermore, the inner half of the facet is supplied by the sinuvertebral n. (ramus meningeus nervorum spinalium). In cases of transmitted pain in this nerve the patient will complain about leg and back pain. This transmitted facet pain radiates into the myotomes and sclerotomes more than into the dermatome [6, 64] (see Chapter: Spinal Anatomy).

Indications for Interventional Procedures

Pain caused by degenerative changes of the facet joints with signs of early hypertrophic spondylarthrosis without compression of the segmental nerve can be treated with the blocking or

Table 16.6. Indication for facet blocks or denervation of the facets.

- Pseudoradicular pain at the cervical, thoracic, and/or lumbar spine;
- locking and changes due to abnormal strain on the facet joints;
- degenerative changes of the facet joints;
- as an addition to periradicular therapy

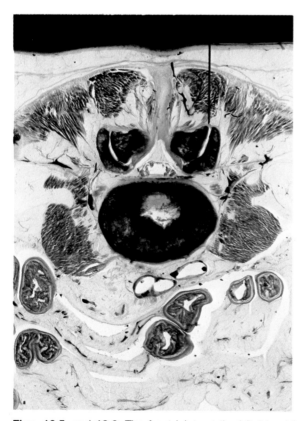
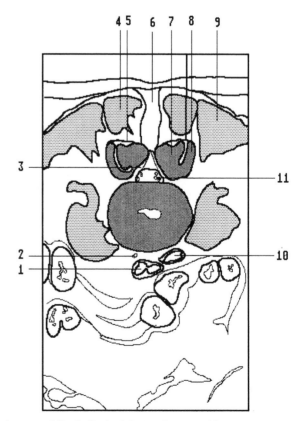

Figs. 16.5. and **16.6.** The facet joints at the L3-4 level (anatomy and illustration). *1* Aorta; *2* sympathicoabdominale ganglion; *3* epidural space; *4* a medial tract of the back muscles; *5* capsula of the facet joint; *6* interspinous ligament; *7* superior articular process L4; *8* inferior articular process L3; *9* lateral aspect of the back muscles; *10* vena cava; *11* cauda equina.

denervation of these facets. If compression of the nerve root is also present, a periradicular treatment (PRT) can be performed (Table 16.6.).

Technique for Facet Blocking

With the patient in the prone position, a CT scan of the posterior portion of the affected facet joint is performed. After measuring the depth and angle for the puncture, a 22-G needle is advanced to the facet joint. Then either a diagnostic provocation test with a physiologic salt solution for pain or a diagnostic blockade is performed. The position of the needle tip and the distribution of the medication are checked using 0.5–1 ml contrast medium. Then 3–5 ml of a local anesthetic is injected followed by the careful injection of 1 ml Triamcinolonacetonide (10 or 40 mg) or 1.5–2 ml of 96% ethanol. CT scans are performed during and after the injection to check the exact distribution of the injected solution (Figs. 16.7.–16.10.).

Findings

From March 1, 1986 to March 1, 1989 a total of 171 patients were treated for pain in the lumbar facet joints. Of the total of 171 patients, 102 patients were treated prior to March 1, 1988. A maximum of six joints were blocked (L3-S1), with an average of three joints per patient. A total of 513 joints were treated in the 171 patients.

After their treatment, 81% of 102 patients (treated before March 1, 1988) stated that immediately after therapy they had no complaints of pain on the treated facets. 13% of the 102 patients required treatment of the opposite side or other facet joints. After this therapy, they were pain-free. After three months, the average success rate (% of patients pain-free) was 79%, after one year 67% and after two years 65%. An additional observation was a distinct improvement, but not being pain-free, in 21% after three months, 17% after one year and 15% of all patients after two years. Recurrent pain after three months was seen in 12% of the patients and after one or two years the rate of recurrent pain remained at 18% of the total therapy group.

From March 1, 1988 to March 1, 1989 31% of the 69 patients had a combination of a disc prolapse with hypertrophy of the facet joints. Therefore they had a combination of periradicular therapy and denervation of the facets.

Complications/Side-Effects

In 2% of the 513 treatments an aching and burning back pain occurred after therapy, which was resolved after two treatments with a mixture of a local anesthetic and corticosteroids.

Instrumentation and medication for denervation of the facet joints	
Needle	10-15 cm 22-G needle DCHN 22-10.0-S1 or DCHN 22-15.0-S1 (Cook)
Local anesthetic	3-5 ml Mepivacaine 1%
Ethanol for injection 96%	1.5-2 ml
Contrast medium	Iopromide 0.4 ml

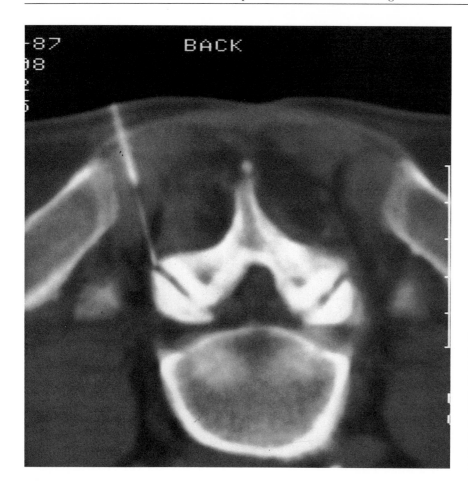

Fig. 16.7. After advancement of the guide needle, the interventional needle is advanced through the guide with the tip at the facet joint. The needle tip must not be advanced into the joint in order to avoid cartilage damage by the alcohol.

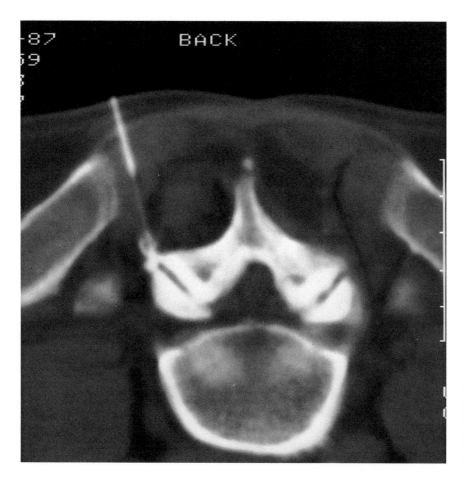

Fig. 16.8. To document the needle position a diluted contrast agent is injected. This contrast spreads in a cap-like fashion dorsally over the joint space. It is important that no contrast agent extends into the joint space.

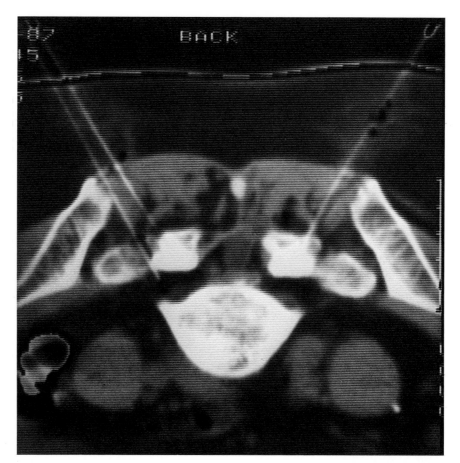

Fig. 16.9. CT scan of a combined procedure of periradicular therapy at L5/S1 level on the left with a bilateral facet block. The interventional needle (on the left and lateral to the other needle) is guided past the facet joint laterally. The tip is now in the intervertebral foramen.
The tips of the two other interventional needles rest directly on the facet joints. The small hyperdense structure seen bilaterally in the tissue are a result of air and/or medication injected.

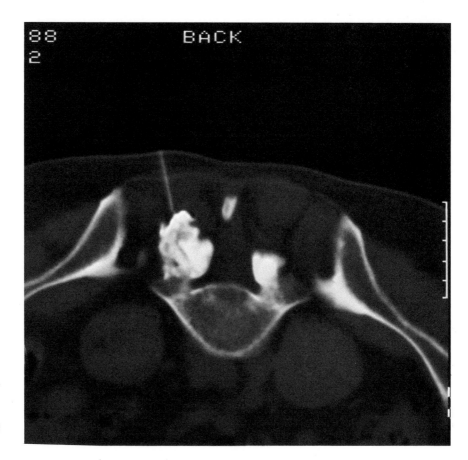

Fig. 16.10. CT scan of a distinct hypertrophic spondylarthrosis at segment L5/S1 level. A hyperdense contrast agent cap is seen just posteriorly to the joint.

B. Periradicular Therapy (PRT)

For patients with continued pain after an unsuccessful disc operation and other patients with different forms of low back pain the clinic has begun a new form of therapy called CT-guided periradicular therapy (PRT). In this therapy, a needle, 0.7 mm, is advanced under CT guidance to the intervertebral foramen in the region of the disc or in the case of a postdiscectomy syndrome to the area of scar tissue, and an injection of medication (see Table Medication for PRT) is administered.

The results of this method are very convincing. For the patient to have a permanent pain reduction or to be pain-free, approximately six to eight separate treatments have to be administered. PRT can result in restoration of the nerve function and resolve minor motor pareses. In almost all post-operative patients treated with PRT, a repeated disc operation was avoided.

So far over 1000 patients have been treated in this manner.

Pain Symptoms

In the evaluation of pain it is fundamental to differentiate between acute and chronic pain. Acute radicular pain remains constant in localization. It is characterized by a sharp and superficial pain of high intensity shooting into the extremity. Associated paresthesias may be absent.

The next chronic stage is characterized by sensation deficits, dull pain, with or without signs of numbness which may extend to weakness. The neurological alterations are often confined to the segmental distribution ("radicular pain"), but may be overlapped by other abnormalities, i.e. a multi-segmental prolapse, spondyloarthrosis or diabetic neuropathy.

The symptoms and the examinations for each radicular segment are listed in Tables 16.7. and 16.8.

Indications for Periradicular Therapy

The original indication for PRT was to treat pain and neurological deficits resulting from a postdiscectomy syndrome or scar formation after disc surgery. Other treatment possibilities for a postdiscetomy syndrome are shown in Table 16.9. After good results for the above indications, PRT was used in patients with disc prolapses for preoperative treatment of nerve root edema. Now, the most common indication for PRT is disc prolapse at any region of the spine. PRT before surgery can result in a shorter convalescence period. The second indication for PRT was chronic disc prolapses that were treated preoperatively. It was found that by using PRT the operative waiting list could be reduced and recoveries without surgery were possible. However, in these patients follow-up examinations during therapy must take place in order to diagnose a hidden lesion or deterioration of symp-

Table 16.7. Cervical root syndrome.

Localization	Associated muscle	Pain provocation	Reflex
C3-4 Shoulder to midline	diaphragm	occasionally by elevation of the scapula	
C5 Neck, shoulder, lateral arm	deltoid m. biceps m. of arm	abduction in shoulder joint	biceps reflex – C5-6
C6 Neck, shoulder radial arm, thumb	biceps m. of arm brachioradial m.,	flection at elbow flection of hand	biceps reflex – C5-6
C7 Neck, shoulder, posterior arm, 2nd and 3rd finger	triceps m. of the arm, round pronator m., greater pectoral m., muscles of the ball thumb, occasionally flexor muscles of the finger, finger extensor muscles on the ulnar side	extension at elbow joint, extension of the hand	triceps reflex – C7-8
C8 Neck, parts of shoulder, ulnar forearm, 4th and 5th finger	hypothenar, ulnar small hand muscles	stretching, closing and extension of the hand	triceps reflex – C7–8

Table 16.8. Lumbar nerve root syndrome.

Localization	Associate muscle	Pain provocation	Reflex
L1–L2 Dysesthesia above and below inguinal ligament			
L3 Dysesthesia in anterior inner thigh	Iliopsoas m., m. quadriceps m. adductor muscles	Extension at knee joint	Patellar reflex: L2–4
L4 Dysesthesia lateral from L3 across patella up to the anterior medial portion of tibia	Quadriceps m.	Extension at knee joint, lifting of foot	Patellar reflex: L2–4
L5 Dysesthesia from outside of knee joint across lateral tibia to the big toe	Long extensor m. of the great toe anterior tibial m., m. extensor muscle of the little finger gluteus med. m.	Hip joint abduction, step gait	1. Posterior tibial reflex 2. Patellar and Achilles reflex inconspicuous
S1 Dysesthesia from the bending side of thigh across lateral-posterior tibia to the lateral arch of foot	Triceps m. of the calf, short peroneal m., gluteus maximus m.	Festinating gait, gluteal and ischiocrural muscles	Achilles reflex

Table 16.9. Therapy possibilities for the postdiscectomy syndrome.

– Periradicular therapy	– Neurolysis
– Intrathecal application	– Repeat discectomy
– Electrostimulation of posterior cords	– Foraminectomy
– Facet denervation	– Osseous decompression
– Physiomechanic measures	– Spondylodesis

Indications for periradicular therapy (PRT)
Disc prolapse Pain caused by scars after disc surgery Spinal stenosis Lateral recessus stenosis Foramina stenosis Paralysis or sensory deficits through compression of the nerve roots

toms. A narrow spinal canal as well as lateral recessus stenosis or intervertebral foramen stenosis (Figs. 16.22.–16.26.) are further indications for PRT. In these cases, PRT can often postpone a back operation or if an operation is necessary it can prepare the patient to an optimum. In some cases with PRT there is a good long-term level of success, although, depending on the extent, spinal stenosis is often an area difficult to treat. Osseous compression of the foramina can also have favorable results after PRT.

Periradicular therapy is an important part of a step-by-step plan for interdisciplinary therapy of spinal diseases. PRT is in the area between conservative therapy and the different operational procedures (including percutaneous nucleotomy).

Unlike the percutaneous nucleotomy, PRT is practicable at all levels of the spine. From the beginning of 1986 to December 1988, PRT was performed on a total of 370 patients. The youngest patient was 19, the oldest patient was 84 years old. The average age was 51 years (Fig. 16.27.). In 133 patients (36%) PRT was conducted in the cervical spine, in 16 patients (4.3%) in the thoracic spine, and the remaining 221 patients (59.7%) were treated in the lumbar spine.

Table 16.10. Localization of PRT (n = 370).

Lumbar spine	221	59.7%
Thoracic spine	16	4.3%
Cervical spine	133	36.0%

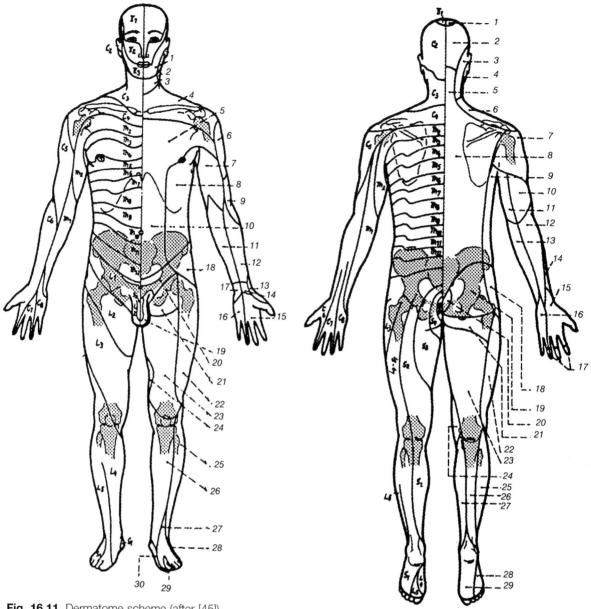

Fig. 16.11. Dermatome scheme (after [45]).

Fig. 16.11a. *1* N. trigeminus; *2* N. auricularis magnus; *3* N. transversus colli; *4* Nn. supraclaviculares; *5* Rr. cutanei anteriores nn. intercostalium; *6* N. cutaneus brachii lateralis superior; *7* N. cutaneus brachii medialis; *8* Rr. mammarii laterales nn. intercostalium; *9* N. cutaneus antebrachii posterior; *10* Rr. cutanei anteriores nn. intercostalium; *11* N. cutaneus antebrachii medialis; *12* N. cutaneus antebrachii lateralis; *13* R. superficialis n. radialis; *14* R. palmaris n. mediana; *15* N. medianus; *16* Nn. digitales palmares communes; *17* R. palmaris n. ulnaris; *18* N. iliohypogastricus (R. cut. lat.); *19* N. ilioinguinalis (Nn. scrotales anteriores); *20* N. iliohypogastricus (R. cutaneus anterior); *21* N. genitofemoralis (R. femoralis); *22* N. cutaneus femoris lateralis; *23* N. femoralis (Rr. cutanei anteriores); *24* N. obturatorius (R. cut.); *25* N. cutaneus surae lateralis; *26* N. saphenus; *27* N. peronaeus superficialis; *28* N. suralis; *29* N. peronaeus profundus; *30* N. tibialis (Rr. calcanei)

Fig. 16.11b. *1* N. frontalis (V₁); *2* N. occipitalis major; *3* N. occipitalis minor; *4* N. auricularis magnus; *5* Rr. dorsales nn. cervicalium; *6* Nn. supraclaviculares; *7* N. cutaneus brachii lateralis superior; *8* Rr. dors. nn. spin. cervic., thorac., lumb.; *9* Rr. cutanei laterales nn. intercostalium; *10* N. cutaneus brachii posterior; *11* N cutaneus brachii medialis; *12* N. cutaneus antebrachii posterior; *13* N. cutaneus antebrachii medialis; *14* N. cutaneus antebrachii lateralis; *15* R superficialis n. radialis; *16* R. dorsalis n. ulnaris; *17* N. medianus; *18* N. iliohypogastricus (R. cut. lat.); *19* Nn. clunium superiores; *20* Nn. clunium medii; *21* Nn. clunium inferiores; *22* N. cutaneus femoris lateralis; *23* N. cutaneus femoris posterior; *24* N. obturatorius (R. cut.); *25* N. cutaneus surae lateralis; *26* N. suralis; *27* N. saphenus; *28* N. plantaris lateralis; *29* N. plantaris medialis.

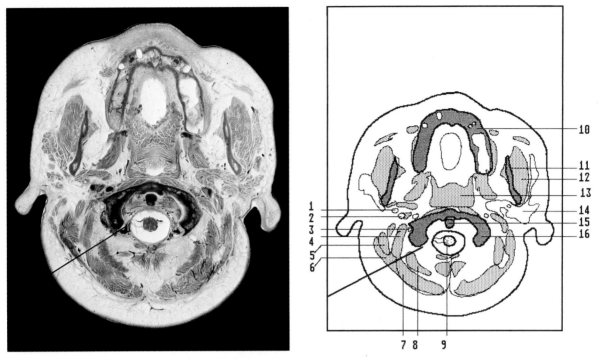

Figs. 16.12. and **16.13.** Periradicular therapy C1/C2 (anatomy and illustration). *1* External carotid artery; *2* jugular vein; *3* vertebral artery; *4* splenius muscle of the neck; *5* sternocleidomastoid muscle; *6* splenius muscle of the head; *7* semispinal muscle of the head; *8* superior oblique muscle of the head; *9* marrow; *10* alveolar process of the maxilla; *11* ramus mandibulae; *12* masseter m.; *13* soft palate; *14* parotid gland; *15* dens of the axis; *16* arch of the atlas.

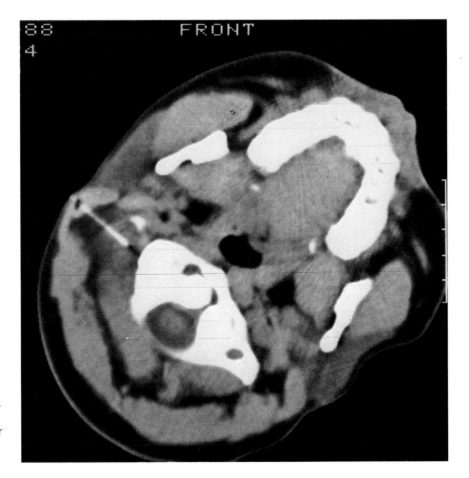

Fig. 16.14. Periradicular therapy in segment C1/C2. The position of the needle tip is identified by the linear artifact in front of the needle.

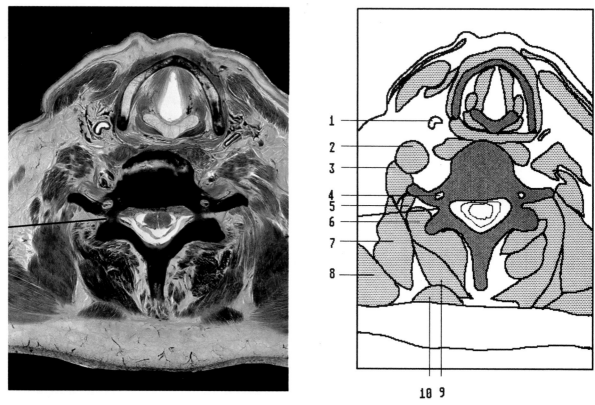

Figs. 16.15. and **16.16.** Periradicular therapy C4/5 (anatomy and illustration). *1* Carotid artery; *2* anterior scalene muscle; *3* middle scalene muscle; *4* vertebral canal and vertebral artery; *5* m. iliocostalis cervicis; *6* semispinal muscle of the neck; *7* m. longissimus cervicis and m. levator scapulae; *8* trapezius muscle; *9* splenius muscle of the head; *10* rhomboid muscle.

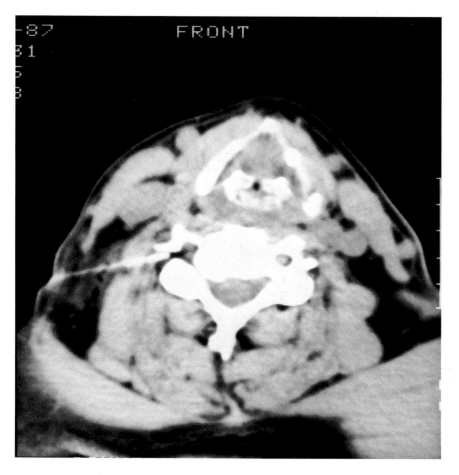

Fig. 16.17. Periradicular therapy C4/5. The puncture is performed posterior to the sternocleidomastoid m. and external jugular vein. The needle tip (to be identified by the artifact in front of the needle) is positioned in the neuroforamen near the vertebral artery and the intervertebral plexus. The large vessels (common carotid artery and internal jugular vein) are shifted anteriorly due to the extension and rotation of the head.

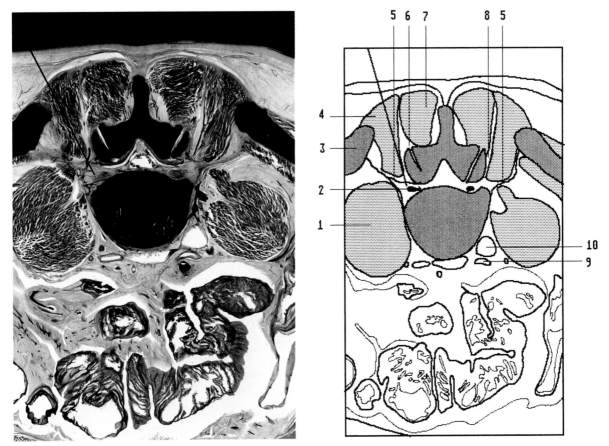

Figs. 16.18. and **16.19.** Periradicular therapy L4/5 (anatomy and illustration). *1* Iliopsoas muscle; *2* spinal ganglion; *3* pelvic crest; *4* m. iliocostalis lumborum; *5* iliolumbal ligament; *6* facet joint L4/5; *7* back musculature (medial tract); *8* segmental artery and vein; *9* common iliac artery; *10* common iliac vein.

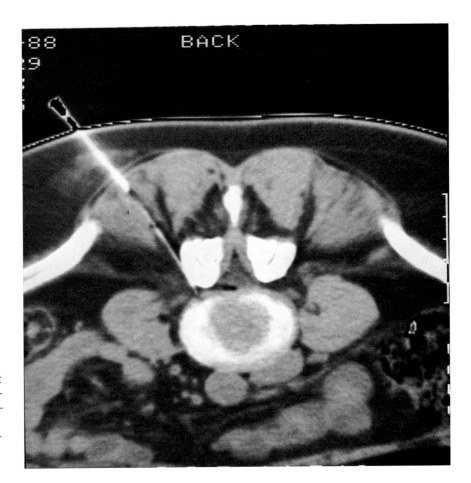

Fig. 16.20. Periradicular therapy L4/5. The needle tip is medial to the segmental nerve L4 in the intervertebral foramen. Exact perineural and epidural distribution of the injection solutions in the spinal canal (hyperdense linear perineural change of density) are identified.

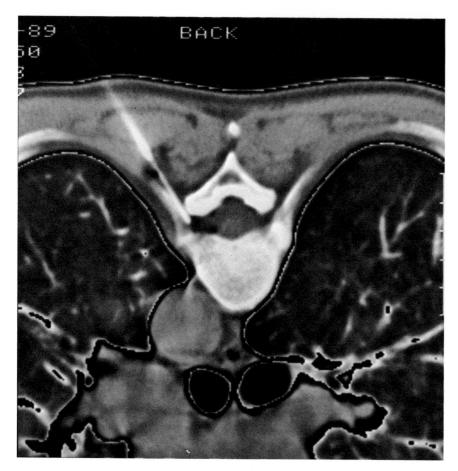

Fig. 16.21. Periradicular therapy at the thoracic spine region. The intervention needle is carefully advanced relatively far into the intervertebral foramen medial of the rib. The needle tip is at a distance of 1 mm from the segment nerve. The distribution of the medication mixture is seen as a hyperdense (black) area. Note should be made of the distribution of the medication anterior and posterior to the nerve and the epidural distribution. The indications of PRT surpass the indications for percutaneous nucleotomy as well as those for conventional nucleotomy. CT control during the puncture and after the injection of the medication is absolutely necessary in order to avoid complications [12].

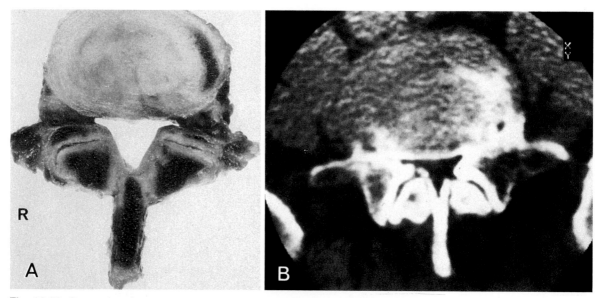

Fig. 16.22. Comparison between a spinal canal of normal width (A) and an osseous spinal stenosis (B). In both figures lateral recess stenosis is identified.

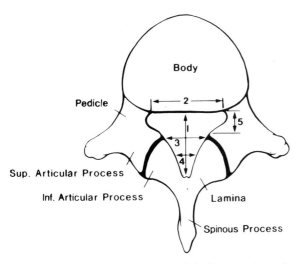

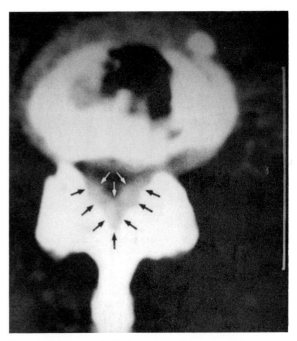

Fig. 16.23. Important measurements in the spinal canal. *1* Sagittal radius – relatively narrow 10–12 mm, extremely narrow < 10 mm; *2* interpedicular distance – pathological < 15 mm; *3* area of spinal canal – pathological < 15 mm; *4* ligamentum flavum – pathological > 5 mm; *5* lateral recessus – no stenosis 5 mm, probable stenosis 3 mm, confirmed stenosis < 2 mm.

Fig. 16.25. Three-fold stenosis in this case of hypertrophy of both ligamenta flava (black arrows). This results in spinal stenosis (white arrows) due to ligament hypertrophy and prolapse of the degenerative disc.

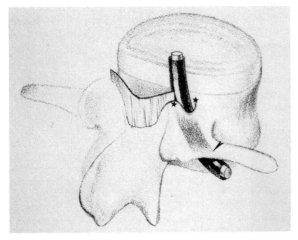

◀ **Fig. 16.24.** Drawing of the spinal nerve in the lateral recess. The two asterisks mark the width of the recess (No. 5, in Fig. 16.23.). If the recess is displaced by degenerative changes or by a disc prolapse, a nerve compression will result.

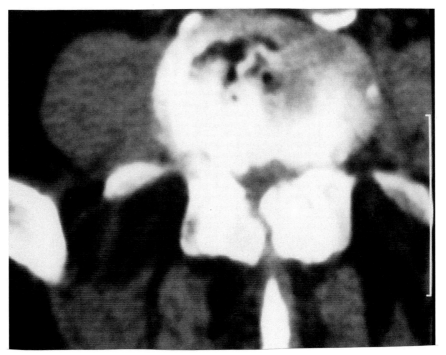

Fig. 16.26. Osseous spinal stenosis resulting from hypertrophic spondylarthrosis and disc prolapse in a massive disc degeneration.

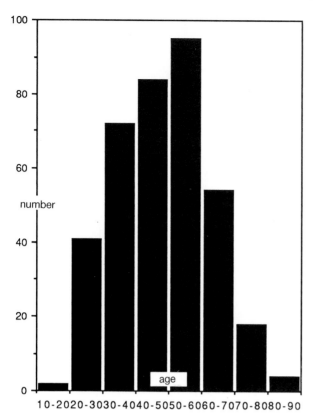

Fig. 16.27. Age-distribution of 370 patients with PRT.

PRT Technique

First, a CT scan of the affected level is obtained. Then, a CT-guided puncture with a coaxial needle set (Fig. 16.28.) to the inferior aspects of the intervertebral foramen is performed from a posterolateral approach under local anesthesia. The exact angle and the depth of the puncture can be ascertained from the CT monitor. After checking the position of the needle tip a mixture of crystal suspension of corticosteroids, local anesthetic and oxypolygelatine is injected.

After each individual step a CT scan is obtained to avoid an injury to the nerve root and avoid injecting this medication in the wrong area. After the injection, the distribution of the medication is checked with a CT scan (Figs. 16.29.–16.40.). The treatment is repeated eight times at intervals of three weeks.

Findings

At the end of the therapy 78% of the patients were pain-free. Three months after termination of the treatment another 5% of the patients showed improvement in their pain. Two years after termination of the treatment 68% of the patients were still pain-free (53 out of 78 patients) (Table 16.11.). Furthermore, there was only a small difference in the results between the different spinal regions (Table 16.12.). After the first treatment, in 15% of cases an alleviation of pain was noted; after the fourth treatment, 72% of the patients experienced a significant decrease in pain.

Table 16.11. Findings after PRT.

Symptoms improvement after first treatment	15%
Symptoms improvement after fourth treatment	72%
No symptoms at the end of treatment	78%
No symptoms three months after treatment	83%
No symptoms two years after treatment (n = 78)	68%
A second vertebra operation after PRT	3%

Table 16.12. PRT success according to location.

No complaints at the end of treatment	
Lumbar spinal column	80%
Thoracic spinal column	82%
Cervical spinal column	84%

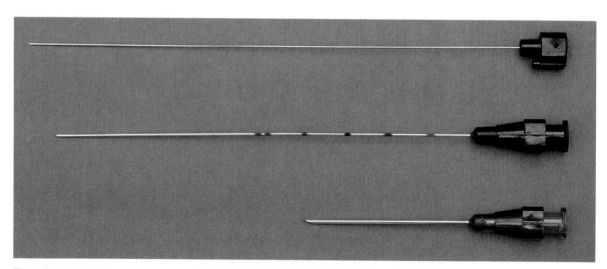

Fig. 16.28. Three-part coaxial Seibel-Grönemeyer interventional needle set.

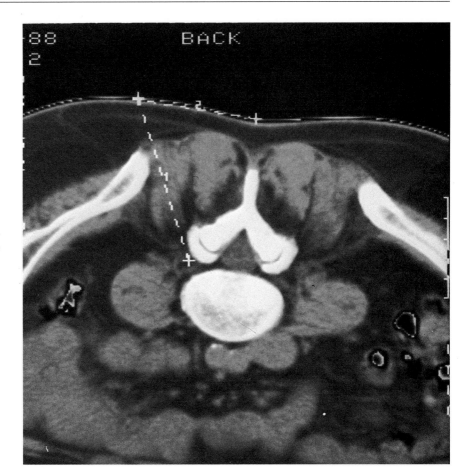

Fig. 16.29. Technical planning for periradicular therapy.
CT scan obtained for distance and angle measurement. Line (1) marks the distance from the skin to the segment nerve in the intervertebral foramen (the nerve is seen just below the cross). Line (2) marks off the distance from the midline to the puncture point on the surface of the skin. The angle between line (1) and line (2) is 68 degrees.

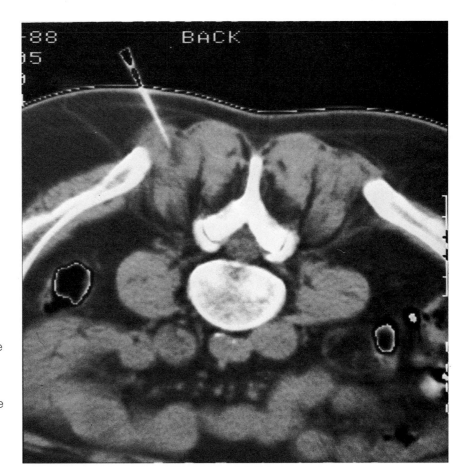

Fig. 16.30. Advancement of the guide needle past the pelvic crest. The needle is now incorrectly directed toward the facet joint. Because only the non-flexible guide needle is present, the angle can be corrected without a new puncture simply by changing the direction of the needle.

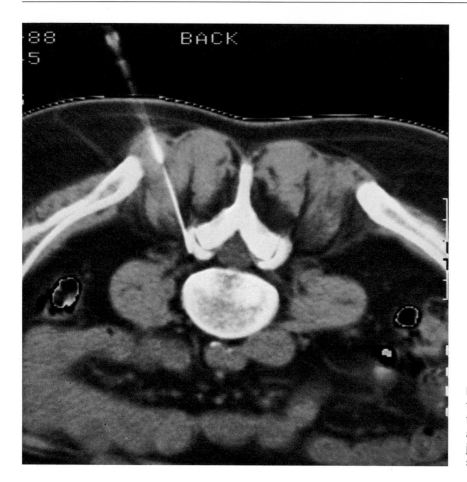

Fig. 16.31. After correcting the external cannula the interventional needle was advanced past the facet joint to 2 mm in front of the segmental nerve.

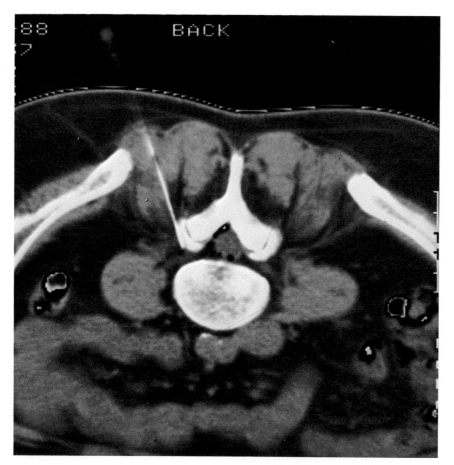

Fig. 16.32. CT scan further advancement of the interventional needle (about 1 mm) and injection of the medication. The solution is distributed in the perineural and epidural space.

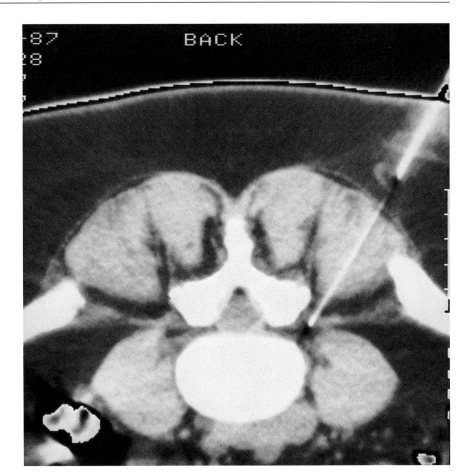

Fig. 16.33. Periradicular therapy at L4/5 on the right. The tip of the interventional needle is 2 mm posterior to the segmental nerve.

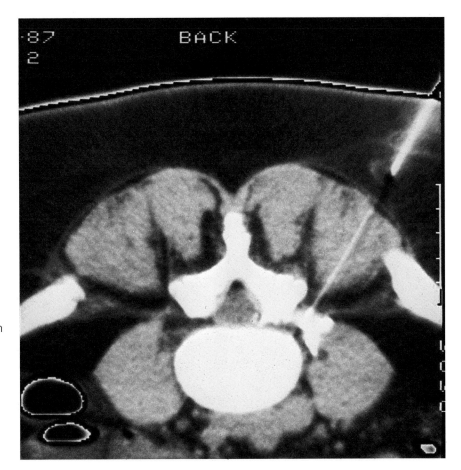

Fig. 16.34. CT scan after injection of the drugs which were diluted with contrast medium. The hyperdense (white) contrast solution spreads peripherally from the perineural area up to the psoas muscle and medially through the intervertebral foramen to the epidural space.

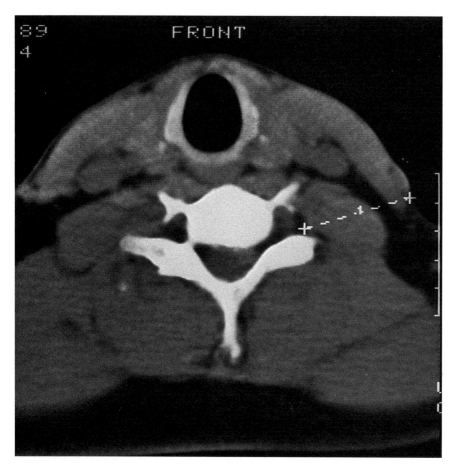

Figs. 16.35.–16.37.
32-year old patient with central and lateral cervical disc herniation at the C6/7 level on the left.
Planning-CT for periradicular therapy at C6/7 (Fig. 16.35.).
The needle should be placed below the external jugular vein and the sternocleidomastoid muscle. The cross-mark inside the intervertebral foramen is located 2 mm lateral to the segmental nerve. This nerve is located directly below the exposed vertebral artery.

Fig. 16.35

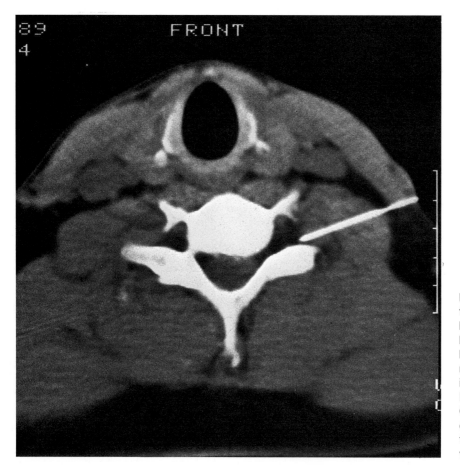

Fig. 16.36. PRT for a central and lateral disc prolapse C6/7 left. The disc herniation is visualized as a hyperdense (gray) half-moon-like structure extending into the spinal canal. PRT was performed at C6/7 on the left. The needle point is at the neural foramen, safely below the vertebral artery.

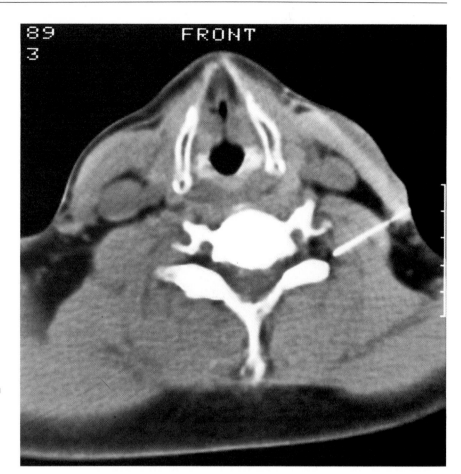

Fig. 16.37. CT scan after the fourth periradicular therapy. The disc herniation is no longer evident. The patient's pain and neurologic deficits are completely resolved after therapy.

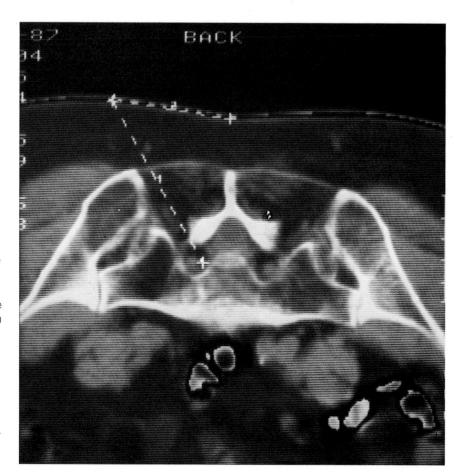

Fig. 16.38. Planning-CT before periradicular therapy at S1/2 level. The distance across the skin from the midline (2) and the distance from the surface of the skin to the segmental nerve (1) were measured and the puncture angle was determined. The cross-mark in the sacral foramen is located directly medial to the spinal nerve. The patient was suffering from a paresthesia with no evidence of neurologic deficits.

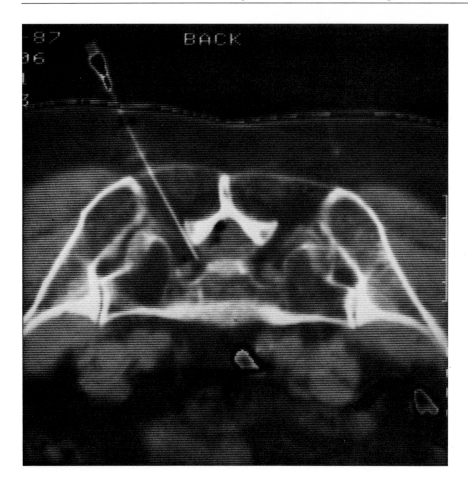

Fig. 16.39. CT scan after periradicular therapy at S1/2. The needle tip was positioned medial to the spinal nerve. The epidural distribution of the medication mixture can be identified.

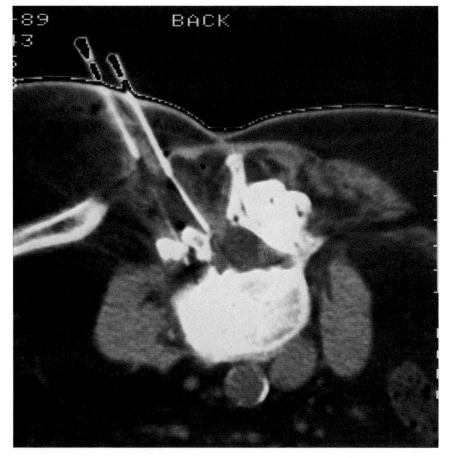

Fig. 16.40. Combination of periradicular therapy and treatment of epidural scar tissue. The patient's status is post a hemilaminectomy and three operations for scar tissue and recurrent herniation.
The needle tip was advanced into the intervertebral foramen which is narrowed by bony structures. The tip of the medial needle is in the extremely hard epidural scar tissue. The medication solution spreads in a semicircular fashion inside the scar-altered lateral dural space. Unless the procedure is performed carefully, an injury to the dura is possible. Prior to PRT the patient had severe pain radiating into the leg. After five treatments at an interval of three weeks each, there was a remarkable alleviation of the patient's complaints (65% improvement).

Complications

Anaphylactoid reactions after the administration of local anesthetics were observed in only two of the patients during PRT. After the usual treatment with antihistamine, corticosteroids, volume replacement and observation, treatment of these patients was continued on an out-patient basis. All of the remaining treatments for these two patients were performed without local anesthetics. The potential complication of an intrathecal injection has not been reported with the use of CT guidance because of the ability to track the needle tip precisely with CT.

Side-effects

The patients in the study had only minimal side-effects caused by the medications used. A short-term segmental nerve irritation was observed in 11 patients who had an initial exacerbation of symptoms, which disappeared within a short time after further treatments (Table 16.13., contra-indications for PRT, Table 16.14.).

Table 16.13. Side-effects after PRT.

Leg cramp	8%
Increase in weight	8%
Acne	4%
Edema	3%
Segmental nerve irritation	3%
Redness and tightness of the facial skin	2%
Petechiae	0.5%
Menstrual irregularities (5 out of 170 females)	3%

The use of a corticosteroid in a crystal suspension significantly decreases the systemic side-effects. If PRT is performed more often than

Table 16.14. Contra-indications for corticosteroid therapy.

1	Peptic ulcer
2	Diabetes, insulin-dependent
3	Adrenal gland insufficiency
4	Active tuberculosis
5	Systemic cortisone therapy
6	Cushing's disease
7	Encephalomyelitis
8	Bacterial sepsis

every three weeks, there will be an increase in the side-effects due to the duration effect of the corticosteroids. In patients that are hypersensitive to corticosteroids, one can reduce the dose without any loss of effectiveness. Other side-effects were a minor increase in weight in 8% of the patients, leg cramps in 8%, acne in 4% and edema in the facial area in 3%. 2% of the patients described a redness and tightness in the skin of the face approximately 24 hours after injection. In two cases petechial hemorrhage was observed and 3% (5 out of 170 of the female patients) experienced irregular menstruation, sometimes with spotting (Table 16.13.). All side-effects had disappeared ten weeks after the last administration of corticosteroids.

Instruments and Medication for PRT	
Needle	15–20 cm 22-G needle DCHN 22-5.000 S1 or DCHN 22-25.0 S1 (Cook)
Local anesthetic	5–10 ml Mepivacaine 1% (Scandicain)
Triamcinolon	10–40 mg (Volon A Crystal Suspension)
Oxypolygelatine	1–3 ml (Gelifundor)

C. Percutaneous Nucleotomy Discectomy (Nucleotomy)

In 1909 disc surgery was successfully intro-duced by Fedor Krause and Oppenheim [50]. In this surgery a complete laminectomy was per-formed by a transdural approach. A mass was removed which the authors believed to be an enchodroma. The clinical symptoms of sciatica had previously been described by Lasègue [30]. In 1934 Mixter and Barr [44] described the degenerative and traumatic changed disc her-niations which trigger sciatica. Then in 1939 Love [37] modified the technique of disc sur-gery to a hemilaminectomy with the surgery en-tirely performed extradurally. Also, Love in 1949 developed the minilaminectomy to sim-plify the operation and preserve the stability of the spine segment. This technique also keeps scar tissue formation to a minimum. Then in 1975 Yasargil [73] was the first to utilize micro-surgical techniques for disc operations (Table 16.15.).

Table 16.15. Development of disc surgery.

1864 Lasègue	Clinical symptoms
1909 Krause/Oppenheim	First laminectomy
1934 Mixter/Barr	Disc hernia as cause of sciatica
1939 Love	Hemilaminectomy
1949 Love	Minilaminectomy
1975 Yasargil	Microsurgery

A decisive change in the treatment of disc pro-lapses was established in 1964 by Lymon Smith [59] who introduced nucleolysis with chymopa-paine. At first there were enthusiastic expecta-tions for this method but currently this tech-nique is limited to a very minor number of indications. In 1975 Hijikata was the first to perform a percutaneous lumbar discectomy [22]. Friedmann [17], Kambin [26] and Sue-zawa [62] have further developed this method. Additionally, Suezawa introduced the discos-copy. For this procedure, Suezawa needed gen-eral anesthesia and required an 11 mm intro-duction cannula to be placed into the spine on each side. Onik [47] devised an entirely new puncture technique in which an automated as-piration probe only 2 mm wide is advanced into the nucleus pulposus and the prolapsed material as well as the nucleus pulposus can be removed. Since 1985 this technique has been performed by Onik under fluoroscopy. Percu-taneous discectomy was introduced in Ger-many by Mayer and Brock [41], Schulitz [55] and Weigand [68].

CT- and Fluoroscopy-guided Percutaneous Nucleotomy

In 1988 with the combination of a digital C-arm with integrated DSA and CT, the authors devel-oped a technique for performing digital sub-straction radiography during the CT proce-dure. For the first time a combined method of digital subtraction X-ray and CT is available (Table 16.16.). This combination has many advantages and may open up a new era of inter-ventional radiology (Fig. 16.41.). With the com-bination method it was possible to accomplish the first CT- and fluoroscopy-guided nucleo-tomy. For percutaneous nucleotomy the automated nucleotome developed by Onik is used. This 2 mm diameter probe is able to absorb disc material via a side window, and via a second internal hollow needle (pneumatically driven) it is able to cut off this disc tissue and flush it into a collection bottle. With this method the removal of between 1 and 5 g of the pro-lapsed disc tissue can be accomplished (Fig. 16.42.).

Table 16.16. Development of percutaneous (therapy for disc prolapse).

1964 Smith	Nucleolysis with Chymopa-paine
1975 Hijikata	Percutaneous nucleotomy
1985 Onik	Automated percutaneous nuc-leotomy
1988 Seibel/ Grönemeyer	CT-guided percutaneous nuc-leotomy

Conditions for PNT

A real advantage of the PNT technique lies in the possibility of accomplishing this operation by using only local anesthesia. Before the proce-dure, a neurologic diagnosis, a lumbar CT with thin slices (at least L3 to S1 must be examined), an A-P and lateral X-ray of the lumbar spine and the coagulation status must be obtained.

Indications

The earliest indication for percutaneous nucleo-tomy (PNT) is after four weeks of non-surgical therapy without sufficient improvement. In the authors' institute periradicular therapy (PRT) is normally performed prior to the percutaneous

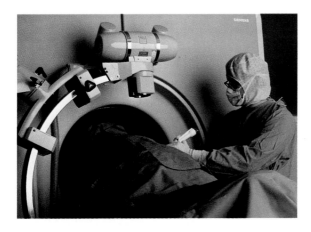

Fig. 16.41. To the best of the authors' knowledge this is the first report of the use of combined procedures with CT (Siemens) and C-arm (OEC diasonics). In this picture a simultaneous CT- and fluoroscopy-guided PNT is shown.

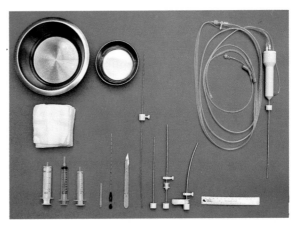

Fig. 16.42. Nucleotomy set (Hugh Co.) From right to left: The nucleotome, curved cannula, straight cannula, cutting-drilling cannula, trocar, scalpel, Seibel-Grönemeyer interventional needle (Cook Co.), guidance cannula, miscellaneous syringes.

nucleotomy. The indications for PNT are disc protrusion or disc prolapse in the lumbar spine, which exhibits segmental neurologic symptoms and morphologic conditions. In PNT patients, pain in the legs should be more pronounced than back pain. The morphologic changes must be well documented by CT or MRI. The authors do not believe that an additional myelogram is necessary when the neurological symptoms coincide with the morphology on CT or MRI. The herniated disc should be at the same level as the remaining disc for the best results.

Indications for percutaneous nucleotomy
Unsuccessful non-surgical therapy for over six weeks and segmental associated findings in disc prolapse or disc protrusion

Contained Disc and Uncontained Disc

In the American literature a distinction is made between contained disc and uncontained disc. Types of contained discs are disc protrusion with a beginning bulge of the annulus fibrosus, a bulge of disc material with impression of the dural sac, a disc prolapse with early destruction of the annulus fibrosus or disc prolapse with subligamental extension (Fig. 16.43.). In an uncontained disc there is a prolapse with herniation through the posterior longitudinal ligament or a prolapse with dislocated sequester. This sequestered disc fragment constitutes a contra-indication for percutaneous nucleotomy. The prolapse with the destruction of the posterior longitudinal ligament remains an indication for percutaneous nucleotomy as long as sequestered disc material is not recognized (Fig. 16.44.).

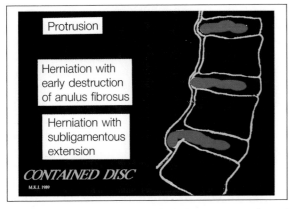

Fig. 16.43. Contained disc: Graphic representation of differential diagnosis for protrusion and prolapse.

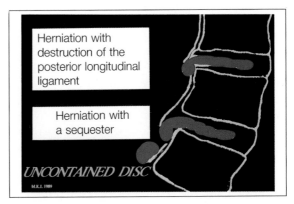

Fig. 16.44. From top to bottom: Uncontained disc: Disc prolapse with perforation of the posterior longitudinal ligament.

Limited Indication and Contraindication

A doubtful indication for PNT is a small inter-vertebral space, a large vacuum phenomenon, severe retrospondylosis, facet syndromes or a narrow spinal canal. A contra-indication for PNT is a massive prolapse with compression of the dura mater and of the cauda equina or a sequestered fragment.

Patients

In 64 patients a CT- and fluoroscopy-guided percutaneous nucleotomy were carried out. The average age of the patients was 45 years. The youngest patient was 25 years, the oldest 66 years old. The most frequent level for percuta-neous nucleotomy was L4/5. In two patients PNT was performed at two levels (Tables 16.17. and 16.18.).

Table 16.17. Age-distribution for PNT (n = 64).

Average age	45 years
Youngest patent	25 years
Oldest patient	66 years

Table 16.18. Localization of PNT (n = 64).

Segment L3/4	2
Segment L4/5	36
Segment L5/S1	26

Technique

PNT is performed with simular instruments to those developed by Onik [48] using the Seld-inger technique. PNT is strictly a puncture method (Fig. 16.45.). To exclude any contra-indication to percutaneous nucleotomy, one requires immediately prior to the procedure another CT scan of the level to be treated. In this scan the morphology of the disc prolapse is again checked to exclude the possibility that the prolapse has formed sequester in the meantime. Then, in the CT (Somatom DRG, Siemens Co.) a scan of the abnormal disc segment is per-formed in the prone position (Figs. 16.46.–16.48.). In this scan the disc is viewed as much as possible in the axial plane. The puncture angle and distance to the skin are determined. At the L5/S1 level the authors' routinely use a 3-D technique.

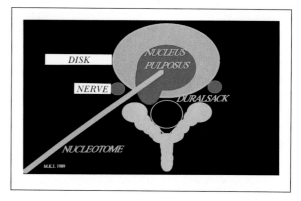

Fig. 16.45. Graphic for better understanding of the puncture technique for percutaneous nucleotomy. The nucleotomy cannula is dorsal to the segmental nerve and lateral to the facet joint. The cannula is advanced into the disc to the middle through the herniated nucleus pulposus.

In this technique the puncture is performed at a slant through several CT slices (Figs. 16.49. and 16.50.). After a planning-CT, local anesthetic is injected into the skin and superficial muscles. A 22-G needle up to 25 cm in length is advanced to the annulus fibrosus by simultaneously advancing with fluoroscopy-control from a digi-tal C-arm (OEC-Diasonics). Local anesthesia of the nerve root must be avoided. The puncture angle has to be selected in such a way that the greatest suction can be applied to the area of the disc prolapse. The puncture needle should be directly guided past the facet joint and under the segmental nerve. This must be controlled by CT. Then, over the 22-G needle a dilator can be advanced right up to the annulus fibrosus. The dilator with the straight cannula or the curved cannula is next advanced to the annulus fibro-sus. These steps are also controlled and docu-mented by CT (Fig. 16.51.). When interposition of tissue between cannula and annulus fibrosus is excluded, a trocar is brought into the nucleus pulposus after removal of the fine needle. After a further control, a hole of 2 mm in diameter is cut with the trephine into the annulus fibrosus. The nucleotome can then be introduced into the nucleus pulposus. All these steps are again carried out under fluoroscopy and CT control (Fig. 16.52.). The entire puncture and introduc-tion phase can be dangerous because of the pos-sibility of injuring the segmental nerve. This is the reason why every step is controlled with CT and/or fluoroscopy. If during the introduction phase a nerve root symptom occurs, the position of the segmental nerve and the possibility of an injury have to be documented. Under CT con-trol the authors did not experience such a com-plication. During the suction phase, by appro-priate manipulation, the entire posterior area of the nucleus pulposus and parts of the prolapse

Figs. 16.46.–16.48. CT- and fluoroscopy-guided percutaneous nucleotomy. Shown is the placement of a 25 cm long needle (22-G) (from the Seibel-Grön-emeyer interventional needle set) into the annulus fibrosus. The needle is in close contact with the facet joint. Note: The segmental spinal nerve which is ventral to the needle, must be identified at all times and avoided. The facet joints are well innervated with pain fibers. For this reason injection of 0.5 ml of 1% Scandicaine at the facets frequently facilitates the procedure.

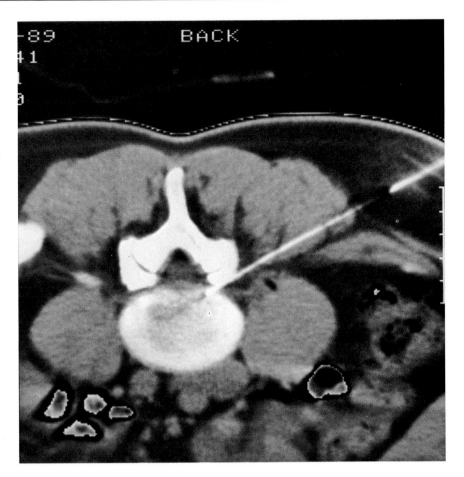

Fig. 16.46

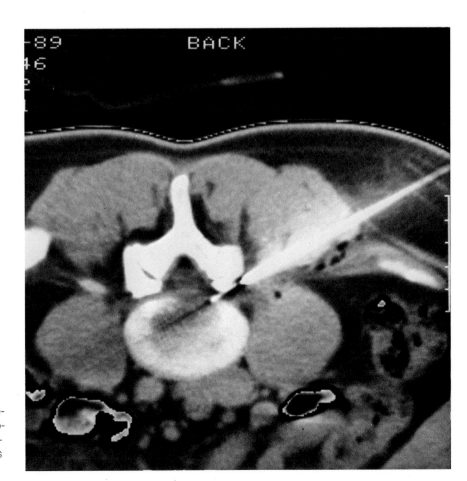

Fig. 16.47. The intrusion cannula, also called the straight cannula, is advanced up to the lateral portion of the facet joint over the interventional needle. A correction of the position of the needle is possible at any time due to its elasticity.

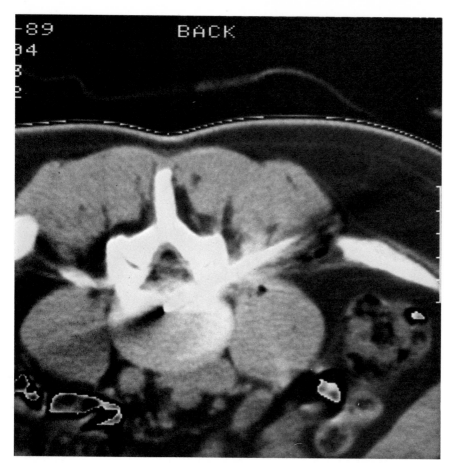

Fig. 16.48. Percutaneous nucleotomy. The tip of the trocar (which is introduced over the straight cannula) of the nucleotomy set is exactly in the mid-line. The trocar is substantially thicker than the interventional needle.

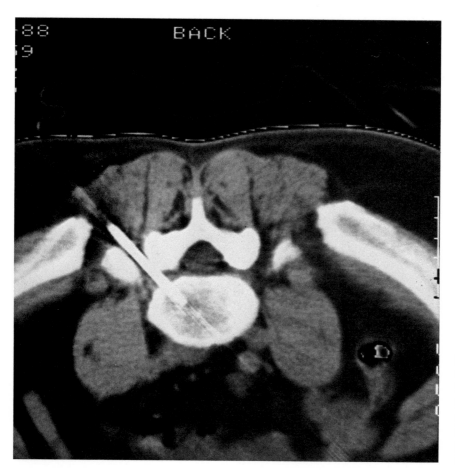

Fig. 16.49. Percutaneous nucleotomy at the L5/S1 level. The trocar tip is in the nucleus pulposus. Also note the relative narrowing between the facet joint and pars lateralis of the first sacral vertebra.

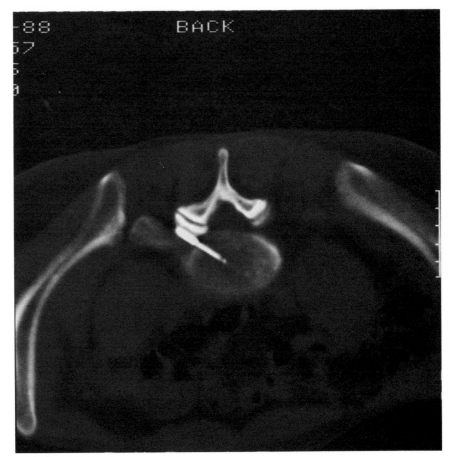

Fig. 16.50. Percutaneous nucleotomy at L5/S1. Three-dimensional puncture technique. Only approximately 1 cm of the intrusion cannula is shown here in the intervertebral foramen. The tip of the curved cannula is drilled into the annulus fibrosus and the tip of the nucleotome is in the center of the nucleus pulposus. At the top of the nucleotome the suction aperture is shown as a point (this scan was filmed using CT bone window).

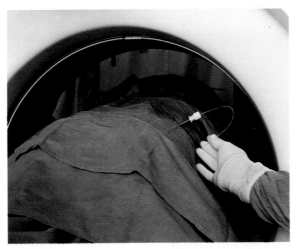

Fig. 16.51. Percutaneous nucleotomy. Manipulating the trocar makes it possible to check on the CT the position of the trocar tip and the straight cannula.

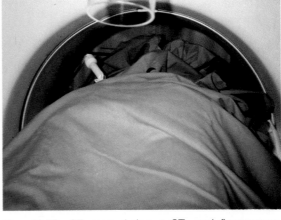

Fig. 16.52. CT scan during a CT- and fluoroscopy-guided nucleotomy. The nucleotome can be seen within the large 70 cm gantry. In the foreground the cone of the C-arm is visible at the upper edge of the gantry.

can be removed. In the patients there was an average suction period of 35 minutes. The entire procedure lasts approximately 50-60 minutes. For the first time by using this technique, it can be verified, both during and after the percutaneous nucleotomy, whether enough material has been sucked off and the subsequent decrease of the prolapse can be visualized (Figs. 16.53.–16.62.).

Findings

In 90% of the PNT patients (32% of the patientsreferred for PNT had one or more of the above contra-indications and were referred for surgery; Figs. 16.63.–16.65.), there was a complete regression of the complaints. Only six patients (9.4%) had unsatisfactory results. Five out of these six patients complained

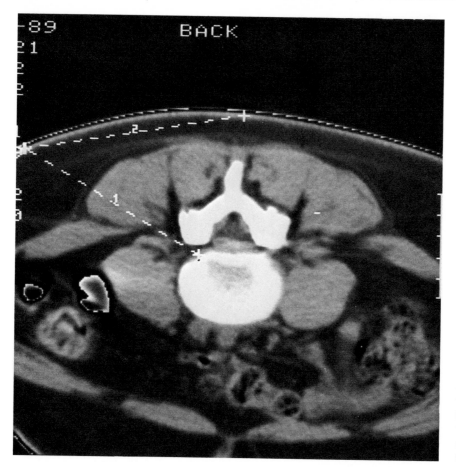

Fig. 16.53. Percutaneous nucleotomy at L4/5. Note the far lateral location of the puncture and the small puncture angle. The authors' modification of the Onik fluoroscopy-guided technique gives them the possibility of small puncture angles for positioning the nucleotome tip. With this method the tip can be accurately placed in the disc near the spinal canal. Thereby the suction can be directed to the region of prolapsed tissue. However, this technique is only possible with the addition of CT. Discrimination of tissue structures in the intervertebral foramen and spinal space requires CT. Therefore there is a danger of nerve damage or a CSF fistula if this technique is attempted with fluoroscopy control only.

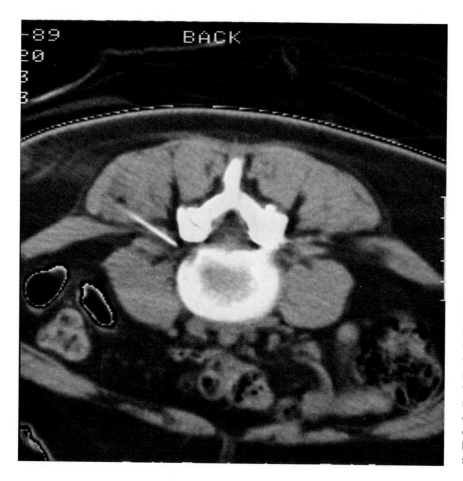

Fig. 16.54. Percutaneous nucleotomy at the L4/5 disc. Three-dimensional technique was used to advance the interventional needle (22-G) directly to the segmental nerve. The nerve is visualized as a linear structure directly anterior to the needle tip. With a blunt tip the nerve can be shifted anteriorly.

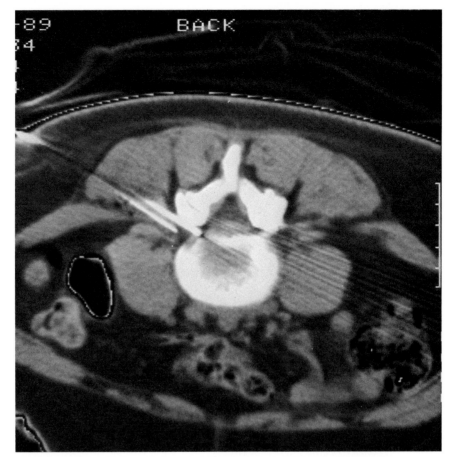

Fig. 16.55. Percutaneous nucleotomy at L4/5. The patient is in the prone position. CT demonstrates two puncture needles. The tip of the anterior needle pulls aside the nerve root L4 and serves as a protection and guide for the advancement of the trocar which is posterior to the guide needle. The trocar is directly in front of the facet joint and in the annulus fibrosus. The thin guidance needle is a 22-G Seibel-Grönemeyer interventional needle.

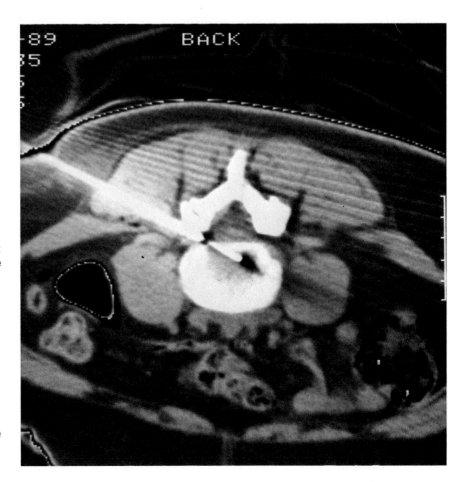

Fig. 16.56. Percutaneous nucleotomy at L4/5 (same patient). After being introduced over the trocar, the straight cannula with its tip in the neural foramen is just at the annulus fibrosus. The tip of the nucleotome is seen in the mid-line.
It is important to note the small puncture angle and the dorsal position of the suction probe which makes a high suction possible in the region of the prolapse. The segmental nerve can be differentiated anteriorly from the straight cannula. By using this technique, the danger of an injury can be minimized.

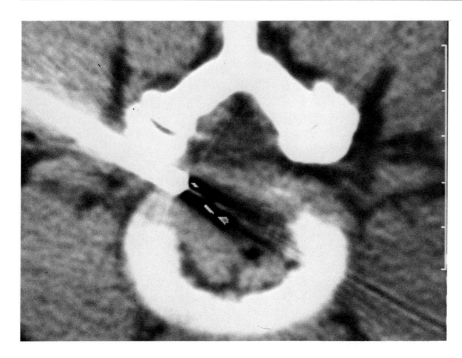

Fig. 16.57. Follow-up CT scan after percutaneous nucleotomy: CT documents a vacuum phenomenon which indicates the successful removal of the nucleus pulposus after therapy.

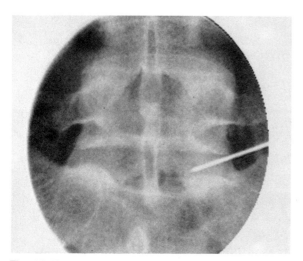

Fig. 16.58

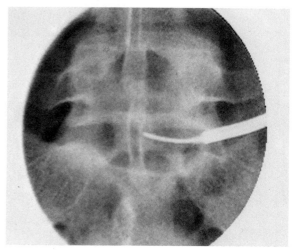

Fig. 16.59

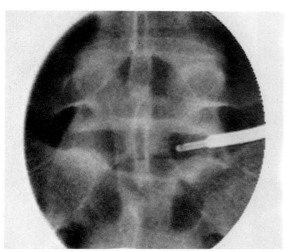

Fig. 16.60

Fig. 16.58. CT- and fluoroscopy-guided percutaneous nucleotomy. Fluoroscopy can provide a P-A view of the spine. This film was obtained with the patient on the CT table and by using a C-arm. The needle tip of the introduction trocar is in the intervertebral foramen.

Fig. 16.59. Compared with Fig. 16.58., the trocar tip had, prior to the procedure, been bent with a pair of special pliers. Without this bend a successful procedure would not have been possible. The tip of the needle now rests in the mid-line.

Fig. 16.60. Fluoroscopy image of the introduction of the nucleotome probe. The point-like low density at the tip of the nucleotome is the suction aperture (see Fig. 16.50.).

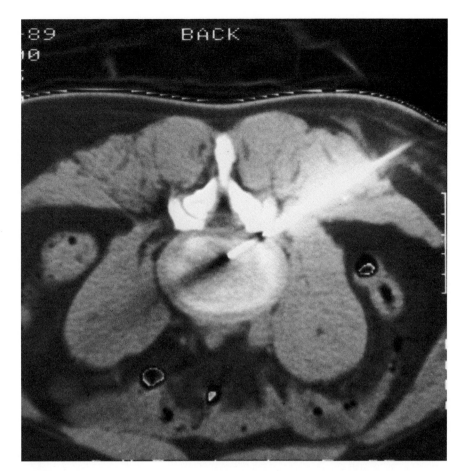

Fig. 16.61. CT- and fluoroscopy-guided percutaneous nucleotomy L4/5. The tip of the nucleotome is in the mid-line anterior to the centrally prolapsed tissue. The tip of the straight cannula is firmly anchored at the edge of the annulus fibrosus; the segmental nerve is uninjured and shown anterior to the straight cannula.

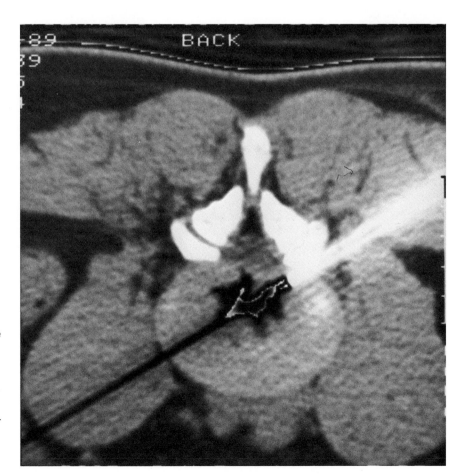

Fig. 16.62. CT scan after CT- and fluoroscopy-guided percutaneous nucleotomy at L4/5. Post-operative vacuum phenomenon is seen anterior to the prolapsed disc tissue in the same patient as in Fig. 16.61. Contrary to fluoroscopy-guided nucleotomy only an immediate determination of a successful suction is possible. In comparison with Fig. 16.61, a distinct decrease of the disc prolapse is visualized.

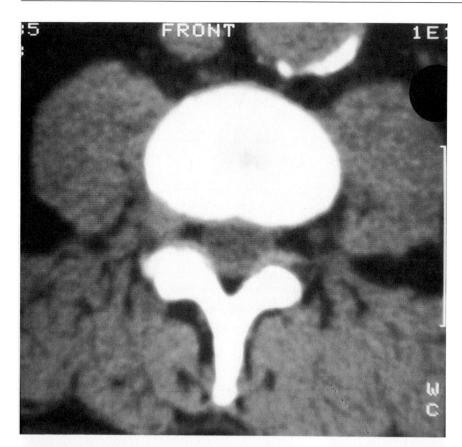

Fig. 16.63. Intra/extra fora-mina disc prolapse on the right side (indication for surgery).

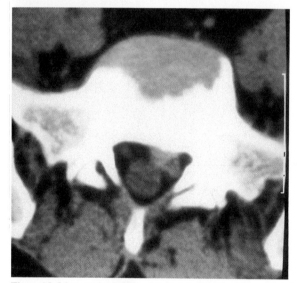

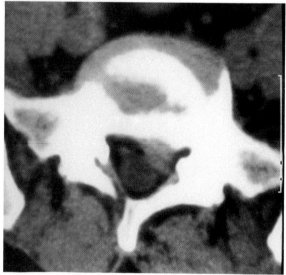

Figs. 16.64a. and **16.64b.** A left-sided sequester which is extending caudally below the first sacral vertebra, with the S1 nerve root shifted laterally. Nerve root swelling and a ventral dura impression can also be seen (these findings are an indication for surgery).

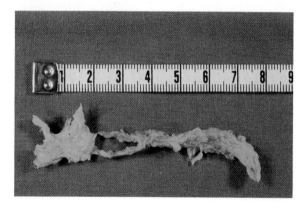

Fig. 16.65. Operative specimen for Fig. 16.63. A part of the sequester has the same appearance as the nerve fibers.

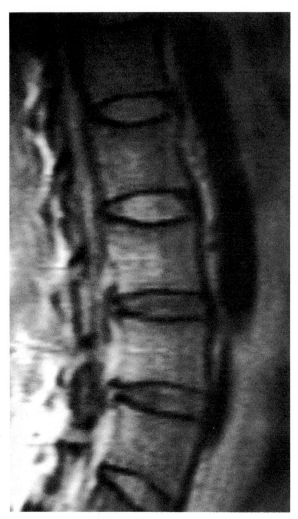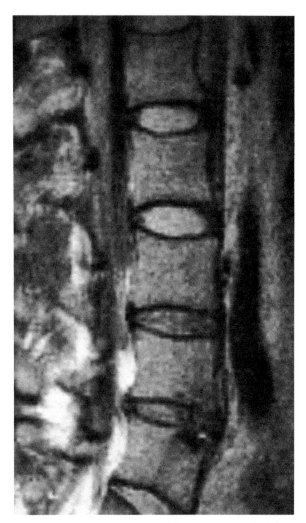

Figs. 16.66. and **16.67.** MRI before (left) and two weeks after percutaneous fluoroscopy-guided nucleotomy in a 33-year old patient with disc prolapse at L4/5 treated outside the authors' institute. After nucleotomy, a distinct reduction of the disc prolapse can be seen, but also a spondylodiscitis with a small fracture at the anterior edge of the fifth lumbar vertebra with separation of the anterior longitudinal ligament can be seen. (The patient was treated in an external center. The authors thank the Institut für Kernspintomographie der Universität Witten/Herdecke, in particular Director Dr. Dr. J. Fischer, who provided the pictures).

about pain in the lumbar spine area after PNT, but had resolution of their sciatica. Only in one of the six patients had the sciatica persisted. On an average 3.5g material were obtained by PNT. The quantity of disc material ranged between 1.9g and 7.9g. A negative or improved Lasègue sign was found in 92% of the patients right after the nucleotomy.

Complications

No complications occurred in these patients after combined CT- and fluoroscopy-guided PNT. By precise documentation of the nerve root in the CT the danger of trauma to the nerve root is almost completely eliminated. Furthermore, the danger of injuring arteries or veins is minimal with the use of CT.

However, with MRI follow-up examinations numerous complications were observed. All of these patients were treated in external medical centers with only fluoroscopy-guided PNT. The following complications were documented: fracture, bleeding, spondylitis and/or discitis and CSF fistula after perforation of the dura.

Side-effects

Among the patients treated there were only a few minor side-effects.
In only 17 patients (26.6%) was irritation of the nerve root observed in the area of the treated segment which began two days after PNT and had regressed after three to five weeks. In four particularly long-term cases (6.3%) after PNT,

Instruments and medication for percutaneous nucleotomy	
Nucleotomy set	Nucleotome (Surgical Dynamics)
Needle	20–25 cm 22-G needle DCHN 22.-20.0/25.0 S1 (Cook)
Local anesthetic	10–20 ml Mepivacaine 0.5% (Scandicaein)

conservative treatment and PRT became necessary. The root symptoms found in these patients were felt to be due to mechanical irritation from pressure on the nerve root during PNT. In these difficult cases, post-procedure MRI was performed to rule out spondylodiscitis as a cause of the pain. Furthermore, in 16% of the cases, after PNT pseudoradicular pain occurred which was treated with a CT-guided block of both facet joints under local anesthetic three times at eight-day intervals.

Combined Treatments

In 31 of the patients who had been treated with PRT, PNT was also performed. In this group of patients, the treatment concept was to combine PNT with PRT. Therefore, normally only two to four PRT sessions, are required in preparation for PNT. The combination of both methods increases the success rate for PNT. PRT as a preparation for disc surgery is also helpful. PNT should also be placed in the step-by-step concept from conservative therapy up to operation. However, especially in cases of chronic complaints or in cases of acute neurologic symptoms, it cannot replace an operation.

Because of the good results after periradicular therapy alone this method is especially suitable for a number of predominantly young patients who wish to return to work as quickly as possible. However, a group of the authors' patients are not free of complaints with periradicular therapy alone. Therefore, in these cases additional measures become necessary, such as facet treatment. In other patients who have a disc prolapse and where a progression of symptoms is suspected, the CT- and fluoroscopy-guided percutaneous nucleotomy are performed earlier than in other cases.

Discussion

For treatment of chronic spine diseases and disc changes there are a number of methods avail-

able in interventional radiology. The previously described methods can achieve resolution of the spine pain syndromes or of neurologic deficiencies in a large number of patients. The treatments can also circumvent an operation. Furthermore, treatment is possible by using these methods for many patients suffering from chronic pain. 22% of the patients who were treated with CT-guided PRT for facet denervation had symptoms for over 10 years. Furthermore, some of the patients had complaints of back pain etc. for 30–40 years.

In chronic pseudoradicular pain conditions and postdiscotomy syndrome, there is immediate pain relief in 79% of the patients after a one or multiple segmental facet denervation [10, 57]. This, however, requires first (as in every back pain patient) an exact pain history and a neurologic examination. Furthermore, A-P and lateral X-rays of the pathological area of the spine and a CT (using thin slices) or an MRI are also required. Only by the use of these examinations can a root compression be excluded. An advantage of MRI is that it enables a review of the entire lumbar spine including the thoracic/lumbar junction in a sagittal view. Also necessary may be one or several injections of corticoids or local anesthetics into the affected joints for a proper diagnosis. This is also discussed by other authors [32, 36, 43, 57, 61]. Contrary to data in the literature which are partially based on results after thermocoagulation, the authors' results in 102 patients after facet denervation are good, with 81% of the patients immediately free of pain and 79% with permanent success after two years. These good results are primarily because of the precise CT-guided positioning of the needle tip and the evaluation of the distribution of medication. Demirel [10], in a study with 27 patients, reported that 44% were complaint-free, 30% showed an improvement and 26% had recurrent pain after three months. He attributes these poor results to an insufficient coagulation of the facet nerves and subsequent nerve regeneration. These effects, in the authors' opinion, are mainly attributed to insufficient morphologic differentiation through the use of fluoroscopy-guidance. These results can be improved by the use of CT guidance. CT-guided facet denervations with alcohol and thermocoagulation are relatively safe procedures which belong to interdisciplinary pain therapy. Indication is given by the presence of pseudoradicular back pain and if the pain can be provoked diagnostically and suppressed by local anesthetics.

In disc herniation, histological examination of posterior roots demonstrated inflammatory-like changes caused by the disc [24, 35]. In 1930 Evans [15] described an alleviation of LBP in 60% of his patients by an epidural injection of a salt solution with procaine. Jones and Barnett in 1955 injected up to 50 mg hydrocortisone in the epidural space [25] using the sacral hiatus for access. In the series of publications that followed, the effectiveness of this method was improved by using intrathecal or systemic high-dosed corticosteroid and long-acting local anesthetics [11, 14, 15, 27]. In this way the pain receptors are diffusely blocked. With the authors' method, however, a segmental and locally directed therapy of the segmental nerve is conducted. The effectiveness of this method most likely has several reasons since three different substances are directly applied perineurally on multiple occasions (as a rule, eight treatments are performed at an interval of three weeks).

Besides the general anti-inflammatory effect, a decrease in exudation and the reduction of algogenic (pain-producing) substances, the high local dose of 40 mg Triamcinolon causes a decreases in nerve root and surrounding tissue swelling with decompression. Since 1953, pre-therapeutic root swelling had already been suspected from the myelogram as the cause of back symptoms [2]. The decrease in nerve root and surrounding soft tissue swelling can be observed in many cases after PRT. The effective mechanism is felt to be the direct local inhibition of the excessive E 2-prostaglandin synthesis [9, 58]. Among others, these prostaglandins influence vascular microcirculation and the release of an ATPase for the development of noradrenalin. They work like acid non-steroid analgesics such as acetylsalicylic acid on the metabolism of the arachidon acid. There they block the phospholipase A which regulates the synthesis of arachidonic acid from phospholipids [75]. Another explanation would be inhibition of the prostaglandin-endoperoxidase synthesis and thromboxan [5, 21, 23].

Good results after post-operative injection of high doses of local dexamethasone and epidural methylprednisolone have been described [7]. It is felt that, additionally, periradicular scar and epidural micro-changes as well as keloid reaction after disc operation are reduced by the direct corticosteroid effect.

The possible side-effects of local cortisone therapy have to be taken into account [58]. To avoid an abscess and meningitis, a sterile and accurate technique is always necessary. To resolve possible systemic cortisone effects further extensive comparative studies will be necessary. Also in these studies local anesthetics and oxypolygelatine should be compared with corticoids in their effects on degenerative changes. Furthermore, discussion of the interchange of triamcinolone acetonide versus the recently developed methylester of triamcinolone, which is only locally effective, should take place.

The injection of 1 to 2 ml oxypolygelatine causes a perineural distribution of the medication and an improved anti-edematous effect due to the osmotic effect of the high carbohydrate concentration. In cases of a sufficiently wide spinal canal and intraforaminal space the possibility of a cushioning effect of the gelatin has to be considered.

The effect of the local anesthetic can be viewed from several standpoints. Local anesthetics take effect directly at the cell membrane and inhibit the sodium-potassium interchange. Also, local anesthetics can have an inhibitive effect directly on the synapses and block the excitation transmission of the nerves. Diffusion takes place in the perineural, epidural, and CSF space [20]. The local pain-reducing effect on the sensory and sympathetic afferent nerves of laminae I to V of Wall's cascade model [66] depends on the localization, type and concentration of the local anesthetic. Due to the distribution effect based on the volume, besides preganglionic sympathetic fibers, postganglionic fibers are also affected in the prevertebral region of the sympathetic trunk [19] (see also Chapter Vegetative Innervation and Chapter Pain Theory). Furthermore, the potentiation of pain from reflexogenic muscle tension and the addition of circulating impulses of the nerves can be effectively interrupted, as well as the ephaptic overturn of efferent sympathetic activity on adjacent nociceptive afferences. This explains why the anesthetic effect often goes far beyond the nerve conduction inhibition effect after local anesthetic injection [74].

The influence on the segmental endorphin metabolism – the presence of encephalins and dynorphin have been proven in laminae I–II and V of the marrow [63] – from the direct application of the utilized medications or from the nerve stimulus by the injection remains hypothetical and has to be examined further.

The vicious circle of nerve root compression – followed by nerve root inflammation – followed by edema of the nerve root – then further compression – then functional disorder, can be interrupted by local anesthetics.

An exact periradicular injection is only possible with CT guidance. Even after nerve irritation (which can occur after injection of the medication), the needle tip can be misplaced under fluoroscopy-guidance. This is not surprising owing to the adjacent location of the lumbar plexus which can be mistakenly injected without CT guidance. Punctures with fluoroscopy-guidance can deviate by as much as 2 cm when documented with CT.

The results of the methods presented in this chapter are amazingly good. Since the authors do not have any long-term results for PNT patients, reference is made to the results of Onik

[48] who has developed this method with fluoroscopy-guidance and can show the largest number of cases. This less invasive therapy concept combined with a prior conservative treatment appears to be significant since a good resolution of the clinical symptoms and CT findings can be achieved [16]. The clinic had acute improvements in symptoms after CT-guided PNT in 91% of patients which is 10% higher than Onik's results. The utilization of CT makes it possible to puncture atraumatically and avoid complications. This is certainly an important factor in the good results. An additional reason for the high success rate is the pre-PNT treatment with three to four PRT sessions. The result of this pre-treatment is a distinct reduction of the enlarged nerve root and its sheath. In most cases this can be demonstrated on a CT scan. After the reduction, a halo effect can often be documented by CT (Fig. 16.68.), in which the nerve root shows a distinct separation of the periradicular fatty margin from the surrounding reactive tissue.

Since 1939, conventional operation with hemilaminectomy has undergone many modifications as far as microsurgical methods are concerned. However, PNT has many advantages over these conventional methods. With PNT, neither the back musculature nor the ligament apparatus are severely traumatized as with the surgical approach. The only trauma with PNT is the introducing of the instruments and a 2 mm hole cut into the annulus fibrosus. Therefore the danger of scar formation is avoided. The authors prefer the automated suction probe developed by Onik to the technique with a clamp forceps or a shaver to remove the nucleus pulposus. The disadvantage of all types of PNT is the fact that dislocated sequesters cannot be removed. Also, massive prolapse with a complete displacement of the nucleus into the spinal canal cannot be treated by PNT. Endoscopic control has no advantage in comparison with the authors' method since only the inner space of the disc can be looked at during or after the nucleotomy, whereas with CT guidance all structures can be examined at any time and even the decompression of the nerve root can be documented.

Only 6.3% of the patients reported radicular symptoms after PNT that required treatment. In all patients with complaints after PNT an MRI was performed. Eight to twelve weeks after PNT, a follow-up CT scan is routinely obtained and in patients complaining of recurrent symptoms an MRI is performed. Only a follow-up MRI can exclude a spondylodiscitis at each stage. This complication did not occur in the authors' patients; however, it was demonstrated at MKI in patients who underwent fluoroscopy-guided PNT at other centers. Important arguments for utilization of computertomography in

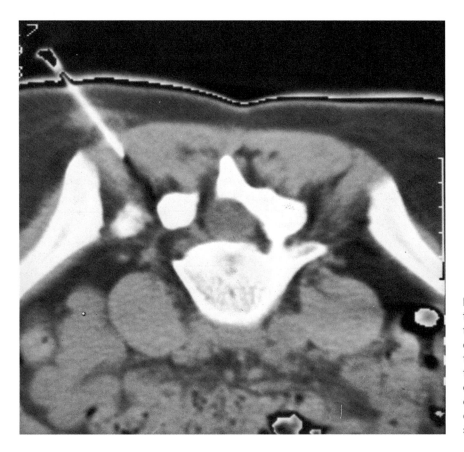

Fig. 16.68. Periradicular therapy at L5/S1 disc. Note the half-moon like hyperdense (black) area around the infraforaminal segmental nerve. This halo effect is often observed after successful therapy and after a decrease in swelling of the segmental nerve.

percutaneous nucleotomy are the precise punctures (1 mm^3) and the ability to avoid injuries to the nerve root, aorta, iliac artery or dura. A further advantage is the possibility of visualizing the disc during and after PNT which allows estimation of the effectiveness of the procedure.

There is no doubt that percutaneous nucleotomy will establish in therapy of disc diseases. The combination of CT and fluoroscopy guidance for PNT is at present the chosen procedure of choice with the least risk and an excellent success rate. A comparison with the success rates of other authors is not possible owing to the low number of patients in this study and the difficulty in comparing the clinical pictures and the criteria for selection. However, pre-treatment with PRT is an important factor in the good results achieved. Due to the relatively easy availability of the equipment and the ease of learning the CT-guided PNT procedure, it should be considered before conventional surgery.

The combination of PRT with PNT is an important addition, since PRT can relieve pain by normalizing nerve function and this can make PNT easier.

Although PRT and PNT are procedures with high accuracy, due to possible complications they should be conducted in an interdisciplinary manner at a location in or near hospital. Both methods have a defined place within the interdisciplinary stage concept between conservative therapy and classic surgery.

Synopsis of the New Treatment Methods for Back Pain

- CT-guided facet denervation is an effective method for treatment of pain caused by degenerative facet joints.
- CT-guided periradicular therapy (PRT) has the widest indication for degenerative diseases of the spine.
- PRT can be applied at any region of the spine.
- PRT is a method for restoration of segmental nerve function.
- The complication and side-effect rate with PRT is low and consists mostly of drug-induced reversible side-effects.
- A sterile procedure is necessary in every interventional back procedure.
- The steroid side-effects are not to be neglected and must be observed. Under certain circumstances complications such as an abscess or meningitis can be made worse with corticoids. This was not observed in any of the clinic's 370 patients. To prevent and treat side-effects and complications, a close inter-

disciplinary cooperation and an intensive theoretical and practical training are necessary.
- Further comparison studies are necessary with regard to the cortisone effects. Triamincinolon-acetonid should, if possible, be replaced by the only locally effective methylester of Triamcinolon. Furthermore, in controlled studies local anesthetics and oxypolygelatin should be compared only with the use of corticoids.
- Two years after PRT 68% of the patients were pain-free.
- PNT can be performed on an out-patient basis.
- PNT is performed with only local anesthesia.
- Depending on the patients, PNT can be performed instead of disc surgery in between 10 and 50% of cases.
- At present, PNT cannot replace disc surgery in every case.
- During and after PNT the abormal level and its morphology can be reviewed by CT.
- PNT does not cause scar tissue as does surgery.
- The side-effects of PNT are minimal.
- After PNT, 70-90% of the treated patients have no complaints of pain.
- Before any treatment of the spine, A-P and lateral and sometimes functional X-rays are necessary.
- CT or MRI should be performed after 4 weeks of unsuccessful non-surgical treatment or in patients with neurologic deficiencies.
- The invasive procedure of myelography is rarely indicated, especially in patients with a negative CT or MIR.
- MRI should be performed in all patients with post-operative complications, postdiscectomy syndrome, or in-patients with complaints after PNT. Furthermore, MRI can be performed before disc surgery.
- The therapy methods described in this chapter are atraumatic and more comfortable for the patients. They can be performed on an out-patient basis. In the step-by-step concept of treatment of spine diseases they are located between conservative therapy and classic disc surgery.
- The methods described in this chapter should be performed in or near a hospital in case of severe complications. Also, these procedures should have an interdisciplinary approach.
- The use of these methods can reduce health costs for the treatment of back pain.

References

1. Auberger H., Biermann E.: Praktische Schmerztherapie. Stuttgart, New York 1988, 15

2. Berg A.: Clinical and myelographic studies of conservatively treated cases of lumbar intervertebral disc protrusion. Acta Chir. Scand. 104 (1953) 124

3. Beyer H.K., Hötzinger H., Oppel U., Tödt Ch.: Wert der Kernspintomographie mit Gadolinium-DTPA bei der Diagnostik des lumbalen Postdiscotomie-Syndroms. Digit. Bilddiagn. 9 (1989) 22–30

4. Biering-Sorensen F.: A prospective study of low back pain in a general population. Scand. J. Rehab. M. 15 (1983) 71–79

5. Blackwell G.J. Flower R.J., Njikamp F.P., Vane J.R.: Phospholipase A2 activity of guinea pig isolated perfused lungs; stimulation and inhibition by antiinflammatory steroids. Br. J. Pharmaco. (1978) 62–79

6. Bogduk N., Long D.M.: The anatomy of the so-called "articular nerves and their relationship to facet denervation in the treatment of low-back pain. J. Neurosurg. (1979) 151–172

7. Brandt F., Kretschmer H.: Der Einfluß von Dexamethason auf die Schmerzsituation nach lumbalen Bandscheibenoperationen. Schmerz 2 (1979) 33–37

8. Brügger A.: Vertebrale radiculäre und pseudoradiculäre Syndrome. Documenta Geigy, Acta rheumatolog. (1960) 18

9. Brune K., Dietzel K., Möller N.: Pharmakologie des Schmerzes, in: Wörz R. (Hrsg.) Pharmakotherapie bei Schmerz. Weinheim 1986, 53

10. Demirel T.: Erfahrungen mit der perkutanen Facett-Neurektomie. Med. Welt 31 (1980) 1018–1020

11. Dilke T.F.W., Burry H.C., Grahame R.: Extradural corticosteriud injection in the management of lumbar nerve compression. Br. Med. J. (1973) 635–637

12. Dougherty J.H., Fraser R.A.R.: Complications following intraspinal injection of steroids. J. Neurosurg. (1978) 1023–1025

13. Ebeling U., Kalbarcyk H., Reulen H.J.: Microsurgical reoperation following lumbar disc surgery, Timing, surgical findings and outcome in 92 patients. J. Neurosurg. 70 (1989) 397–404

14. El Kohoury G.Y., Ehara S., Weinstein J.N., Montgomery W.J., Kathol M.H.: Epidural steroid injection: a procedure ideally performed with fluoroscopic control. Radiology 168 (1988) 554–557

15. Evans W.: Intrasacral epidural injection therapy in the treatment of sciatica. Lancet (1930) 1225–1229

16. Fischer R., Schumacher M., Thoden U.: Verlauf nicht operierter lumbaler Bandscheibenvorfälle. Radikuläre Störungen und computertomographische Befunde. Schmerz 2 (1988) 26–32

17. Friedmann W.A.: Percutaneous discectomy: an alternative to chemonucleolysis? Neurosurgery 13 (1983) 542–547

18. Goald H.J.: Microlumbar discotomy; follow-up of 147 patients. Spine 3 (1978) 2

19. Greene N.M.: Sympathikusblockade bei Spinal- und Epiduralanästhesie. Schmerz 2 (1987) 58–60

20. Gross D.: Diagnostische und therapeutische Lokalanästhesie beim Gesichtsschmerz. In: Pauser G., Gerstenbrand F., Gross D. (Hrsg.) Gesichtsschmerz, Schmerzstudien Bd. 2, Stuttgart, New York 1979, 175

21. Gryglewski R.J., Panczenko B., Korbut R., Grodzinska I., Ocetkiewicz A.: Corticosteroids inhibit prostaglandin release from perfused mesenteric blood vessels of rabbit and from perfused lungs of sensitized guinea pig. Prostaglandins 10 (1975) 343

22. Hijikata S., Yamiagishi M., Nakayama T., Oomori K.: Percutaneous discectomy: a new treatment method for lumbar disc herniation. J. Toden Hosp. 5 (1975) 5–13

23. Hong S.L., Levine L.: Inhibition of arachidonic acid release from cells as the biochemical action of antiinflammatory corticosteroids. Proc. Nat. Acad. Sci. USA 73 (1976) 1730

24. Irsigler F.J.: Microscopic findings in spinal cord roots of patients with lumbar and lumbosacral disc prolapse. Acta Neurochir. 1 (1951) 478–516

25. Jones K.G., Barnett H.C.: Use of hydrocortisone in spinal surgery. South Med. J. 48 (1955) 617–623

26. Kambin P., Sampson S.: Posterolateral percutaneous suction-excision of herniated lumbar intervertebral discs. Clin. Orth. Rel. Res. 207 (1986) 37

27. Kelman H.: Epidural injection therapy for sciatic pain. Amer. J. Surg. 64 (1944) 183–190

28. Kreuscher H.: Chronische Rücken- und Kreuzschmerzen. In: Sehhati Gh. (Hrsg.) Schmerzdiagnostik und Therapie. Bd. 2, Bochum 1986, 211

29. Ladurner G., Jeindl E., Auer L., Justich E., Gallhofer B., Lechner H.: Die Behandlung des lumbalen Diskusprolaps; ein Vergleich chirurgischer und konservativer Langzeitresultate. In: Berger M., Gerstenbrand F., Lewit K. Schmerz und Bewegungssystem, Stuttgart, New York, Schmerzstudien 6 (1984) 332–344.

30. Lasègue C.: Considerations sur la sciatique. Arch. Gen. Med. 4 (1864) 558

31. LaMont R.L., Morawa L.G., Pederson H.E.: Comparison of disc excision and combined disc excision and spinal fusions for lumbar disc ruptures. Clin. Orthop. 121 (1976) 212–216

32. Lenz G., Schulitz K.-P.: Das Facettensyndrom als mögliche Ursache persistierender Schmerzen nach lumbaler Diskotomie – Aufzeigung therapeutischer Möglichkeiten. Orthop. Praxis 16 (1980) 14–19

33. Lewis P.J., Weir B.K.A., Broad R.W., Grace M.: Long-term prospective study of lumbosacral discectomy. J. Neurosurg. 67 (1987) 49–53.

34. Lichtblau H.: Der lumbale Bandscheibenprolaps; klinische Diagnostik – operative Therapie – Spätergebnisse. Münch. med. Wschr. 126 (1984) 939–942

35. Lindahl D., Rexed B.: Histological changes in spinal nerve roots of operated cases of sciatica. Acta Orthop. Scand. 20 (1951) 215

36. Lora J., Long M.D.: So-called facet denervation in the management of intractable back pain. Spine 1 (1976) 121–126

37. Love J.G.: Removal of protruded intervertebral discs without laminectomy. Proc. Staff Meet. Mayo Clin. 14 (1939) 800

38. Mattmann E.: Reoperationen bei operierten lumbalen Diskushernien. Schweiz. med. Wochenschr. 99 (1968) 43–47

39. Mattmann E.: Das Problem der Rezidive nach Operationen lumbaler Diskushernien. Schweiz. Arch. Neurol. Neurochirurg. Psych. 108 (1971) 39–44

40. Mau, H.: Chirurg. 53 (1982) 292–298

41. Mayer H.M., Brock M.: Die perkutane Diskektomie. Dt. Ärztebl. 85 (1988) 632–637

42. Meinig G., Kretschmar K., Samii M., et al.: Spondylodiscitis – lumbar disc removal. Adv. Neurosurg. 4 (1977) 55–58

43. McCulloch J.A.: Percutaneous Radiofrequency Lumbar Rhizolysis (Rhizotomy). Appl. Neurophysiol. 39 (1976/77) 87–96

44. Mixter W.J., Barr J.S.: Rupture of the intervertebral disc with involvement of the spinal canal. New Engl. J. Med. 211 (1934) 210

45. Mumenthaler M.: Neurologie. Stuttgart 1979, 7

46. Oldenkott P.: A study of the medical and social problems involved in cases of prolapse of an intervertebral disc in the lumbar region. Adv. Neurosurg. 4 (1977) 28–32

47. Onik G., Helms C.A., Ginsberg I., Hoaglund F.T., Morris J.: Percutaneous lumbar discectomy using a new aspiration probe: Porcine and cadaver model. Radiology 155 (1985) 251

48. Onik G.: Percutaneous automated discectomy: Technique. In: Onik G., Helms C.A. (eds). Automated percutaneous lumbar discectomy. Rad. Res. Educ. Found. Univ. Cal. Print. Dep. 1988, 77–110

49. Oppel F., Schramm J., Schirmer M., et al.: Results and complicated course after surgery for lumbar disc herniation. Adv. Neurosurg. 4 (1977) 36–52

50. Oppenheim H., Krause F.: Über Einklemmung bzw. Strangulation der Cauda equina. Dtsch. Med. Wochenschr. 35 (1909) 697

51. Rees W.S.: Multiple, bilateral subcutaneous rhizolysis of segmental nerves in the treatment of the intervertebral discsyndrome. Ann. Gen. Prac. 26 (1971) 126–127

52. Salenius P., Laurent L.E.: Results of operative treatment of lumbar disc herniation. A survey of 1886 patients. Acta Orthop. Scand. 48 (1977) 630–634

53. Schepelmann F., Greiner L., Pia H.W.: Complications following operation of herniated lumbar discs. Adv. Neurosurg. 4 (1977) 52–55

54. Schulitz K.P., Lenz G.: Das Facettensyndrom – Klinik und Therapie. In: Hohmann D., Kügelgen B., Liebig K., Schirmer M. (Hrsg.) Neuroorthopädie 11. Berlin, Heidelberg, New York 1984, 543

55. Schulitz K.P., Lenz G.: Perkutane Nukleolyse. In: Günther R.W., Thelen M. (Hrsg.): Interventionelle Radiologie, Stuttgart, New York 1988, 445

56. Shealy C.N.: Percutaneous radiofrequency denervation of spinal facets: Treatment for chronic back pain and sciatica. J. Neurosurg. 43 (1975) 448–451

57. Shealy C.N., Maurer D.D.: Transcutaneous neurostimulation for control of pain. Surg. Neurol. 2 (1974) 45–47

58. Silbernagl St., Despopoulos A.: Atlas der Physiologie, Stuttgart 1979, 48–56

59. Smith L.: Enzyme dissolution of the nucleus pulposus in humans. JAMA 187 (1964) 137–140

60. Spangfort E.: The lumbar disc herniation. A computer-aided analysis of 2504 operations. Acta Orthop. Scan., Suppl. 142 (1972) 5–93

61. Staudte H.W., Hild A., Niehaus P.: Klinische Ergebnisse mit der Facetten-Koagulation des Ramus articularis der unteren Lendenwirbelsäule. In: Hohmann D., Kügelgen B., Liebig K., Schirmer M. (Hrsg.) Neuroorthopädie 11. Berlin, Heidelberg, New York 1984, 551

62. Suezawa Y., Jacob H.A.C.: Percutaneous nucleotomy – an alternative to spinal surgery. Arch. Orth. Trauma Surg. (in press)

63. Thoden U.: Neurogene Schmerzsyndrome. Stuttgart 1987, 22–23

64. Thoden U.: Neurogene Schmerzsyndrome. Stuttgart 1987, 122

65. Thomalske G., Galow W., Ploke G.: Critical comments on an comparison of two series (1000 patients each) of lumbar disc surgery. Adv. Neurosurg. 4 (1977) 22–28

66. Wall W.P.: The dorsal horn. In: Wall P.D., Melzack R. (eds.) Textbook of pain. Edinburgh 1984, 80

67. Wallöe A., Sundén G.: Operations for herniated lumbar discs: a follow-up study 2–5 years after surgery. Spine 11, 6 (1986) 636–637

68. Weigand H., Heyder J.: Perkutane Nukleotomie. In: Friedmann G., Steinbrich W., Gross-Fengels W. (Hrsg.): Interventionelle Methoden der Radiologie. Konstanz 1988, 187–191

69. Weitbrecht W.U., Gilsbach J., Pfaff E., Thoden U.: Langzeitergebnisse verschiedener Operationsmethoden bei lumbalen Bandscheibenvorfällen. Orthop. Prax. 1 (1980) 8–10

70. White A.H., von Rogov P., Zuchermann J., Heiden D.: Lumbar laminectomy for herniated disc: A prospective controlled comparison with internal fixation fusion. Spine 3 (1987) 305–307

71. Wickboldt J., Bushe K.A.: On the technique of clearing protruded lumbar disc – a comparison of two surgical methods. Adv. Neurosurg. 4 (1977) 62–67

72. Williams R.W.: Microlumbar discectomy: a conservative surgical approach to the virgin herniated lumbar disc. Spine 3 (1977) 81–82

73. Yasargil M.G., Delong W.B., Guarnaschelli J.J.: Complete microsurgical excision of cervical extramedullary and intramedullary vascular malformations. Surg. Neurol. 4 (1975) 211

74. Zimmermann M.: Nociception und Schmerz: Physiologische Mechanismen. In: Wörz R., Gross D. (Hrsg.) Kreuzschmerz, Schmerzstudien Bd. 1. Stuttgart, New York 1978, 29

75. Zimmermann M., Seemann H.: Der Schmerz, ein vernachlässigtes Gebiet der Medizin. Berlin, Heidelberg, New York, London, Paris, Tokyo 1986, 9

76. Zimmermann M., Seemann H.: Der Schmerz, ein vernachlässigtes Gebiet der Medizin. Berlin, Heidelberg. New York, London, Paris, Tokyo 1986, 76–79

Further Reading

Auberger H., Biermann E.: Praktische Schmerztherapie. Stuttgart, New York 1988

Braun W., Demirel T.: Einführung in die Schmerzchirurgie, Stuttgart 1982

Grönemeyer, D.H.W., Seibel, R.M.M.: Interventionelle Computertomographie. Wien, Berlin 1989

Thoden U.: Neurogene Schmerzsyndrome. Stuttgart 1987

Cancer and Cancer-Pain Therapy

Chapter 17
New Forms of Interventional Tumor Therapy in Radiology

D.H.W. Grönemeyer, R.M.M. Seibel

Every year in Europe approximately 2 million people develop cancer [6]. In the FRG alone approximately 200,000 people die of cancer every year (1983: 170,000 [1]) and many suffer from inadequately treated severe pain [4]. As far as tumor frequency is concerned, the FRG takes the No. 1 position in Europe and comes 7th in an age-standardized study of 43 industrial nations (USA 22nd and Japan 23rd) [8]. Since the fifties, in the FRG there has been an almost 20% (+ 1% per year) increase in the frequency of tumors in males and in females a decrease of 14% (− 0.5% per year) [8]. However, due to insufficient surveys and statistics on cancer, these figures are disputable. Interestingly, there is a considerably higher risk of falling ill with cancer in blue collar workers, unemployed and foreigners [2, 3]. Therefore, adequate, multidisciplinary strategies are necessary for early diagnosis, treatment, and prevention of cancer.

In this chapter, new possibilities for multidimensional therapy are presented which can be used either in addition to or as an alternative to other conventional methods of cancer therapy.

During the past few years, a trend toward interventional procedures can be observed in local tumor therapy. Predominantly, fluoroscopy-guided and endoscopic methods have been used for these therapies. Also in tumor patients, interventional procedures can be used for the treatment of certain symptoms (i.e. for decompression of the kidney). These drainage techniques for relief of biliary and urinary tract obstruction (i.e. in the case of pancreatic carcinoma or of tumor-caused hydronephrosis) and the percutaneous implantation of endoprotheses are established techniques. Another possibility for interventional therapy is the placement of nutritional fistulae. Furthermore, conventional tumor therapy (i.e. chemotherapy or radiation therapy) can often be performed only after an interventional procedure (see Chapter CT-Guided Drainages).

Other interventional methods have recently been developed in local and regional tumor therapy, such as tumor perfusion with cytostatics and interstitial radiation therapy, using the afterloading technique.

CT-guided local tumor therapy was developed from CT-guided fine-needle biopsy and CT-guided pain therapy. The biopsy and pain methods allow for better patient care, firstly through a faster diagnosis and secondly through the treatment of tumor pain.

A. CT-Guided Tumor Pain Therapy

The diagnosis of cancer incites six types of anxiety in the patient [7]:
1. fear of death;
2. fear of bodily deterioration;
3. fear of insufficient therapy;
4. fear of intractable pain;
5. fear of being helpless;
6. fear of being socially isolated.

Therefore, a fundamental part of each tumor therapy is not to leave the patient alone with his or her fears but to initiate individual strategies for overcoming these fears. Additionally, the pain level can be reduced with more physician time and devotion to the tumor patient.

An intensive detailed history and interdisciplinary examinations are necessary prior to any treatment, especially if new symptoms appear in addition to those of the primary diagnosis. To characterize tumor pain as regards quality, localization and intensity can be very difficult due to the complexity of the pain, the psychological situation, and the pain perceptibility of these tumor patients.

Furthermore, it is not possible to predict whether a tumor will cause pain or what type of pain is caused by which particular tumor. Bone pain and retroperitoneal pain are almost always very intense types of pain. Most of the time, nerve infiltrations, compressions and abdominal obstructions can also result in severe pain. However, tissue tumors and parenchyma tumors often do not produce pain.

In cancer patients, quite frequently new symptoms are assumed to be caused by recurrent tumors or metastases. However, tumor patients, because of the seriousness of their illness, often

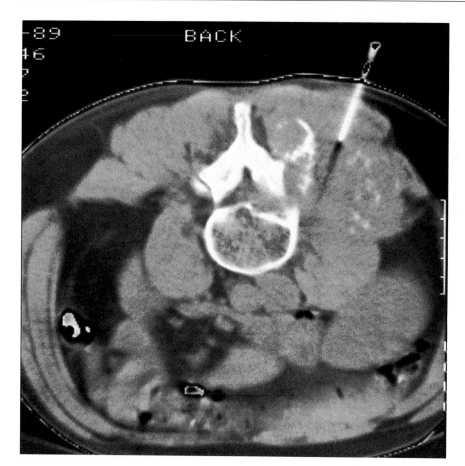

Figs. 17.1.–17.5. 35-year old patient with a renal cell carcinoma. CT scans of intratumoral therapy shows a fan-shaped infiltration of 96% ethanol into a soft-tissue tumor (vertebral metastasis).

Fig. 17.1. CT scan of the tumor, originating in and destroying the vertebral body. The tumor has infil-trated the right back mus-culature and the psoas muscle. The hyperdense areas in the tumor are cal-cified residues of previous alcohol administration. The guide needle was ad-vanced through the lateral portion of the back muscu-lature into the periphery of the tumor.

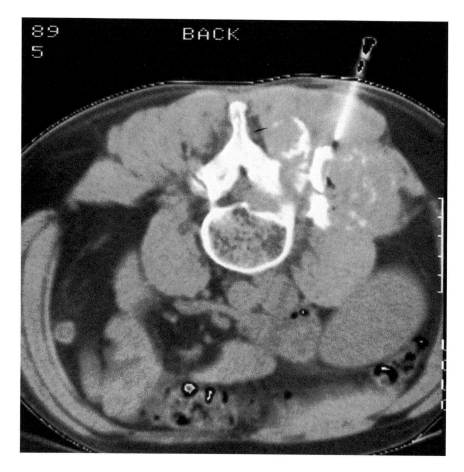

Fig. 17.2. Via an interven-tional needle, contrast medium is injected into the tumor to evaluate the anticipated distribution of the alcohol prior to the intratumoral therapy.

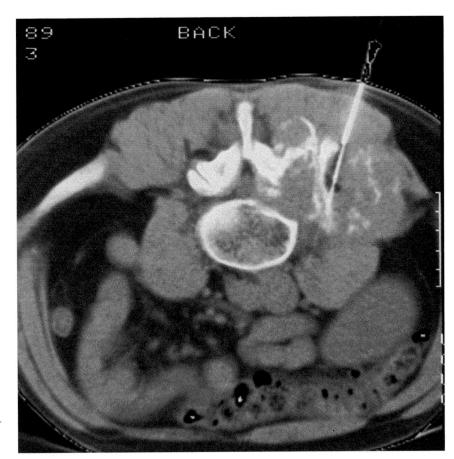

Fig. 17.3. Half-moon shaped distribution of the alcohol in the renal cell metastasis. In comparison with Fig. 17.2., the contrast-medium column has been diluted by the alcohol.

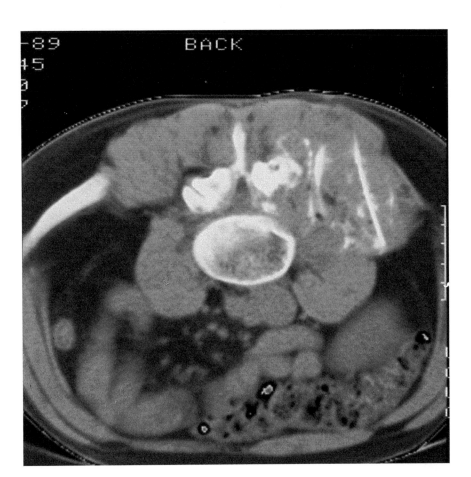

Fig. 17.4. The position of the interventional needle was changed during the same session. Another alcohol instillation was performed in the tumor periphery.

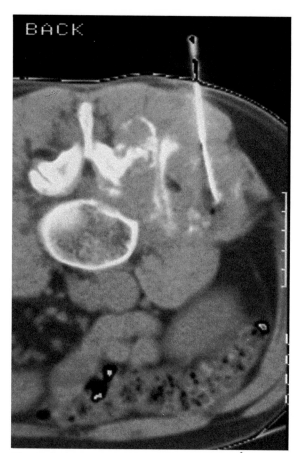

Fig. 17.5. CT scan after another needle position change. A central alcohol injection has been performed.

Table 17.1. Interventional tumor pain therapy.

A   Pain blockades (repeatable)
B   Nerve and/or plexus neurolysis (irrevocable)

A   Pain blockades
   1.   stellate ganglion
   2.   brachiocervical plexus
   3.   brachial plexus
   4.   thoracic sympathetic trunk
   5.   lumbar sympathetic trunk
   6.   periradicular therapy

B   Nerve and/or plexus neurolysis
   1.   peripheral nerve
   2.   cervicobrachial plexus
   3.   thoracic sympathetic trunk
   4.   brachialis plexus
   5.   celiac plexus
   6.   lumbar sympathetic trunk
   7.   precoccygeal and presacral sympathetic trunk

CT-Guided Treatment of the Cervicobrachial Plexus and Neurolysis of the Thoracic Sympathetic Trunk

Tumor infiltration of the cervicobrachial and axillary plexus can cause severe pain. In cases of pain resistance to conventional therapy, a CT-guided pain treatment of a part of the plexus and/or neurolysis of the cervical or thoracic sympathetic trunk can lead to a significant reduction in pain (i.e. case of pancoast tumors with infiltration of the brachial plexus – see Chapter 15). Furthermore, in patients with lung tumors, a CT-guided thoracic sympathetic trunk neurolysis can eliminate the tumor pain (see Chapter 16).

CT-Guided Neurolysis of the Celiac Plexus

An important development in the treatment of upper abdominal pain is celiac plexus neurolysis. All visceral pain fibers of the upper abdominal region traverse this plexus. Therefore, it is possible to achieve permanent elimination of pain by carrying out a single neurolysis of the entire plexus in these patients.

The authors have conducted a total of 188 CT-guided neurolyses of the celiac plexus for tumor pain. As their basic disease process the majority of the patients had a pancreatic or gastric carcinoma with celiac plexus infiltration while the next most frequent group had metastases with direct infiltration of the plexus. The authors have also successfully used the celiac plexus neurolysis for liver metastases with capsular pain. Permanent elimination of pain was achieved in 80% of patients after celiac plexus neurolysis. There are several ways to access the celiac plexus (see Chapter 18). The anterior route is preferred but the morphologic findings

have the tendency to somatize their problems due to their justified or unjustified fears and strained psycho-social situation. This can lead to psychosomatic illnesses such as gastric ulcers, biliary colic or functional disorders like muscle stiffness, facet locking etc. These illnesses occur in cancer patients more frequently than in the general population. Besides this, tumor patients are predisposed to non-malignant second and third illnesses (such as angina pectoris, disc prolapse and other similar illnesses). These alterations are often treated inadequately or not recognized at all. This can lead to negative psychological reactions in the patient. Furthermore, tumor accompanying functional disorders or illnesses such as mycosis genitalis, pneumonia, and infection of the urinary tract have to be considered since they can lead to tumor-associated pain.

Therefore, every doctor dealing with oncologic patients must have a comprehensive knowledge of the different pain patterns and differential diagnosis of malignant diseases. The possibilities for interventional CT-guided tumor pain therapy are shown in Table 17.1.

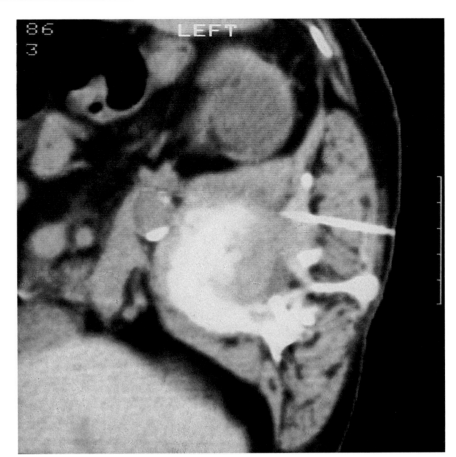

Fig. 17.6. CT scan of a bronchial metastasis in the lateral process and vertebral body. The needle tip is in the lateral portion of the metastatic lesion in the vertebral arch. The CT scan was performed after an injection of 2 ml 96% ethanol. The elimination of the sympathetic trunk may be necessary if infiltrated by tumor, if spinal column metastases are present, or in cases of segmental nerve infiltration.

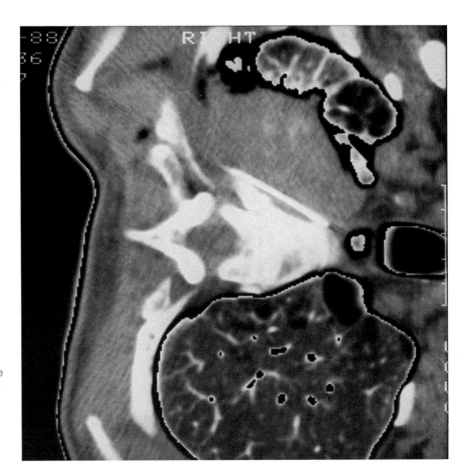

Fig. 17.7. CT scan of an extensive pleural mesothelioma. The needle is advanced by means of a 3-D technique and the tip is in the area of the thoracic sympathetic trunk. Because of severe pain, the thoracic sympathetic trunk was destroyed. Two treatments with 2 ml 96% ethanol each were necessary for complete neurolysis.

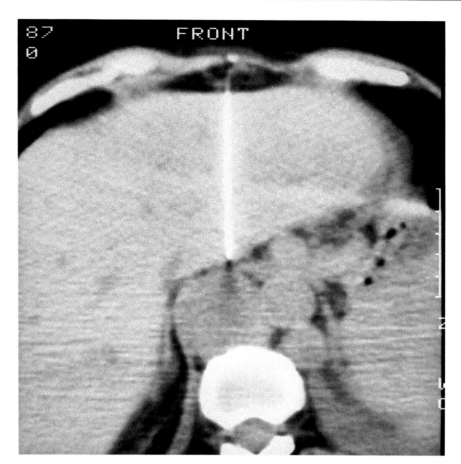

Figs. 17.8. and **17.9.** 56-year old female patient with a renal cell carcinoma. In the same session the celiac plexus and deep thoracic sympathetic trunk were destroyed.

Fig. 17.8. A transhepatic access route was chosen for the neurolysis of the celiac plexus. The puncture was made through the left liver lobe. The needle tip protrudes 1 mm beyond the liver capsula. Note the distribution of the alcohol.

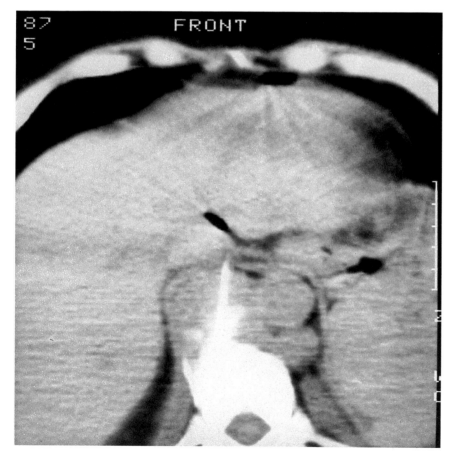

Fig. 17.9. After neurolysis of the celiac plexus, during the same treatment session, the needle was advanced through the infra-diaphragmatic metastasis to a distal thoracic ganglion. After contrast injection, the diffuse distribution of the contrast demonstrates that the needle tip is not in the vena cava. Therefore, a neurolysis of the thoracic sympathetic trunk could be performed. Another lymph node metastasis can be seen on the left, posterior to the aorta. The hyperdense areas anterior to the diaphragm are signs of the alcohol injection used for elimination of the celiac plexus.

Figs. 17.10. and **17.11.** Bilateral neurolysis of the lumbar sympathetic trunk for metastatic renal cell carcinoma in a patient with severe tumor pain. The tumor is prevertebral and has shifted the abdominal vessels anterolaterally to the right.

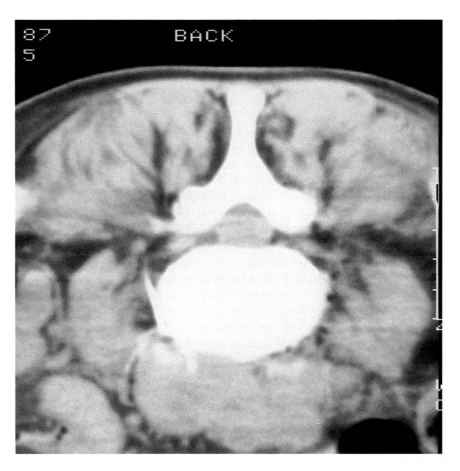

Fig. 17.10. The potential for pain reduction using neurolysis of the lumbar sympathetic trunk in a vertebral body breast metastasis is demonstrated in this patient. After one treatment the pain was considerably reduced. An important point in neurolysis, in the case of patients with pathologic anatomy, is that CT guidance is necessary, as in this case.

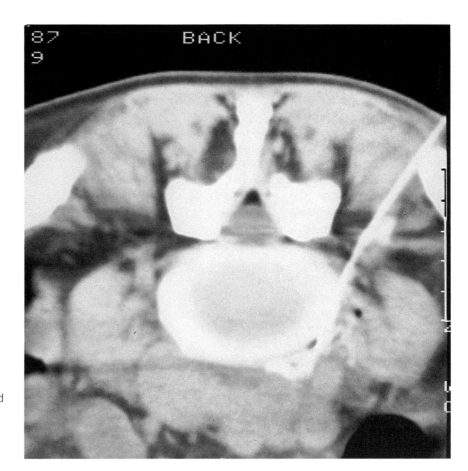

Fig. 17.11. The needle tip is in the region of a lumbar sympathetic ganglion. The anticipated distribution of alcohol within the region of the ganglion is documented by the contrast dissemination. For needle placement a three-dimensional technique was used.

of the planning-CT are always evaluated and the access route is selected by the safest approach, i.e. trans-hepatic, para-gastral, trans-gastral or even infra-colic. The plexus is destroyed with 20 to 50 ml of 50% ethanol. This therapy normally results in immediate elimination of pain. Complications did not occur in the clinic's neurolysis patients. The reasons for recurrence of pain, after previously being pain-free, are – as already described – either regeneration of the nerves within the region of the plexus or tumor infiltration of the surrounding nerve structures (see Chapter 18). In these patients, the procedure is repeated. Also, in patients with metastases into the mediastinum from the abdomen, celiac plexus neurolysis can be followed by a thoracic sympathetic trunk neurolysis.

CT-Guided Neurolysis of the Lumbar Sympathetic Trunk

As with the celiac plexus, the lumbar sympathetic trunk plays a substantial part in tumor pain. The original indication for lumbar sympathetic trunk neurolysis was to increase the circulation in the lower extremities (see Chapter 17). Neurolysis of the lumbar sympathetic trunk may be required for alleviation of tumor pain in cases of tumor infiltration of the sympathetic trunk, lumbar vertebrae metastases or infiltration of segmental nerves by tumor. For neurolysis of the sympathetic trunk the authors prefer a posterolateral translumbar approach. The exact position (1 mm³) of the needle tip can be documented with CT. With this precise control of the needle tip, most complications can be avoided.

CT-Guided Neurolysis of the Precoccygeal Sympathetic Trunk

The authors performed neurolysis of the presacral and precoccygeal plexus in patients with pain from a tumor infiltrating into the pelvis (mostly by colorectal or gynecological carcinomas). This procedure can be performed precisely and with minimal complications by using CT guidance. The interventional needle is seen in its entire length. The needle tip is in the region of a lumbar sympathetic ganglion. The anticipated distribution of the ethanol is established by the contrast medium and is in the correct area for therapy. This neurolysis technique for pain therapy should only be performed with CT guidance. The differentiation of the tumor from the shifted vessels is not possible with ultrasound or fluoroscopy. Only with

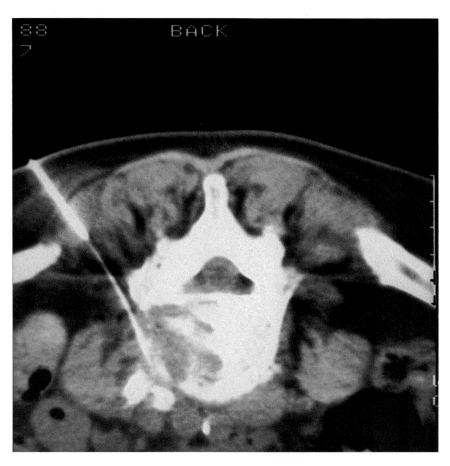

Fig. 17.12. The interventional needle is seen in its entire length. The needle tip is in the region of a lumbar sympathetic ganglion. The anticipated distribution of the ethanol is documented by the contrast medium and is in the proper area for therapy. This neurolysis technique for pain therapy should only be performed with CT guidance. The differentiation of the tumor from the shifted vessels is not possible with ultrasound or fluoroscopy. Only with CT guidance is the risk of an unintentional intramural or intravascular alcohol injection minimized. This patient was nearly painfree following treatment.

Figs. 17.13.–17.16. In these scans, the patient is undergoing therapy for a bone metastasis in the ilium from a colorectal carcinoma. An extensive soft-tissue tumor can be seen in the region of the iliopsoas muscle.

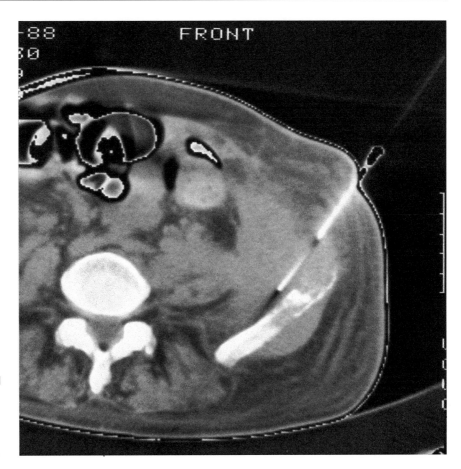

Fig. 17.13. The interventional needle was advanced from an anterolateral approach for 14 cm through the soft-tissue tumor. The needle tip is in the periphery of the tumor posteriorly.

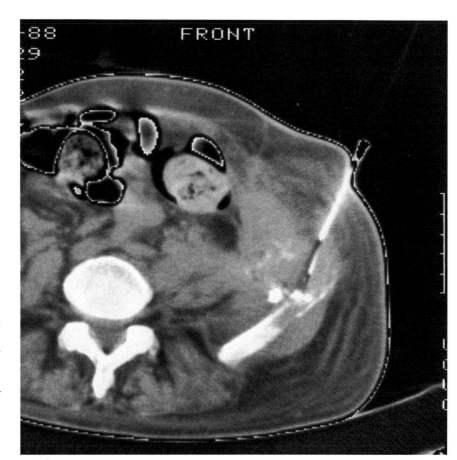

Fig. 17.14. After evaluation of the contrast-medium distribution, ethanol was injected into the medial part of the tumor. The needle was then shifted to another position in the tumor. An additional ethanol injection was performed in this second region.

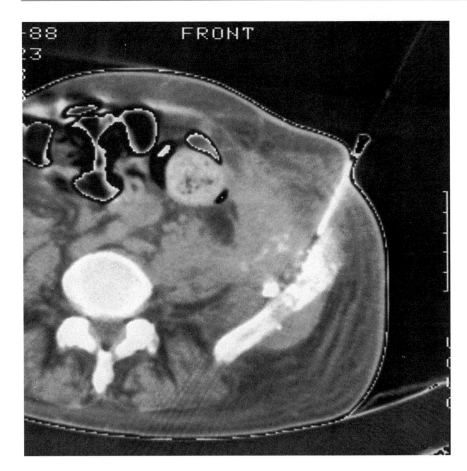

Fig. 17.15. The needle tip is now seen in the peripheral part of the tumor. The ethanol appears as multiple small hyperdense pearl-shaped areas on CT.

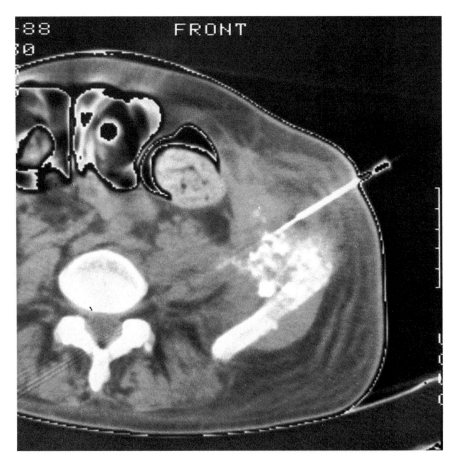

Fig. 17.16. Lastly an injection of ethanol into the anterior peritumoral area was performed. All of the above figures demonstrate that, by careful attention in procedure and CT guidance, the alcohol can be injected without major complications. This requires that for each step only small amounts of alcohol are used. After being treated on four different occasions, this patient was pain-free.

Figs. 17.17.–17.19.
67-year old patient with destruction of the acetabulum and a pathological fracture caused by prostatical metastases. As in the case of fracture fissure anesthesia the interventional needle is advanced into the pathological fracture. Alcohol injections were performed several times. After four treatments with 5 ml alcohol each, calcification and stabilization of the fracture were observed. After 2 months the patient was able to walk again without pain.

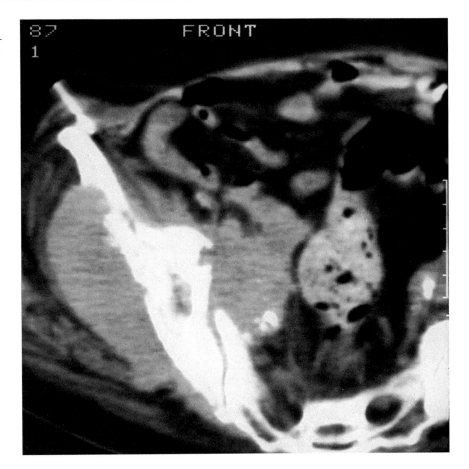

Fig. 17.17

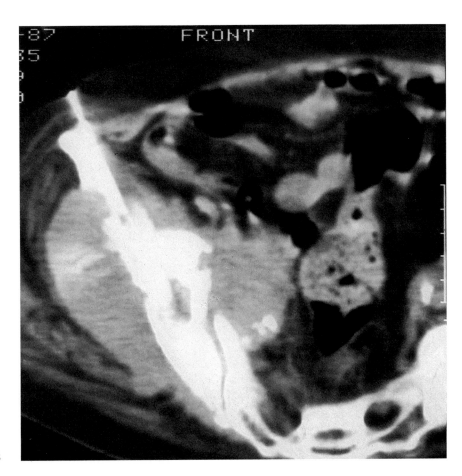

Fig. 17.18

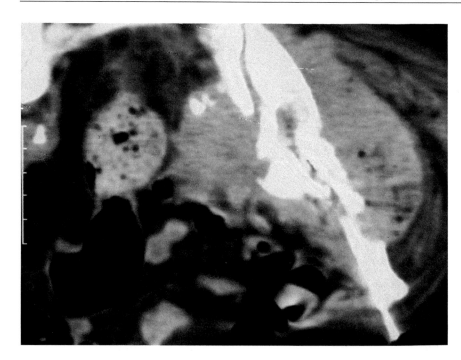

Fig. 17.19

CT guidance is the risk of an unintentional intramural or intravascular alcohol injection minimized. This patient was nearly pain-free following treatment. Contrary to the neurolysis of the lumbar sympathetic trunk and celiac plexus, presacral and precoccygeal plexus therapy always requires multiple treatments. Normally the therapy is performed on four separate occasions. Each time 5-8 ml alcohol is injected into the plexus. The combination of lumbar sympathetic trunk neurolysis with presacral and precoccygeal sympathetic trunk neurolysis made a chordotomy unnecessary in patients with typical pelvic-leg pain caused by tumor invasion into the iliac region (see Chapter 19).

B. CT-Guided Tumor Therapy

After achieving good results with pain therapy, the authors decided to perform intra- and peritumoral therapy in patients in an advanced state of malignancy. Precondition for this treatment protocol was prior radiation therapy or chemotherapy without success. Also included were patients for whom a systemic chemotherapy or radiation therapy was contra-indicated. Either 96% ethanol or Mitoxantron (an intracyclin that is well tolerated after local injections) was used in the tumor therapy. In total intra- and/or peritumoral therapy was performed in 71 patients (Table 17.2.).

Table 17.2. CT-guided tumor therapy (n = 71).

Mitoxantron (Novantron®)	30 patients
96% ethanol	41 patients

Indications

Large tumors at stage 1M were treated with intra- and/or peritumoral therapy after exhausting the conventional therapeutic approach. Further indications are in patients with tumor pain and neurologic deficits caused by a rapidly expanding tumor. Also, bone metastases which can fracture or lead to immobilization of the patient are further indications which show good results after therapy (Tables 17.3. and 17.4.).

Table 17.3. Indications for CT-guided tumor therapy.

Tumor patients at stage 1M
– Pain
– Neurologic deficits
– Danger of fracture
– Danger of immobilization
– Severe side-effects from systemic analgesics

Table 17.4. Prerequisites for CT-guided tumor therapy.

Tumor patients at stage 1M
1 Unsuccessful treatment with:
   radiation therapy
   chemotherapy
2 No other therapy possible

Figs. 17.20.–17.22.
58-year old female patient
with a breast carcinoma
and osteolytic metastases
with fracture of the right ala
of the ilium.

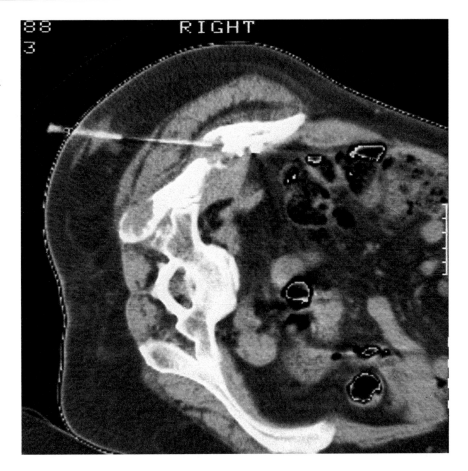

Fig. 17.20. The tip of the
interventional needle has
been advanced into the
fracture.

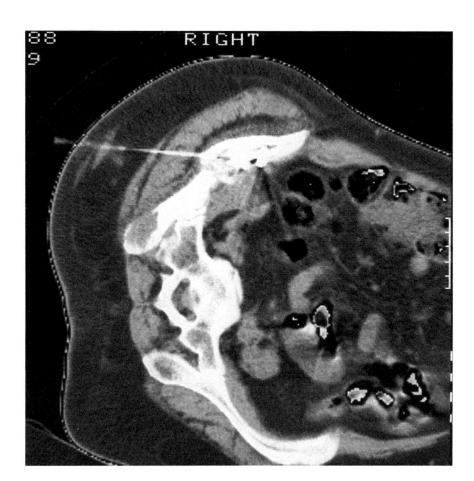

Fig. 17.21. After the contrast-medium injection,
3 ml alcohol was injected.

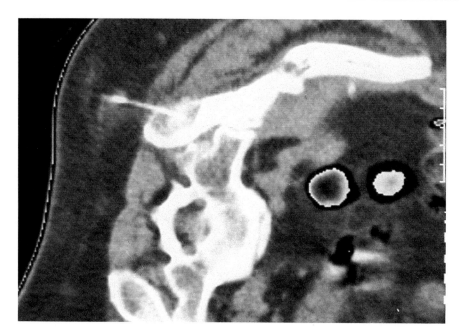

Fig. 17.22. CT scan four weeks after therapy. The fracture fissure is now narrowed. The patient stated that her pain was reduced by 85%. The three-dimensional advanced interventional needle is visualized in another osteolytic metastasis. 2 ml Novantron was injected.

Patients

During the period from March 1, 1986 to February 28, 1989, a total of 71 tumor patients in late stages of their illness had been treated. The youngest patient was 29 years, the oldest 81 years old. The average age was 64 years (Table 17.5.). Besides the intra- and/or peritumoral therapy, pain therapy was additionally performed in all patients using only one method or a combination of different pain-therapeutic methods (Figs. 17.1.–17.42.).

Additionally, 291 tumor patients were treated with pain therapy only. The results of the different therapy methods for tumor pain are described in the pain therapy chapters. In total, 362 tumor patients had been treated (Table 17.6.).

These therapies were performed in the regions where the primary tumor and/or the metastases had been discovered (Tables 17.7. and 17.8.).

Table 17.5. Age of the patients undergoing CT-guided tumor therapy.

Youngest patient	29 years
Average age of patients	64 years
Oldest patient	81 years

Table 17.6. Number of tumor patients in each therapy method.

Tumor and pain therapy	71 patients
Pain therapy only	291 patients
Total number of patients	362 patients

Table 17.7. Tumor localization in 362 patients.

Localization	Patients
Extracranial trigeminal region	3
Cervicobrachial plexus	38
Mediastinum	4
Thoracic wall	17
Pancreas, hepatic porta	188
Renal fossa	8
Retroperitoneum	21
Peritoneum	15
Pelvic floor	20
Skeleton	23
Lumbosacral plexus	25
Total	362

Table 17.8. Tumor etiology.

Tumor	Frequency
Glomus tumor	3
Breast carcinoma	33
Pancoast tumor	28
Small cell bronchial carcinoma	17
Squamous cell carcinoma	15
Mesothelioma	9
Pancreatic carcinoma	82
Lymphoma	12
Hypernephroma	34
Urinary bladder carcinoma	6
Gastric carcinoma	54
Colon/rectal carcinoma	17
Liver metastases	9
Metastases with infiltration of celiac plexus	43
Total	362

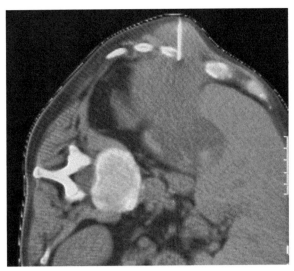
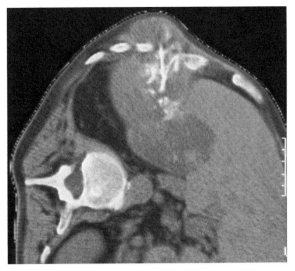

Figs. 17.23. and **17.24.** Large malignant histiocytic metastasis with rib destructions and intra- and extra-abdominal growth. **Fig. 17.23.** The needle tip is at the inferior portion of the rib. After injection of 3 ml ethanol, a hyperdense border is seen around the needle tip. **Fig. 17.24.** The next step is intratumoral therapy with 5 ml alcohol. The distribution of the contrast medium alcohol mixture is well demonstrated by CT.

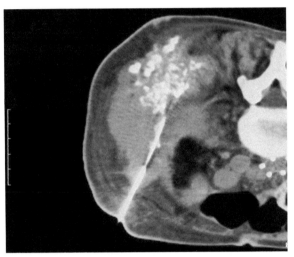
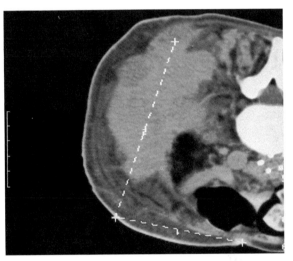

Figs. 17.25. and **17.26.** A large renal cell metastasis is well illustrated. **Fig. 17.25.** Planning-CT for intra- and peritumoral treatment. The needle tip has to be advanced to a depth of 15 cm to be at the correct level for treatment. **Fig. 17.26.** As the needle is withdrawn, the injection of approximately 6 ml Mitoxantron was performed in several fractions into an area approximately 4 × 5 cm along the periphery of the tumor. The injection was performed into the tumor tissue without complications. The risk of an intravasal injection is minimal when using the CT technique.

Technique

After accurate definition of the tumor area in contiguous non-contrast and contrast CT scans, the center of the region to be treated is determined. If possible, a reconstruction in another plane is performed for better localization. After measuring the depth to the center of the injection and the puncture angle, a guide needle is advanced. Following this, the 22-G therapy needle is placed through the guide needle. After local anesthesia, an injection of diluted contrast medium is performed to document the distribution of the medication. In 41 patients, this was followed by the instillation of 96% ethanol. In 30 patients Mitoxantron was injected instead of alcohol. Depending on tumor size, 1.5–12 ml of alcohol or 1–8 mg of Mitoxantron was injected. It is important to achieve an almost homogeneous distribution of the medication in the tumor. For very large tumors, only the tumor areas which are felt to be responsible for the patient's complaints are treated. A repetition of the therapy is carried out after three to four weeks. Between four and ten separate treatments are performed in every case.

After the first and subsequent therapies, liquefied necrosis is a common finding. This necrosis should be removed with a catheter using CT guidance before performing the therapy.

Side-effects

The drugs which were used can cause considerable damage to the surrounding healthy tissue. However, the authors did not observe any serious side-effects in their patients. Also, no relevant systemic side-effects developed either, especially after Mitoxantron. In only three patients did they observe a minor myelotoxicity with minimally reduced thrombocyte and granulocyte values. Furthermore, vomiting, stomatitis or hair loss did not occur in any of the patients.

Preliminary Results

71 patients had intra- and/or peritumoral therapy, some up to ten separate treatments, at intervals of two to four weeks. In addition to the tumor therapy, pain therapy was necessary in all patients. This consisted of a single type or a combination of different pain-therapeutic procedures. On average, these pain therapies were performed six separate times. Although it is not the aim of a palliative therapy to achieve a reduction in tumor size, in 25% of the patients a reduction of up to 50% was observed. More important was the palliative effect of the pain reduction, stabilization of vertebral body metastases, and decompression of the dural sac. Intraspinal metastases were also successfully treated. In these cases, the authors conducted a therapy with Mitoxantron only in order to avoid any complications through a misplaced injection of alcohol. In eight out of ten patients with metastases and unstable spinal column they were able to achieve stabilization. Furthermore, in tumors which normally respond poorly to chemotherapy (i.e. hypernephroid kidney carcinomas, pancreatic carcinomas or colorectal carcinomas), it was possible to obtain good results. The number of cases for each tumor type and each location treated is too small for a complete evaluation at this stage.

In a controlled study which is being conducted at present, it will be explored whether there are any advantages from the use of a combination therapy with alcohol and Mitoxantron in comparison with an exclusive alcohol or Mitoxantron therapy (Table 17.9.).

Table 17.9. Results after CT-guided tumor therapy (n = 71).

Free of complaint	80%
Tumor reduction (< 50%)	25%
No change in size of tumor	58%
Tumor progression	17%

Summary

With effective pain and local tumor therapy on an out-patient basis, together with extensive psycho-social care, the quality of life of cancer patients can be improved. The less invasive CT- and MRI-guided tumor therapies can be utilized either in addition to or as an alternative to the conventional tumor therapy methods for advanced malignancies. By combining CT guidance with fluoroscopy and/or digital radiography, the procedure is improved and permits an on line three-dimensional view of the region to be treated. The CT-guided methods discussed here have good patient tolerance and a lack of serious systemic side-effects. The distribution of the medication used can be evaluated with CT. This is especially important in the case of abnormal anatomy. Due to the minor side-effects observed, even patients in a poor state of health and with a low Karnofsky index can be treated successfully (Table 17.10.), even with CT-guided laser therapy (Figs. 17.33.–17.34.). The complete discussion can be found in chapter 18.

Table 17.10. Advantages of CT-guided percutaneous tumor therapy.

Accurate needle placement (1 mm^3)
Differentiation of abnormal anatomy
Minimal danger of injuring surrounding structures
Accurate control and documentation of the medication distribution
Minimal systemic side-effects
Very sick patients can be treated

References

1. Daten des Gesundheitswesens, Schriftenreihe des Bumi. f. Jug. Fam. Ges., Stuttgart Bd. 152 (1983) 188–90
2. Ewers U.: Krebserkrankungen bei Arbeitern und Angestellten im Spiegel der Daten der Deutschen Rentenversicherungsträger. Öff. Ges. Wes. 45 (1983) 561–571
3. Koch E., Klopfleisch R., Maywald A.: Die Gesundheit der Nation. Köln (1986)
4. Porges P.: Der Karzinomschmerz. Schmerz 2 (1988) 59–65
5. Robra B.P., Schwartz F.W., Kramer P.: Zur Entwicklung der Mortalität in der Bundesrepublik Deutschland 1952–1979, 1. Mitteilung: Gesamtmortalität und altersstandardisierte Mortalität an Herz-Kreislaufer-krankungen und Krebs. Öff. Ges. Wes. 45 (1983) 47–52
6. Schara J.: Tumorschmerz. Schmerz-Pain-Douleur 2 (1986) 41–42
7. Schara J.: Gedanken zur Betreuung terminaler Kranker mit Krebsschmerz. Schmerz 2 (1988) 151–160
8. Segi institute of cancer epidemiology: age-adjusted death rates for cancer for selected sites (A-classification) in 43 countries in 1977, Nagoya 1982

Figs. 17.27. and **17.28.**
This patient has an extensive metastasis to the pelvic wall with sciatic nerve infiltration from a recurrent rectal carcinoma (center of picture). After completion of intra- and peritumoral therapy, the patient was free of complaints and no sciatic nerve deficit occurred (combination therapy with ethanol and Mitoxantron).

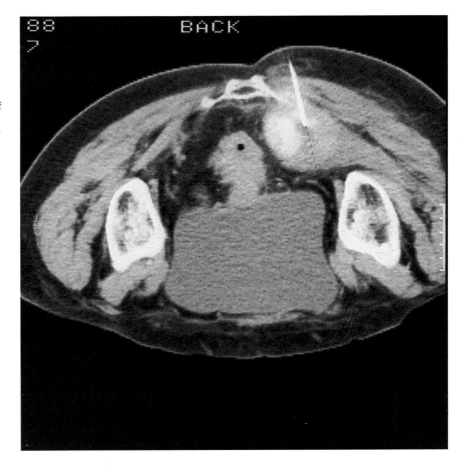

Fig. 17.27. CT scan with the needle tip in the tumor shows the intratumoral distribution of the medication.

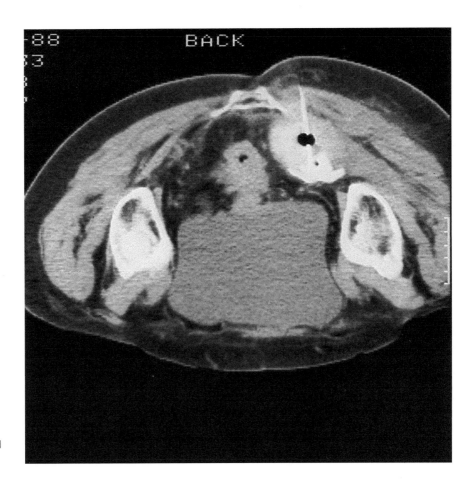

Fig. 17.28. The needle tip was advanced into the peritumoral region and a contrast medium was injected for documentation. The arch-shaped distribution of the contrast around the tumor is observed.

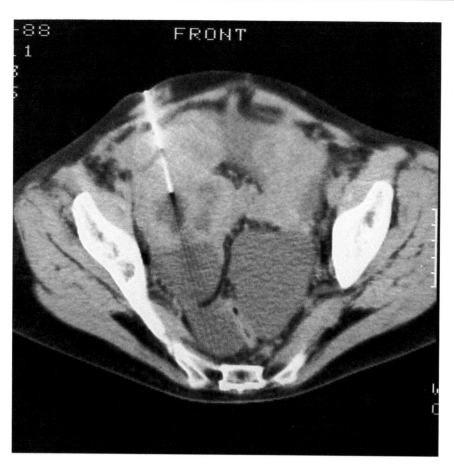

Figs. 17.29.–17.34. Intratumoral therapy in a 65-year old female patient with a large renal cell metastasis. The patient had the beginning of an obstructive ileus. At intervals of 2 weeks, 5 to 10 ml ethanol and 10 ml Mitoxantron were injected into the tumor. Together with the local anesthetics, a total injection of 30 to 50 ml is normal for this type of tumor therapy. Beginning with the second therapy and prior to each subsequent treatment, approximately 30 ml of liquid necrosis were aspirated from the tumor.

Fig. 17.29. The tip of the interventional needle is at the edge of necrotic area which was produced by earlier intratumoral treatment.

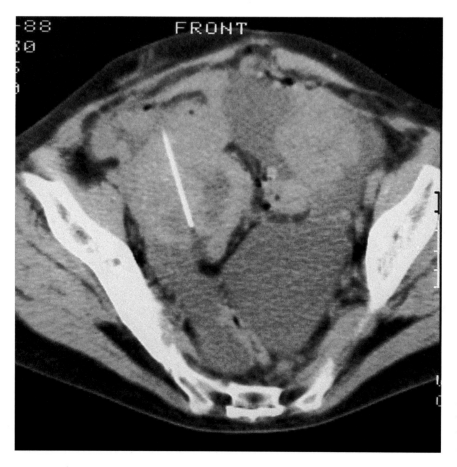

Fig. 17.30. CT demonstrates the advancement of the interventional needle to the periphery of the metastasis in the three-dimensional technique.

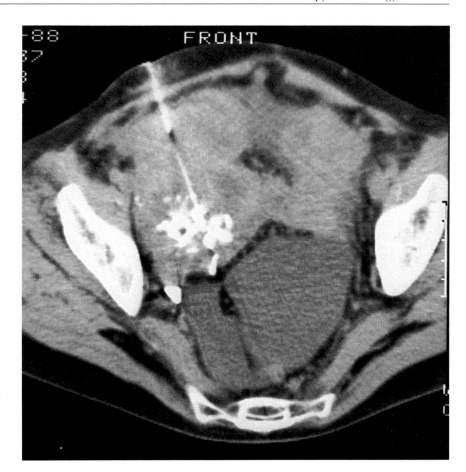

Fig. 17.31. The injection of contrast medium documents the potential distribution of Mitoxantron and alcohol.

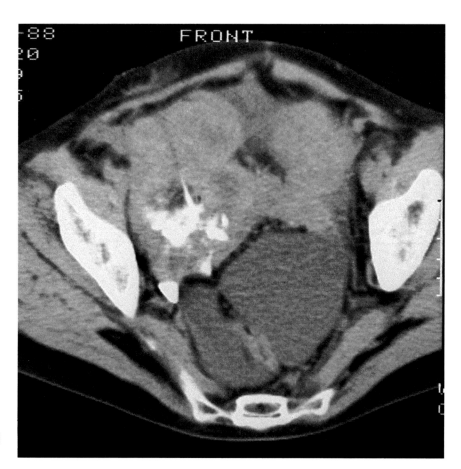

Fig. 17.32. Above the contrast medium is a dome-like hyperdense area. This area represents the injected alcohol.

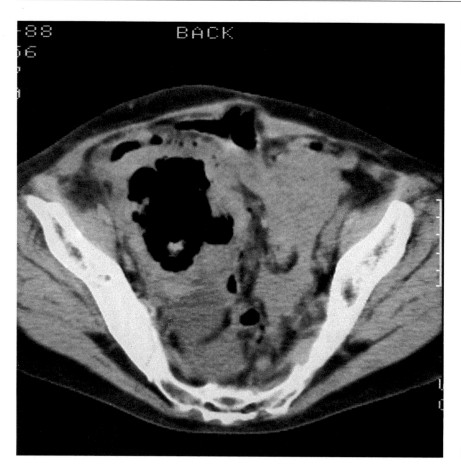

Figs. 17.33. and **17.34.**
CT scan shows a large
gas-filled zone of necrosis
after therapy. A CT guided
laser therapy (Hot-tip-laser).

Fig. 17.33. Laser therapy.

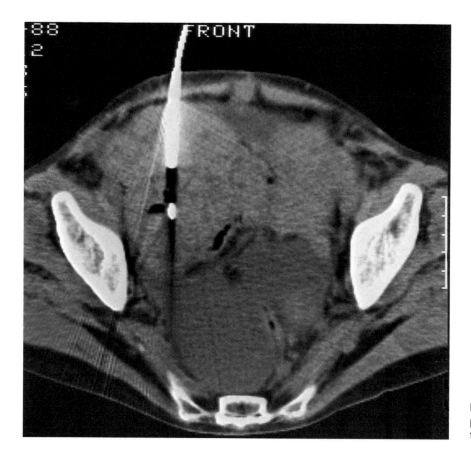

Fig. 17.34. The laser is
placed in the center of the
tumor.

Figs. 17.35.–17.42.
31-year old patient with a large renal cell metastasis with diffuse destruction of the vertebral body and displacement of the thecal sac. The following scans were obtained between October 1988 and March 1989.

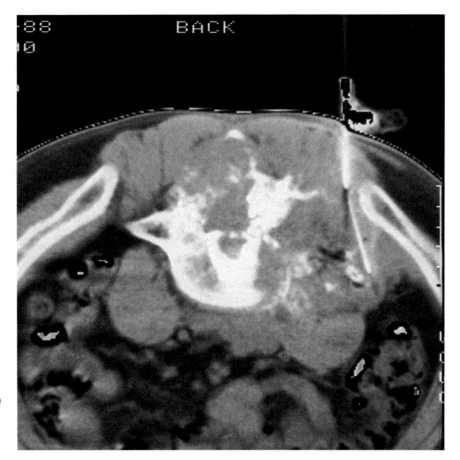

Fig. 17.35. In a special technique the interventional needle is advanced into the lateral aspect of the soft tissue metastasis and 3 ml of alcohol is injected.

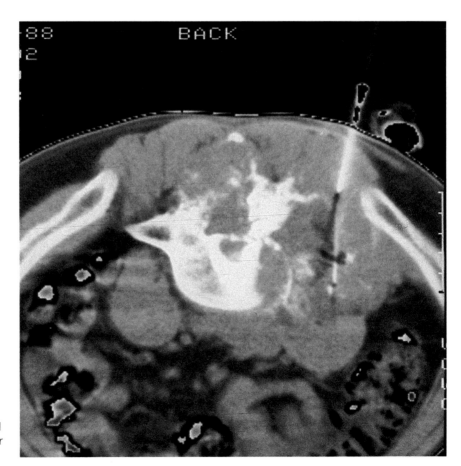

Fig. 17.36. Change of needle position with injection of another 3 ml of alcohol into the tumor center.

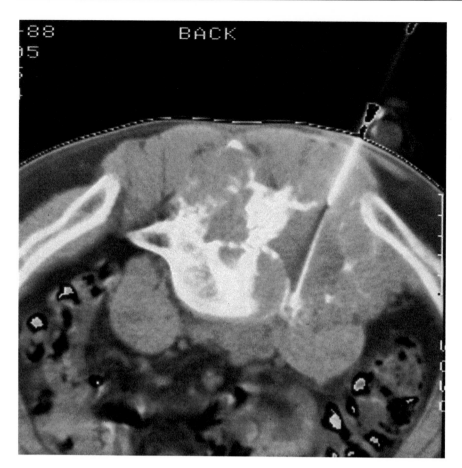

Fig. 17.37. In the third step, the medial side of the tumor is treated with 96% ethanol, followed by a neurolysis of the lumbar sympathetic trunk.

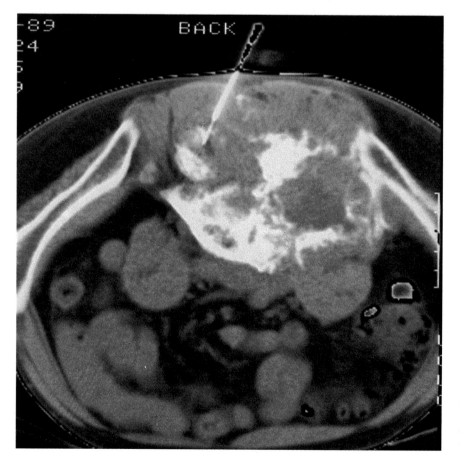

Fig. 17.38. In January 1989 the left vertebral arch was treated with 2 mg Mitoxantron.

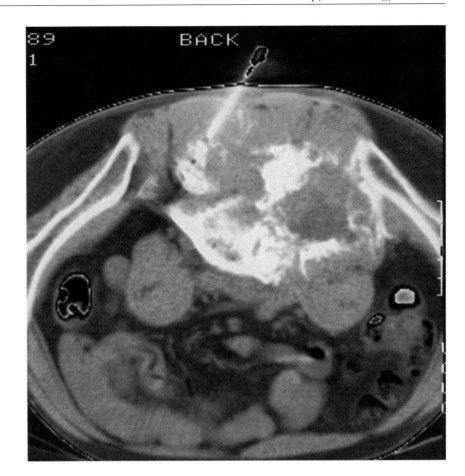

Fig. 17.39. Injection of Mitoxantron into the vertebral arch.

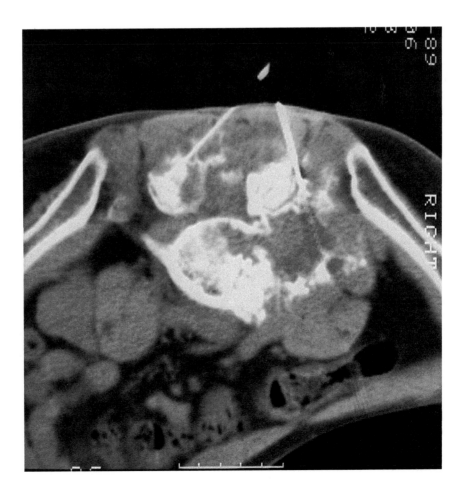

Fig. 17.40. March 1989. Injection of 2 ml Mitoxantron into the right vertebral arch. The left interventional needle was advanced, lateral to the facet joints, into the tumor periphery and 2 ml of alcohol was injected.

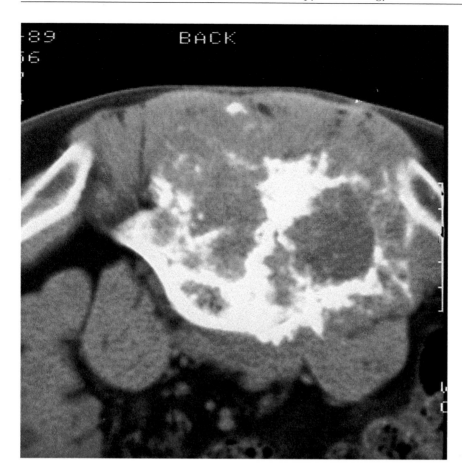

Fig. 17.41. In comparison with the scans of October 1988 (Figs. 17.35.–17.37.), osseous bridging has occurred with subsequent stabilization in this region. Note the double-arch-shaped calcification of vertebral bodies to the ala of the ilium.

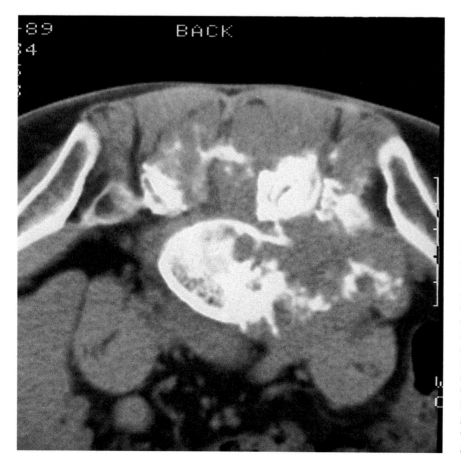

Fig. 17.42. In comparison with October 1988, there has been a reduction in the size of the tumor and a decompression of the spinal canal. The left epidural fat and the dural sac can be distinguished again. This procedure led to a pain reduction of approximately 95%. Five months after the beginning of therapy and after 6 treatments, the patient was able to walk again without pain.

Chapter 18
CT-Guided Cervical Blockades and Methods of Cancer Therapy for Lesions of the Cervicobrachial Plexus

D.H.W. Grönemeyer, R.M.M. Seibel

Introduction

Therapeutic effects of local anesthesia have been known since 1884. At that time Koller [18] reported the clinical use of cocaine topically in the eye. In 1892 Schleich observed the therapeutic effect to locally applied cocaine for low back pain [32]. In 1904, novocaine was first synthesized by Einhorn [11].

In 1925, Mandl [23, 24] was the first to perform a stellate ganglion block from a posterior approach. Demarez [10] also described this technique in 1937. Then, in 1955 Reischauer [30] modified the same technique for stellate ganglion block by performing the injection from a posterior approach between C6 and C7 instead of between C7 and T1. The lateral approach to the stellate ganglion was first used in 1934 by Leriche and Fontane [21] and then by De Sèze in 1953 [33]. In 1943 Herget [15] reported a temporary block of the stellate ganglion from an anterior approach.

The indication and technique for the conventional block of stellate ganglion are described in many publications and manuals [1–6, 17]. A technique for blocking the superior cervical ganglion was first reported by Orsoni [28]. CT-guided techniques have, to the best of the authors' knowledge, not been described so far in the literature.

Painful changes in the shoulder-arm region can have many causes and until now treatment has followed the methods described by Kaeser [16]. These methods are partially established and partially new. Causes of this type of pain can range from lesions in the nerve roots of the middle or lower cervical area to pseudo-radicular symptoms due to alteration of the vertebral facet joints or other changes resulting in muscular tension. Furthermore, plexus lesions resulting from impingement of cervical ribs or fibrous lesions are possible.

In the majority of cases the cause of the pain is brachial plexus compression and/or infiltration by a malignant process or hypertrophic scar growth after surgery or radiation. Other causes include neuritis of the brachial plexus, lymphedema after surgical removal or axillary lymph nodes or lesions after shoulder or clavicular surgery. The most commonly affected roots are C7, C8, and T1 [3, 4].

Anatomy

The *sympathetic trunk* of the neck consists of three pairs of ganglia (Figs. 18.1. and 18.2.) (see also Chapter Autonomic Nervous System):

1. *Superior cervical ganglion.* This ganglion is located in the region of the second and third cervical vertebrae at an angle between the vertebral body and the transverse process. This is the largest of the sympathetic cervical ganglia.
2. *Middle cervical ganglion.* Located at the level of the 4th and 5th cervical vertebral body.
3. *Stellate ganglion.* Normally this ganglion lies on the head of the first rib 1 cm lateral to the costovertebral joint in front of the longus colli muscle. However, a wide variation exists in the localization of the stellate ganglion. It is composed of the inferior cervical ganglion and the superior thoracic ganglion (ganglion thoracale 1). The stellate ganglion is sheathed in by 2 fasciae: anteriorly by the same fascia that surrounds the carotid artery and posteriorly by the prevertebral fascia [17].

The *brachial plexus* is composed of nerve bundles originating from C4-T2. After traversing the gap between the anterior and middle scalene muscles, the brachial plexus separates into the following nerve roots: axillary n., musculocutaneous n., radial n., median n. and ulnar n. This occurs at the level of the first rib. These nerve bundles run together in a sheath with the axillary artery and vein.

Differential Diagnosis of Pain Syndromes

Cervicobrachial Plexus

Especially fast-growing bronchial carcinomas that spread into the apex of the lung (pancoast tumors) often infiltrate into the vertebrae, ribs and into the supraclavicular cavity. These

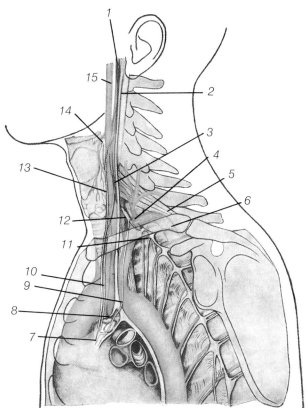

Fig. 18.1. Cervicothoracic ganglion (stellate ganglion) in the topography of the superior thoracic aperture after Rohen J.W.: Topographische Anatomie, Kurzlehrbuch für Studierende und Ärzte, published by F.K. Schattauer, Stuttgart, New York, 1984, 231, Fig. 151).
1 Superior cervical ganglion; *2* left vagus n.; *3* middle cervical ganglion; *4* thyreocervical trunk; *5* brachial plexus; *6* left subclavian a.; *7* cardiac plexus; *8* recurrent laryngeal n.; *9* inferior cardiac branch of the vagus n.; *10* middle cardiac branch of the vagus n.; *11* and *12* cervicothoracic ganglion (stellate ganglion) and subclavian loop, inferior cervical ganglion and superior thoracic ganglion; *13* superior cardiac branch of the vagus n.; *14* superior thyroid a.; *15* ext. carotid a.

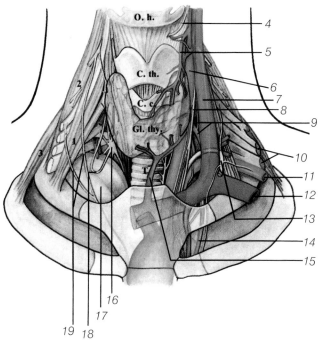

Fig. 18.2. Relation of the brachial plexus and stellate ganglion to the surrounding vessels and muscles after Rohen J.W.: Topographische Anatomie, Kurzlehrbuch für Studierende und Ärzte, published by F.K. Schattauer, Stuttgart, New York, 1984, 233, Fig. 152).
1 Anterior scalene muscle; *2* medial scalene muscle; *3* posterior scalene muscle; *4* superior laryngeal n.; *5* superior thyroid a. and n.; *6* common carotid a.; *7* internal juglar v.; *8* vagus n.; *9* inferior thyroid a. with ascending cervical a.; *10* brachial plexus; *11* subclavian a.; *12* subclavian v.; *13* thoracic duct; *14* internal thoracic a. and v.; *15* inferior thyroid a.; *16* cervicothoracic ganglion; *17* cervical pleura; *18* subclavian loop; *19* phrenic n. with accessory phrenic n.

tumors can also infiltrate and damage the cervicobrachial plexus and the cervical sympathetic trunk. Other tumors can also extend to this area such as pleuramesotheliomas, breast carcinomas and head and neck tumors.

Early symptoms of infiltration such as equilateral Horner's syndrome with miosis, ptosis, enophthalmos and anhidrosis in the upper part of the body as well as pain in the shoulder girdle radiating down into the finger tips are present in about 75% of the patients. Pancoast tumors frequently first infiltrate the cervicothoracic sympathetic trunk and lower portion of the brachial plexus (C8 and T1). The patients first experience a change in the sensation of the 5th finger and the ring finger followed by an inferior plexus paralysis (Klumpke's paralysis). Later stages of infiltration can lead to Sudeck's atrophy (reflex sympathetic dystrophy).

Lymph node metastases from carcinomas such as breast or bronchial or hypertrophic post-operative scar after mastectomy or radiation-induced scar tissue can lead to painful compressions of the vessel-nerve sheath with or without lymphedema. In breast cancer patients, a lesion of the brachial plexus is often associated with lymphedema in the ipsilateral arm. The clinical symptoms with these tumors, metastases and plexus infiltration (by a Hodgkin or a non-Hodgkin lymphoma) are not as typical as for a pancoast tumor. The prognosis in a patient with a brachial plexus lesion from malignant tumors in the sense of "neuritis carcinomatosa" is generally poor.

Patients characterize pain from arm plexus lesion as an intense tearing pain, often extending down to the ulnar side of the forearm and hand. This pain is perceived to be superficial in location. The early appearing dysesthesias and paresthesias are later replaced by hypesthesia and weakness leading to paralysis of flexorus digitorum and other hand muscles. Another symptom is reflex sympathetic dystrophy with dull, burning pain which can involve the entire extremity, scapular region and anterior chest wall. With progressive growth of the tumor, infiltration into the proximal part of the plexus can also be observed.

Radiation Damage to the Arm Plexus

Pain caused by radiation therapy tends to be a diffuse pain with a slow onset which cannot be precisely localized. This can intensify and may lead to severe attacks of pain. The cause of this pain is a connective tissue proliferation with scar enveloping and compressing the nerves. The intensity of the pain often increases with time and can be followed by the development of paralysis and loss of feeling in the affected area. A complete arm-plexus paralysis is fairly rare.

Lymphedema

In a patient with a plexus lesion, discomfort from lymphedema must be differentiated from the symptoms of radiation therapy. Furthermore, there is the possibility that both changes can appear simultaneously. In lymphedema, the lymph transport is hampered and a doughlike, albumin-rich edema results. The increasing tissue pressure can cause pain leading to a heavy arm and a decrease in motion of the affected extremity. This often causes excessive strain in the shoulder joint and its musculature, which leads to a stiff shoulder with a dull, nagging pain. With increasing size of the arm, a burst pain may result.

Indications and Contraindications for Therapy

The combination treatment of the stellate ganglion (see Chapter Tumor Therapy) and the brachial plexus is the optimum form of therapy for shoulder-arm pain in patients with a tumor infiltrating into this region. In cases of inflammatory, degenerative or post-operative alterations in the shoulder girdle only treatment of the brachial plexus should be attempted.

The solitary stellate ganglion treatment is indicated in general vasomotor disorder of the arteries and vein, i.e. by reflex sympathetic dystrophy, Volkmann's ischemia contracture, thoracic outlet syndrome and by thrombophlebitis or thrombosis of the upper extremity. Also

Table 18.1. Indications for treatment of the cervical sympathetic trunk after Gross [14].

1 Stellate ganglion
- Tumor pain
- Herpes zoster
- Post-herpetic neuralgia
- Pain caused by radiation or surgically induced scar
- Thoracic outlet syndrome
- Volkmann's contracture
- Osteoporosis pain
- Thrombophlebitis – thrombosis
- Lymphedema
- Phantom pain
- Reflex sympathetic dystrophy

2 Superior cervical ganglion
- Atypical facial pain
- Post-herpetic neuralgia
- Trigeminal neuralgia
- Reflex sympathetic dystrophy
- Facial nerve parlysis with lagophthalmus (Hare's eye)
- Unilateral facial spasm

phantom pain, the acute stage of herpes zoster, as well as post-herpetic neuralgia and pain caused by scar tissue, can be treated by this method.

The treatment of the superior cervical ganglion is useful in post-herpetic neuralgia, pain caused by disruption of postganglionic sympathetic nerve fibers and by the indications shown in Table 18.1. These techniques are not indicated in patients with coagulation disorders.

Technique

Interventional cervical blockade techniques are performed predominantly with CT guidance or with a combination of CT and fluoroscopy or DSA (see Chapter Combination Methods). The cervical spinal column is scanned in the prone or supine position. The treatment of the superior cervical ganglion takes place at the level of C2-3. On the other hand, the stellate ganglion is treated in the region of the transition from the cervical to the thoracic spinal cord (Figs. 18.3.-18.5.).

The procedure is as follows: After identification of the area overlying the ganglion, a determination of the puncture point, the puncture angle and the distance to the skin is made. Following local anesthesia in the skin a coaxial two-needle system with a 22-G fine needle with stylet is advanced into the ganglion to be blocked or to its immediate vicinity. The puncture point for the superior cervical ganglion is anterolateral, while for the stellate ganglion the puncture point is posterior, lateral or anterolateral. The lateral approach to the stellate ganglion has the

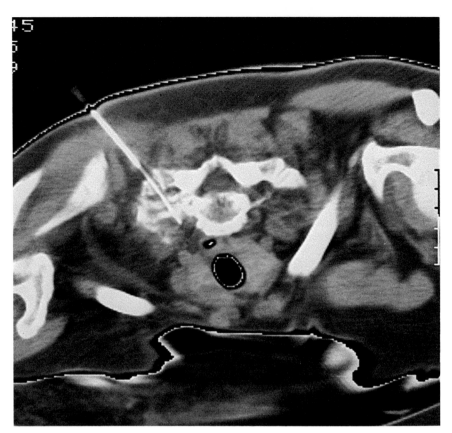

Figs. 18.3.–18.5. CT-guided stellate ganglion in a female patient with lymph edema and severe left shoulder pain after radiation. The block is performed with the patient in the prone position. The needle is advanced through the guiding needle and from posterolateral to anteromedial direction. In Fig. 18.3. the needle tip is just 1 mm lateral to the vertebral a. and v.

Fig. 18.3

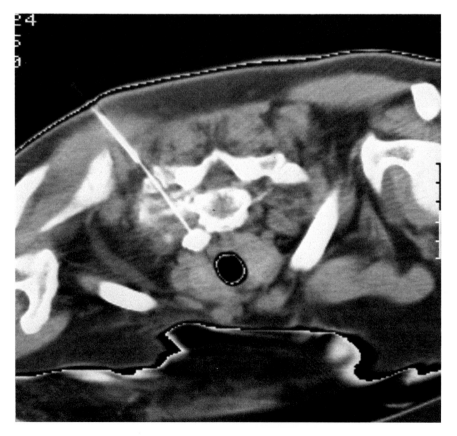

Fig. 18.4. The needle is advanced just anterior to the longus colli muscle and 0.2 ml of a dilute contrast agent is injected. The contrast medium is distributed in the perineural and perivascular fatty tissue. Anteriorly the contrast medium reaches the common carotid a. and the internal jugular v. This is the correct distribution of the contrast.

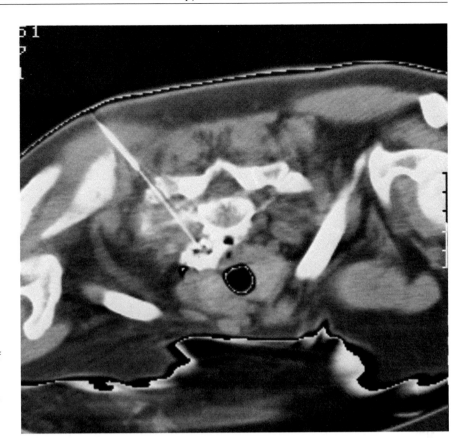

Fig. 18.5. Distribution of the medication and contrast medium in the perineural and perivascular region. After the injection of 2 ml of local anesthetic, the contrast area has been expanded. The hyperdense medication is observed around the needle tip.

longest distance from the skin to the ganglion. The authors prefer the anterolateral approach for stellate ganglion blockade. Knowledge of the exact location of the carotid and vertebral arteries is mandatory, since in many cases they are located only 1 to 2 mm away from the puncture needle (Figs. 18.6.–18.8.).

Following this, 2-3 ml of a short and long-acting local anesthetic (mixture 1:2) is injected around the ganglion. To extend the anesthesia effectiveness and for local tumor therapy, 10 mg Volon-A (cortical steroid) can be added. Distribution of the medication is verified with a dose of a diluted contrast medium. In cases where this procedure is part of tumor therapy, it will normally be combined with an intra- and peritumoral therapy (Figs. 18.14.–18.17.) (see Chapter Tumor Therapy).

For the brachial plexus block and treatment different approaches are often possible. CT documentation and measurement of the puncture depth and the puncture angle are all performed as usual. The therapy can be performed by either the:

1 interscalene approach (paravertebrally at the region of the spinal nerves forming the brachial plexus);

2 supraclavicular approach (above the first rib, at the perforation point of the brachial plexus through the gap between anterior and middle scalene muscles).

The authors prefer a modified, more laterally located supraclavicular approach (Figs. 18.18. and 18.19.). After identification of the plexus the needle is advanced in several steps as described above for the stellate ganglion block. As soon as the needle tip is in the region of the plexus, diluted contrast medium is injected (Figs. 18.9.–18.11.).

The anesthetic, consisting of a 30 ml mixture of a 1% Mepivacaine solution with 0.25% Bupivacaine solution (mixture 1:1), is injected. Treatment of the shoulder-arm syndrome by block of the plexus should consist of a combination of a stellate ganglion block and a brachial plexus block, with a mixture of short- and long-acting local anesthetics. A local cytostasis with Mitoxantron (Lederle) or cytotoxic effective 96% ethanol (Pfrimmer) is appropriate in intra-tumoral therapy (see Chapter Tumor Therapy) (Figs. 18.9.–18.11.).

Patients

In this chapter the authors have dealt predominantly with pain and tumor therapy in patients with shoulder-arm pain with or without infiltration of the brachial plexus. Up to December 1988, they had a total of 189 CT-guided cervical blockades (Table 18.2.). Since that time, additional treatments have been conducted for the same indications as previously discussed in this

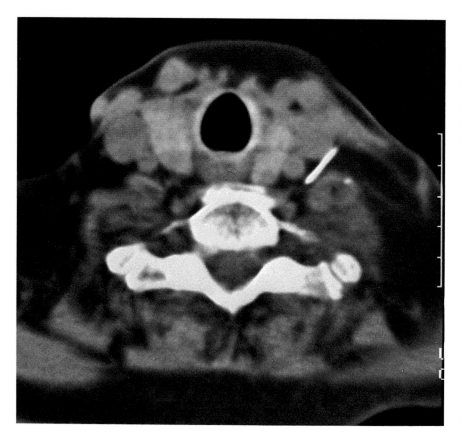

Figs. 18.6.–18.8. Stellate ganglion block from antero-lateral approach. Three-dimensional puncture technique: only the anterior third of the puncture needle is shown which is next to the internal jugular v. and carotid a.

Fig. 18.6

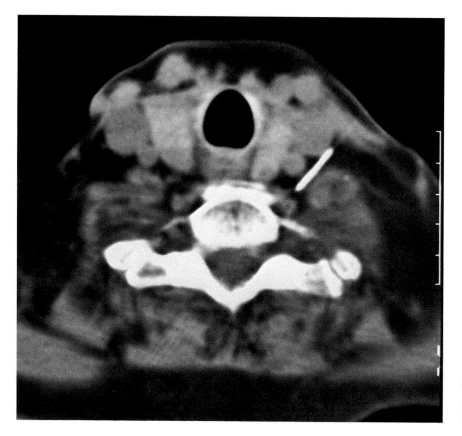

Fig. 18.7. The puncture needle is advanced for 2 mm. The tip is now at the stellate ganglion which appears as a peak-like process on the longus colli muscle. Above it, the vertebral a. and v. can be seen. The distance from the needle tip to the vertebral a. is 2 mm.

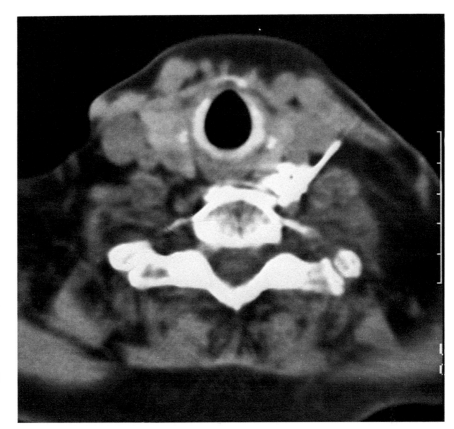

Fig. 18.8. CT scan after injection of 0.2 ml of dilute contrast agent. The contrast flow around the muscle and the vessels. An unintentional vascular injection or intramural injection is ruled out by the contrast distribution present.

Figs. 18.9.–18.11. Partial destruction of the brachial plexus. In this patient, the plexus has been infiltrated by breast cancer. The interventional needle is first advanced centrally into the tumor. After local anesthesia, 1 ml of alcohol is injected. The CT scan demonstrates a hyperdense area in the tumor around the needle tip (Fig. 18.9.).

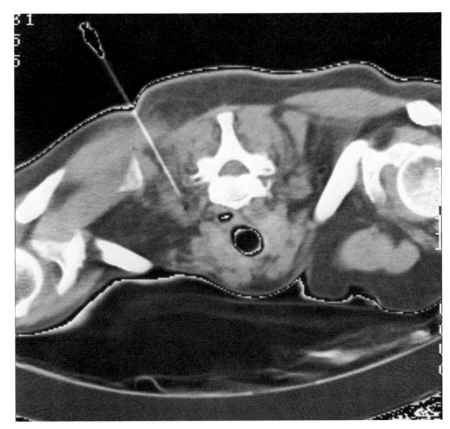

Fig. 18.9

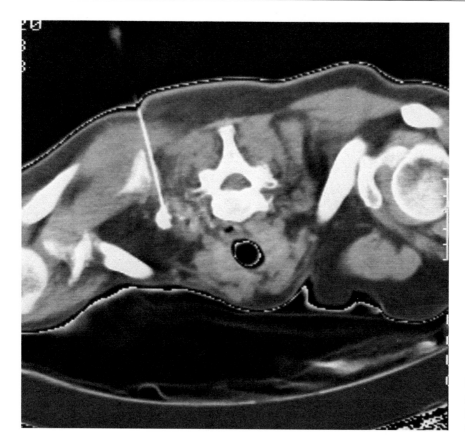

Fig. 18.10. The fringe areas of the tumor are emphasized with contrast medium.

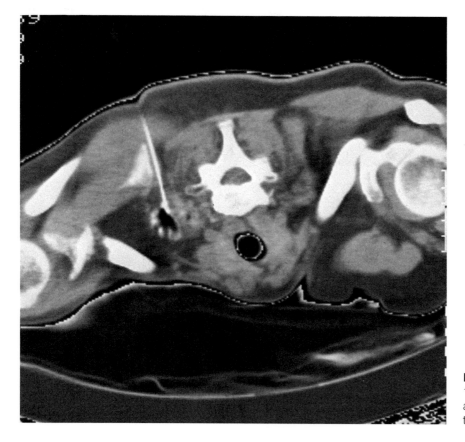

Fig. 18.11. Distribution of 1 ml alcohol (hyperdense area ahead of the needle tip).

chapter (Table 18.1.). Stellate ganglion block were performed in 38 tumor patients for pain therapy or lymph edema caused by tumor infiltration.

Six comparative studies for pain therapy were conducted (Tables 18.3. and 18.4.). The patients studied were recruited from conventionally treated female breast cancer patients with brachial plexus infiltration or from patients with pancoast tumors. They were placed into one of six groups.

Group 1: In this group of 6 female patients (a total of 30 treatments) stellate ganglion block with 2-3 ml local anesthetic were performed.

Group 2: 6 patients (a total of 32 treatments) were treated with electrostimulation of the stellate ganglion for 20 minutes at 2 Hz using an IPENS-apparatus (BioHoloPens) from BHT (technique as in Figs. 18.6.–18.8.) (see Chapter Electrostimulation).

Group 3: 6 patients (28 treatments) were treated only with brachial plexus block using 30 ml of a mixture of short- and long-acting local anesthetics.

Group 4: With these 7 patients (30 treatments) the authors simultaneously performed a stellate ganglion block, brachial plexus block and an intra- and peritumoral injection of 3 to 5 mg Mitroxantron (Lederle) (Figs. 18.14.–18.17.).

Group 5: 7 patients (26 treatments) had a stellate ganglion block, a brachial plexus block and intratumoral therapy with 2 ml 96% ethanol (Pfrimmer) (Figs. 18.9.–18.11., Figs. 18.18.–18.21.).

Group 6: This group contained only patients with lymphedema after mastectomy and postoperative radiation without signs of tumor infiltration into the plexus. All six patients had a

Table 18.2. Total number of CT-guided cervical sympathetic treatments (n = 189).

Tumor pain	38 patients	178 treatments
Acute herpes zoster	2 patients	6 treatments
Phantom pain	1 patient	5 treatments

Table 18.3. Therapy methods for tumor pain (n = 178).

Group 1	Stellate ganglion block only	6 patients	30 treatments
Group 2	Electric stellate block only	6 patients	32 treatments
Group 3	Brachial plexus block only	6 patients	28 treatments
Group 4	Stellate block + brachial plexus block + Mitoxantron intratumoral	7 patients	30 treatments
Group 5	Stellate block + brachial plexus block + 96% alcohol	7 patients	26 treatments
Group 6	Stellate block + brachial plexus block + Volon A into the scar tissue	6 patients	32 treatments
		38 patients	**178 treatments**

Table 18.4. Tumor etiology (n = 38).

Group 1	n = 6	Breast carcinoma	3 Female
		Pancoast tumor	3 Male
Group 2	n = 6	Breast carcinoma	4 Female
		Pancoast tumor	3 Male
Group 3	n = 6	Breast carcinoma	3 Female
		Pancoast tumor	3 Male
Group 4	n = 7	Breast carcinoma	3 Female
		Pancoast tumor	4 Male
Group 5	n = 7	Breast carcinoma	3 Female
		Pancoast tumor	4 Male
Group 6	n = 6	Breast carcinoma	6 Female

combination of a stellate ganglion block, (Figs. 18.6.–18.8.), brachial plexus block (Figs. 18.12. and 18.13.) and an injection of 40 mg Volon A (Squibb) around the brachial plexus (32 treatments).

The patients not included in one of the six groups were two patients treated (six times) for an acute herpes zoster, and 1 patient treated (5 times) for phantom pain.

In these three patients, the therapy consisted of a cervical block combined with periradicular therapy (PRT) and brachial plexus block.

The patients' ages ranged from 35 to 82 years. In all cases neurologic and radiologic diagnoses were carried out prior to treatment. Furthermore, all tumor patients had completed treatment with conventional methods.

Complications

Major complications of a cervical sympathetic treatment (Table 18.5.) or brachial plexus block (Table 18.6.) did not occur in this study. Serious complications can, however, develop without CT guidance, such as by an unintentional intravascular injection [3, 4, 17]. Major CNS-alterations with convulsions [1, 4, 12, 17] can occur. Other potential complications include intradural injection resulting in high spinal anesthetic [3, 4, 17], pneumothorax and post-procedure aneurysms [7, 25]. Unilateral paralysis of the recurrent laryngeal nerve is regularly produced for some hours by stellate blockade [4, 17]. Bilateral simultaneous stellate ganglion blocks should never be performed due to the possibili-

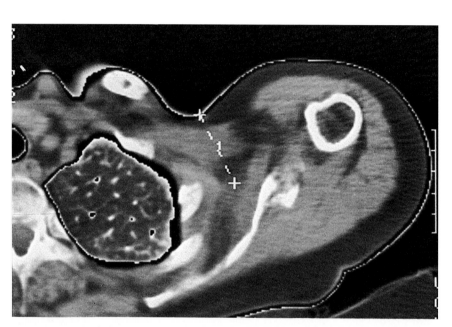

Figs. 18.12. and **18.13.** Planning CT scan and completed puncture of the inferior brachial plexus. This patient has an infiltrating breast cancer after postoperative radiation. The distribution of the local anesthetic and 40 mg Volon A around the needle tip is documented.

Fig. 18.12

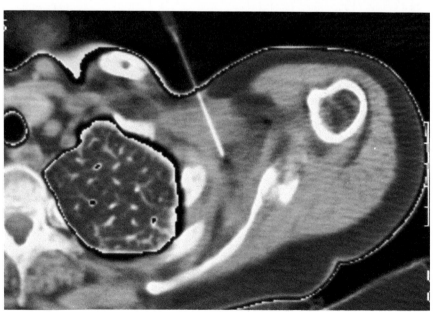

Fig. 18.13

Figs. 18.14.–18.17. Combined procedure for a stellate ganglion block, carried out simultaneously with intratumoral therapy in a patient with brachial plexus infiltration by metastatic breast cancer. In this three-dimensional puncture technique, the interventional needles are not shown in their entire length.

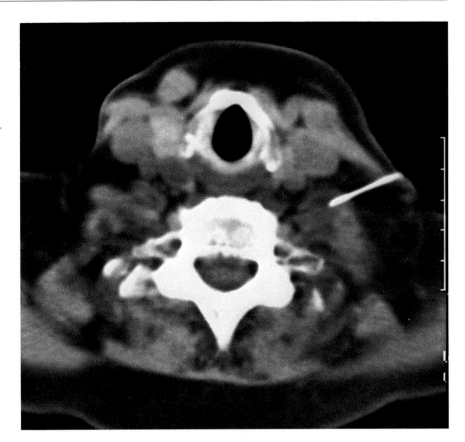

Fig. 18.14. The needle tip is in the infiltrating tumor at the region of the superior brachial plexus.

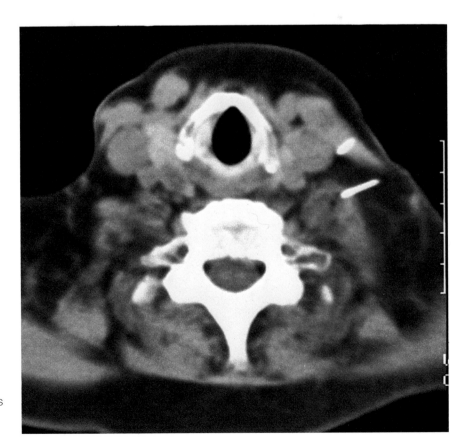

Fig. 18.15. After injection of local anesthetic into the tumor area, another interventional needle is advanced from an anterior approach. The needle tip is just lateral to the jugular vein.

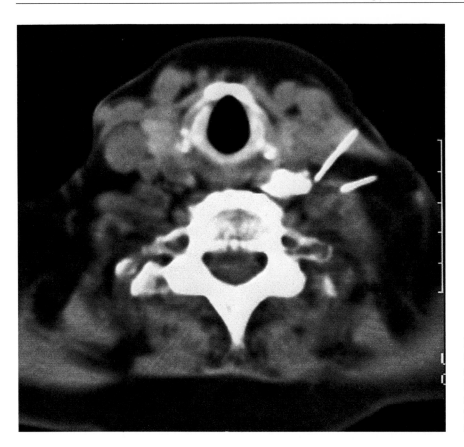

Fig. 18.16. A CT scan to check the position of the second needle tip after an injection of a dilute contrast medium shows it just in front of the stellate ganglion.

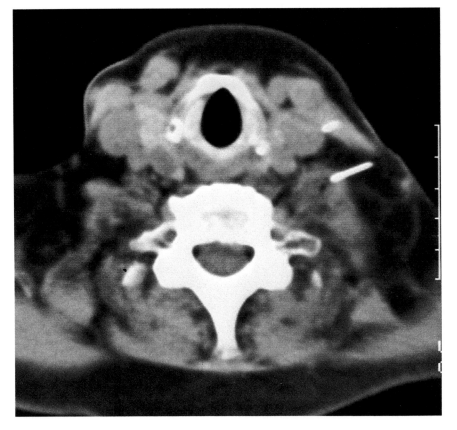

Fig. 18.17. In this scan one can understand the ease of unintentionally puncturing the jugular v. or the carotid a. The needle tip rests at the lateral wall of the jugular v. Therefore, extreme caution in the introduction and advancement of the needle is absolutely necessary. Furthermore, a millimeter by millimeter evaluation of the location of the needle tip may by necessary.

Figs. 18.18. and **18.19.**
Partial neurolysis of the
brachial plexus. Infiltration
of the brachial plexus by
breast cancer metastasis in
a 56-year old female pa-
tient. The needle tip is in
the posterolateral region of
the metastatic mass.

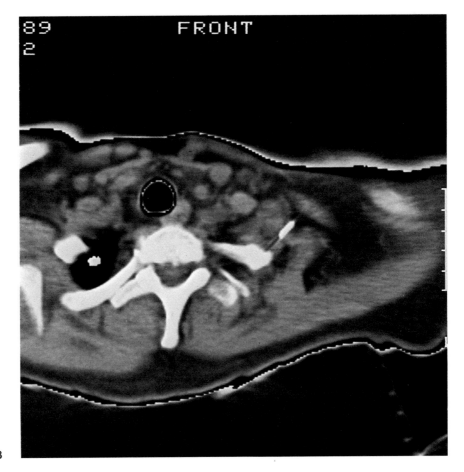

Fig. 18.18

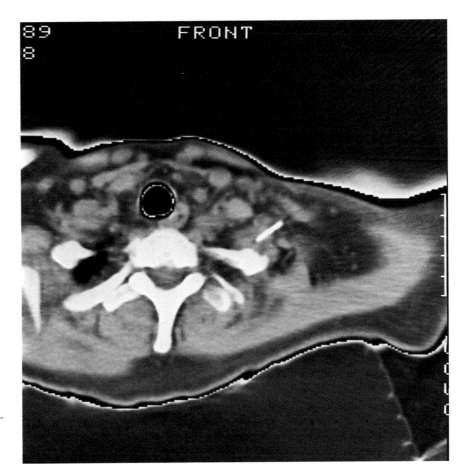

Fig. 18.19. CT scan after
alcohol injection. The alcohol is recognized by the hypodense area in the region
of the tumor and brachial
plexus.

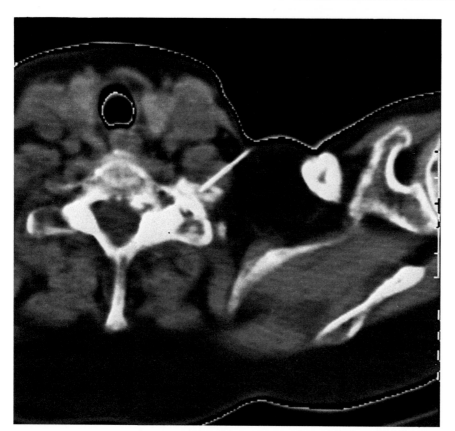

Figs. 18.20. and **18.21.** 63-year old female patient with breast cancer metastasis in the superior brachial plexus. An onion-skin appearance of the contrast and alcohol is seen on CT after the procedure is completed.

Fig. 18.20. The interventional needle is advanced medially to the lateral portion of the tumor and a careful injection of constrast medium and alcohol is performed.

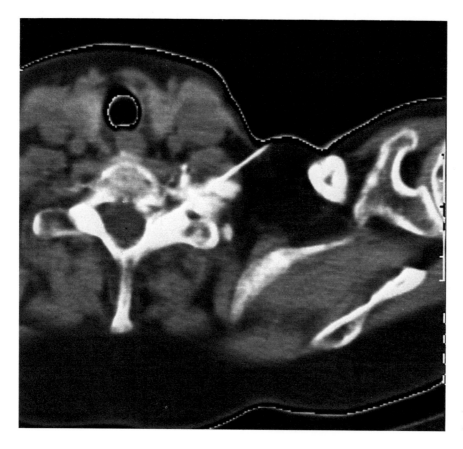

Fig. 18.21. CT scan after a quadruple injection of alcohol. The increasing distribution of the contrast medium can be recognized.

Table 18.5. Complications reported after stellate ganglion block without guidance.

Intravascular injection
Intradural injection
Pneumothorax
Vertebral aneurysm
Carotid aneurysm
Esophagal injections

Table 18.6. Complications reported after brachial plexus block without CT guidance.

Intravascular injection
Intradural injection
Pneumothorax
Subclavian artery aneurysm
Direct injury of a nerve

ty of a subsequent bilateral recurrent nerve block and its attendant respiratory compromise. Other reported complications include unintentional esophagal puncture, paralysis, large subclavian hematomas, and pneumothoraxes after brachial plexus block [3, 4, 25].

Side-effects

Approximately 2 to 5 minutes after each stellate ganglion block, Horner's syndrome appears (miosis, ptosis, enophthalmos) [2-4, 17]. Anhidrosis and a temperature increase in the arm and in the face can also be found on the ipsilateral side. These side-effects are due to the sympathetic blockade and should not be interpreted as complications.
Unilateral blockage of the nose (due to engorgement of the nasal mucosa) and conjunctival engorgement point toward a successful block but these symptoms can also appear with imperfect sympathetic blocks. Motor paralyses of varying degrees may develop after a brachial plexus block. These paralyses disappear after a few hours. The above symptoms and unilateral recurrent laryngeal nerve paralysis along with associated hoarseness and dyspnea will disappear within a day.

Results

Pain was described using a 10 grade visual analog scale. The result was termed good only if, after the first therapy, the patient was free of

pain for more than one day, and after repeated treatment (s)he had either no pain or significantly less pain. The result was termed moderate if, after the treatment, the patient was pain-free for more than 7 hours, but there was still significant pain remaining at the end of the treatment. Therapy was deemed unsuccessful if there was no change in the pain when compared with the beginning of the treatment. Reduction of tumor size was not a stated goal of this therapy but was observed in 29% of all tumor patients. In these cases the tumor volume was reduced by about one third.

An average of 4.68 treatments (n = 178) was performed per patient with an interval of 3 weeks between each treatment. Of the 146 stellate blocks in tumor patients, 30 treatments were only stellate ganglion blocks with local anesthetic (group 1). The success rate in this group was unsatisfactory (Table 18.7.). In 2 patients (a total of 8 treatments), good reduction in shoulder-arm pain for 23 to 27 hours was reported. In these cases it was discovered that a mixture of short- and long-acting local anesthetics (1 ml Scandicaine 1% and 1 ml Bupivacaine 0.25%) with 10 mg Volon A produced the longest pain-free intervals. Moderate success was produced in 2 patients (13 treatments) of group 1, i.e. there was a reduction of pain for 8 to 10 hours only. In another 2 patients (a total of 9 treatments), the clinic had poor results (no effect).

In 20 patients (a total of 88 treatments) (groups 4 to 6) the arm plexus was treated simultaneously with a mixture of 15 ml Scandicaine 1% and 15 ml Bupivacaine 0.25%. All seven patients (30 treatments) in group 4 were treated with an intratumoral injection of 3-5 mg Mitoxantron (Lederle). In all seven patients (26 treatments) in group 5, intra- or peritumoral injections with 2–5 ml 96% ethanol were performed. Six patients (32 treatments) in group 6 were treated for lymphedema with injections of 40 mg Volon A into the scar tissue, in addition to stellate and plexus blocks.

In all patients, immediately after any of the combination treatments (groups 4, 5 and 6) either an elimination or decrease in the pain was experienced. A temporary motor paralysis was often present in all cases except in those with alcohol injection. This paralysis disappeared within one day.

Substantially better results were found in group 4 than in group 1. Good results were achieved in four patients (57,1%), after 17 treatments (x [average number of treatments per patient] = 4.2) in group 4.

Good results were also found in groups 2 and 3, in three patients (50%), each with 13 (x = 4.3) and 12 treatments (x = 4) respectively.

Table 18.7. Treatment results (n = 178).

Group	Total treatments	Number of Patients	Good Treatments ($\bar{x}$)	Good Number of Patients (%)	Moderate Treatments ($\bar{x}$)	Moderate Number of patients (%)	Poor Treatments ($\bar{x}$)	Poor Number of patients
Group 1	n = 30	6	n = 8 (4)	2 (33.3%)	n = 13 (6.5)	2 (33.3%)	n = 9 (4.5)	2 (33.3%)
Group 2	n = 32	6	n = 13 (4.3)	3 (50%)	n = 14 (7)	2 (33.3%)	n = 5 (5)	1 (16.7%)
Group 3	n = 28	6	n = 12 (4)	3 (50%)	n = 11 (5.5)	2 (33.3%)	n = 5 (5)	1 (16.7%)
Group 4	n = 30	7	n = 17 (4.2)	4 (57.1%)	n = 8 (4)	2 (28.6%)	n = 5 (5)	1 (14.3%)
Group 5	n = 26	7	n = 18 (3.6)	5 (71.4%)	n = 4 (4)	1 (14.2)	n = 4 (4)	1 (14.3%)
Group 6	n = 32	6	n = 22 (5.5)	4 (66.6%)	n = 4 (4)	1 (16.7%)	n = 6 (6)	1 (16.7%)
Total	178	38	90 (x = 4.27)	21	54 (x = 5.16)	10	34 (x = 4.91)	7
%	100%	100%	50.5%	55.2%	30.3%	26.3%	19.1%	18.4%

In group 5, there was a good treatment result in 5 patients (71.4%) after 18 treatments (x = 3.6). In group 6, 4 female patients (66.6%) had good results after 22 treatments (x = 5.5), and the lymphedema decreased by 30 to 40% in all patients.

Moderate improvements in pain were found in two patients (28.6%) (8 treatments, x = 4) in group 4, one patient (14.2%) (4 treatments, x = 4) in group 5, one female patient (16.7%) with 4 treatments (x = 4) in group 6, and finally in two patients (33.3%) with 14 (x = 7) or 11 treatments (x = 5.5) respectively in groups 2 and 3. Poor results were found in each group in one or two patients (see Table 18.7.).

Discussion

Altogether the results of this study are most encouraging. In 21 of 38 patients (55.2%) with an average of 4.2 treatments per patient, a significant long-term pain reduction was achieved. Furthermore, satisfactory results (moderate pain reduction) were found in 26.3% (10) of the treated patients.

Group 1 had unsatisfactory results (only 33.3% of this group had good pain reduction). In these tumor patients the treatment of their shoulder-arm syndrome was by the sole use of stellate ganglion blocks. This is consistent with the experience of other authors [27]. Interestingly, better results were achieved with a brachial plexus block alone than with a stellate ganglion block alone (50% significant long-term pain reduction and 33.3% moderate pain reduction). In treating pain, reflex sympathetic dystrophy, or causalgia due to a tumor, CT-guided brachial plexus block should be the first therapy measure used. This therapy should be attempted prior to use of the stellate ganglion block alone. IPENS-electrostimulation therapy, group 2 (50% good results in treatment), is also very promising and should increasingly be included in therapy for this type of pain. Electrostimulation therapy can also be used with other therapeutic methods. A disadvantage of this method is the considerable amount of time which is required for the procedure. The results of the stellate ganglion block could be significantly improved if used simultaneously in combination with the brachial plexus block.

Both the combination of short- and long-acting local anesthetics and the intratumoral injection of a local cytostatic agent (Mitoxantron) will also improve results. The treatment success was convincing in the case of four patients (group 4) after an average of 4.1 treatments per patient. In this study, systemic side-effects were not a problem with Mitoxantron.

The best results were seen after injecting 2 ml of 96% ethanol into the tumor infiltrated regions and simultaneously performing ganglion and plexus block (with good results in five patients [71.4%] after 18 treatments in group 5). An important part of the tumor therapy is that 2/3 of the injection goes into the tumor center and 1/3 is administered into the peritumoral area. The fairly good result of the treatment with alcohol is in all probability based on the destruction of small sensory nerve branches. However, in one patient a permanent partial motor paralysis was observed. At first the patient was relieved, due to the decrease in his pain, but acceptance of the paralysis was difficult for this patient and required a high degree of psychological support. For this reason treatment with Mitoxantron is normally preferred in areas with motor innervation. Further comparative studies are needed to determine the proper dilution of alcohol injected and also the best combination of alcohol and Mitoxantron. Additionally, it is still not clear as to the optimal volume of alcohol required in order to achieve best results in reducing the size of each type of tumor. The tumor size was reduced by an average of 29% in this treatment group. In a review of Japanese and American studies, in the case of smaller tumors, a reduction of up to 100% can be achieved by injecting a small amount of high grade alcohol.

The effect of a further dilution of alcohol will have to be reviewed in future, as well as the combination of alcohol and local cytostatic drugs. Furthermore, the relationship of the injected volume with the reduction of tumor size in different tumor types is still not clear. The curative use of an intratumoral tumor alcohol injection in small hepatocellular carcinomas has been shown by the Chinese [34]. Also an Italian group [22] had similar findings in small liver and abdominal tumors. In the above studies a reduction of tumor size of up to 100% [22] in tumors of less than 2 cm were reported. Other experimental and clinical studies have pointed in that direction [9, 13, 19].

Although serious side-effects are possible even with careful use of these medications, neither the present nor other authors have reported any side-effects [22, 34]. Other local treatments, such as the implantation of cytostatic particles [26], heat therapy after alcohol injection [29] and the use of lasers, will be examined in future.

One point should be emphasized: in tumor pain therapy, one should always strive to use combination therapy. Also, tumor size reduction in palliation is not the most important factor. It is the patient's perception of pain that is the most important factor in determining the therapy for his or her pain. This is also true for the treatment of shoulder-arm syndrome in breast cancer patients with lymphedema of the affected arm, without tumor infiltration of the plexus.

The successful treatment of four out of six female patients after a total of 22 treatments, with significant pain reduction and diminution of lymphedema in group 6, is an optimistic sign for this therapy in these patients.

The logical extension of these treatment methods is the CT- and fluoroscopy-guided insertion of a permanent catheter in the region of the stellate ganglion or the brachial plexus. The first successful tests of this treatment were performed at MKI (Figs. 15.22. and 15.23.). Sterile technique is crucial in order to avoid abscesses, spondylitis and other inflammatory processes.

It is important to remember that there is a vast variation in the localization of the stellate gangli-on plexus. This explains the different treatment results in the literature without using CT guidance. Also with these blind punctures there is the danger of perforating the vertebral or carotid artery. Even with a negative aspiration test the position of the needle tip cannot be determined with certainty. It may rest intramurally and project only minimally into the lumen. Furthermore, aneurysms have been reported with this technique [7, 25]. Even the smallest injection of local anesthetics in one of these two arteries can result in serious complications with immediate convulsions [3, 4, 7, 17]. For these reasons some authors recommend the use of a total of only 2-5 ml of a local anesthetic in non CT-guided procedures [12, 25]. However, for a safe stellate block without CT, because of the variable position of the stellate ganglion, 6-10 ml local anesthetic is recommended [17]. For a complete cervicothoracic sympathetic blockade, up to 15 ml of local anesthetic is necessary. A CT-guided block should be used especially when pathologic anatomy is present, i.e. tumors or scar tissue. Furthermore, with normal anatomy the CT-guided injection technique is safer for the patient. With this technique a very small volume of 2 ml of local anesthetic is sufficient for a good block.

CT guidance is also the method of choice for use in combination with an intratumoral treatment, especially when the cervical ganglia have been infiltrated or dislocated by tumor. Under CT guidance the ganglia can be blocked accurately and local cytostatic medications such as Mitoxantron or alcohol administered (see Chapter Tumor Therapy).

The injection of a suspension of cortisone crystal to intensify the blockade, or as an inhibitor of scar tissue proliferation, is also possible with this technique. Prior to the therapy, an injection of contrast agents is performed to document the possible local distribution of the medication. This will help to avoid an unintentional injection into nerves or vessels. Other complications that have been described in the literature, such as intradural administration or the danger of a pneumothorax, are much less likely with this CT-guided technique.

In conclusion, the results of the present study are encouraging. Also, another advantage of the CT-guided technique is that it can be performed on an outpatient basis and is much less stressful for the patient than other methods which is especially important for seriously ill or terminal patients. However, it should not be forgotten that these methods are very difficult, they require utmost precision, and in the interest of the patient should be practised in or near a hospital.

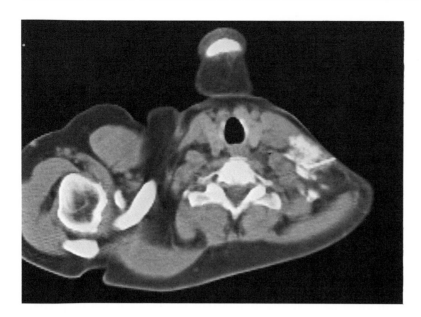

Figs. 18.22. and **18.23.** 44-year old female patient, status post an operative procedure for shoulder-arm stiffness, now experiencing extreme shoulder pain and requiring around-the-clock opiates. A 2-French catheter has been positioned in the superior brachial plexus. To stabilize the catheter, it was placed under the skin at a distance of approximately 10 cm and the catheter was fixed to the skin at the entrance point with an ethylene suture.

Fig. 18.22. After 20 days the tip of the catheter had slipped out of the brachial plexus. The incorrect position of the catheter tip is demonstrated by the diffuse distribution of the contrast medium into the surrounding tissue.

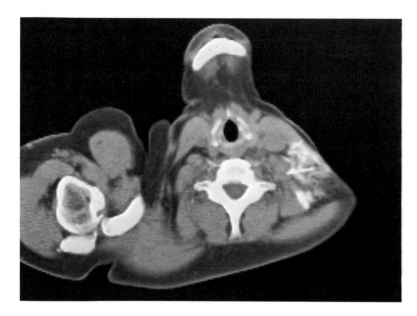

Fig. 18.23. CT scan after repositioning of the catheter tip into the plexus. The catheter was in place for a total of approximately 6 weeks. Daily, a mixture of 15 ml Scandicaine 1% and 15 ml Bupivacaine 0.25% was injected through an antibiotic filter. During this period of time the patient did not complain of pain and was even able to do range of motion exercises in water. After the treatment period, the pain sensations were reduced by 60%. Further pain treatment in this patient required only a low dose of oral analgesics. Opiates were no longer needed.

Summary

1. A stellate or brachial plexus block for tumor pain therapy should be performed using CT guidance.
2. An improvement of this CT-guided method is possible with the simultaneous combination of CT and fluoroscopy with a C-arm.
3. Therapy with only fluoroscopy-guidance should not be used due to inaccurate localization and poor tissue differentiation. Furthermore, the blind puncture technique should never be used.
4. The injection of medication should only be carried out under CT guidance to minimize the danger of serious complications caused by unintentional intravascular or intradural injections.
5. Partial motor paralysis can occur in the region of the brachial plexus with intratumoral alcohol therapy. Normally this paralysis disappears after some hours.
6. With CT guidance a significant reduction in the volume of local anesthetics is possible in comparison with blind punctures or fluoroscopy-guided methods. The complications can range from aneurysms and convulsions to paralysis after an intradural injection.
7. A prolongation of the pain-free interval occurs by combining short- and long-acting local anesthetics and by the local administration of Volon A.
8. When shoulder-arm pain is caused by tumor, or infiltration into the brachial plexus, a stellate ganglion block alone is not sufficient.

9. The combination of a stellate block and brachial plexus block with intratumoral therapy with Mitoxantron or alcohol results in very good pain reduction.

10. The use of local cytostatics requires further large-scale and multicenter studies before any conclusions can be reached concerning their efficacy.

11. The pain caused by breast cancer metastasized into the brachial plexus and lymphedema after mastectomy and/or radiation can be successfully treated with a combination of stellate ganglion block and brachial plexus block and local injection of Volon A.

12. The interventional methods for pain therapy using local anesthetics and corticoids should also be used with curative therapy. These procedures can be performed on an out-patient basis.

13. Interventional percutaneous electric nerve stimulation (IPENS) is noteworthy. However, it is a time-consuming addition to local anesthesia and further research is needed to determine the actual benefits.

14. The great success of the methods presented here justifies the cost of these high-tech imaging devices for the above indications. This is patient-friendly, with a high rate of success and a decrease in complications, when compared with other types of therapy.

References

1. Ariani J., Parmley J., Ochsner A.: Fatalities and complications after attemps at stellate ganglion block. Surgery 32 (1952) 615

2. Allen G., Samson B.: Contralateral Horners syndrome following stellate ganglion block. Can. Anaesth. Soc. J. 33 (1986) 112

3. Auberger H., Nisel Ch.: Praktische Lokalanästhesie. Stuttgart (1982) 85–88

4. Auberger H., Biermann E.: Praktische Schmerztherapie. Stuttgart (1988) 85–87

5. Boas R.A.: The sympathetic nervous system and pain relief. In: Swerdlow M. (ed.): Relief of intracable pain. Amsterdam 1981, 222

6. Boas R.A., Hatangdi V.S.: Chemical sympathectomy-techniques and responses. In: Yokota T., Dubner R. (eds.): Current topics in pain research and therapy. Proceedings of the international symposium on pain. Amsterdam 1983, 259

7. Bonica J.J.: The management of pain. Philadelphia 1953

8. Braun H.: Über einige örtliche Anästhetica (Stovain, Alypin, Novacain). Dtsch. med. Wschr. 31 (1905) 1667–1671

9. Burgener F.A. Steinmetz Sh.D.: Treatment of experimental adenocarcinomas by percutaneous intratumoral injection of absolute ethanol. Invest Radiol 22 (1987) 472–478

10. Demarez D.: Note à la technique de l'infiltration du ganglion étoilé par voie posterieure. Echo méd. du Nord (1937) 240

11. Einhorn A.: Siehe Gross. D. [14]

12. Eschrich I.: Sympathikusblockaden in der Praxis, in: Pongratz W. (Hrsg.): Therapie chronischer Schmerzzustände in der Praxis, Berlin 1985, 156–157

13. Fujisawa T., Hongo H., Yamaguchi Y. et al.: Intratumoral Ethanol injection for malignant tracheobronchial lesions: a new bronchofiberscopic procedure. Endoscopy 18 (1986) 188–191

14. Gross D.: Therapeutische Lokalanästhesie. Stuttgart 1985, 192–209

15. Herget R.: Einfache Technik zur zeitweiligen Ausschaltung des Ganglion stellatum. Chirurg 15 (1943) 680

16. Kaeser H.E.: Schulterarmschmerzen aus der Sicht des Neurologen. In: Kocher R., Gross D., Kaeser H.E. (Hrsg.): Schmerzstudien 3, Stuttgart (1980) 151–153

17. Katz J., Renck H.: Thorakoabdominale Nervenblockaden, Lehrbuch und Atlas. Weinheim 1988, 128–129

18. Koller C.: Vorläufige Mitteilung über lokale Anästhesie am Auge. Klinische Monatsblätter, Augenheilkunde 22 Beilagenheft (1884) 60

19. Kozak B.E., Keller F.S., Rosch J., Barry J.: Selective therapeutic embolization of renal cell carcinoma in solitary kidneys. J. Uro. 137 (1982) 1223–1225

20. Lambret O.: Technique de la Chirurgie du sympathique. Paris, 1953, Siehe Gross D. [14].

21. Leriche R., Fontaine R.: 1. Anaesthesie isol du ganglion étoilé. Presse med. 41 (1934) 845

22. Livraghi T., Festi D., Monti F. et al.: US-guided percutaneous alcohol injection of small hepatic and abdominal tumors. Radiology 161 (1986) 309–312

23. Mandl F.: Die Wirkung der paravertebralen Injektion bei Angina pectoris. Arch. klin. Chir. 136 (1925) 495–518

24. Mandl F.: Die Anwendungsweise der paravertebralen Injektion. Berliner klin. Wschr. 4 (1925) 2356–2358

25. Mastroianni A.: The effects of stellate ganglion block. Schmerzdiagnostik und Therapie. Band 2 Bochum (1986) 80–93

26. Miyazaki Sh., Takeuchi Sh., Sugiyama M. et al.: Effect of implanted ethylene-vinyl alcohol copolymer matrices containing 5-fluorouracil on Ehrlich ascites carcinoma. J. Pharm. Pharmacol. 37 (1985) 64–66

27. Nolte H.: Zur Therapie des Nacken-Schulter-Arm-Syndroms aus der Sicht des Anästhesisten in: Kocher R., Gross D., Kaeser H.E.: Schmerzstudien 3, Stuttgart 1980, 154–159

28. Orsoni J.: zitiert nach o. Lambret et al. [20].

29. Rama B.N., Prasad K.N.: Ethanol. A heat sensitizer on neuroblastoma cells in culture. Cancer 57 (1986) 1140–1144

30. Reischauer F.: Die cervikalen Vertebralsyndrome. Eine vorläufige Bilanz der Kliniker. Stuttgart 1955. Siehe Gross D. [14].

31. Schleich C.L.: Schmerzlose Operationen. Berlin 1906. Siehe Gross D. [14].

32. Schleich C.L.: Infiltrationsanästhesie (lokale Anästhesie) und ihr Verhältnis zur allgemeinen Narkose (Injektionsanästhesie). Verhandl. d. Dtsch. Ges. f. Chir. 21 (1892) 121

33. Sèze De: Die Stellatumanästhesie nach De Sèze, Neuralmedizin 1, Stuttgart 1953, 47. Siehe Gross D. [14].

34. Sheu J.Ch., Huang G.T., Che D.Sh. et al.: Small hepatocellular carcinoma: intratumor ethanol treatment using new needle and guidance systems. Radiology 163 (1987) 43–48

Chapter 19
Percutaneous Neurolysis of the Celiac Plexus

H.H. Schild, R.M.M. Seibel, D.H.W. Grönemeyer

Introduction

The suitability of neurolysis of the celiac plexus for pain therapy has been known for many years; as early as 1919 a celiac plexus block had been described by Kappis. He used bony landmarks for orientation regarding the localization of the plexus [14]. In the years that followed, such blockades were performed intraoperatively, percutaneously, with and without fluoroscopy-control, sonography-guided and finally CT-guided. Today, the CT-guided procedure is, because of its accuracy, the technique for celiac plexus blocks.

Anatomy

The celiac plexus (also known as solar p.; cerebrum abdominale; abdominal brain; Vieussen's ganglion) is the name for the upper and largest of the autonomic nerve plexi which extends in front of, and alongside, the aorta. It also extends around the celiac artery trunk (see Chapter 12). On both sides of the celiac plexus there is an average of three interspersed ganglionic nodes, almost always located beside or below the celiac artery trunk.

The celiac nerve plexus contains afferent and efferent visceral sympathetic and interlaced preganglionic parasympathetic fibers. These nerves supply the pancreas, liver, gall bladder, kidney, pelvis, ureter, small intestine, large intestine (up to the transverse colon), and other abdominal structures (Table 19.1.) [1–3, 5, 15, 19, 20, 21].

Indications

A celiac plexus blockade is indicated for therapy of chronic pain which can no longer be alleviated by other treatment. The major causes of this type of intractable pain are diseases of the epigastric organs. However, successful plexus blockades have also been performed for pain caused by diseases of other abdominal organs as well as retroperitoneal structures.

The most common patient for this therapy is one with pancreatic carcinoma or chronic pancreatitis. Other patients for this palliative therapy have a wide variety of diseases (i.e. liver metastases, lymphomas, Crohn's disease, carcinomas of the bile ducts and gall bladder, kidney, stomach, colon, rectum, uterus and ovaries) [2, 3, 6, 8, 10, 11, 16–19].

Patients

CT-guided destruction (neurolysis) of the celiac plexus was performed in 190 patients whose average age was 67 years. The pain in most of these patients was due to an infiltration of the celiac plexus by a pancreatic carcinoma or gastric carcinoma. Two patients with chronic pancreatitis had neurolysis after repeated blockades which did not result in a sufficient improvement in pain (Table 19.2.).

Table 19.1. Segments of sympathetic innervation after Mandl [15].

Heart	Stellate ganglion, bilateral Thoracic T1–4
Lungs, bronchi	Stellate ganglion, bilateral T1–5
Pylorus; duodenum	right T6–8
Stomach, lesser curvature	bilateral T6–7
Stomach	bilateral T6–8
Gall bladder	right T9–10
Appendix	right T12–L1
Right kidney	right T12–L2
Left kidney	left T12–L2
Pancreas	left T8–T10

Table 19.2. Indications for celiac plexus neurolysis (n = 190).

Pancreatic carcinoma	82
Gastric carcinoma	54
Metastases with direct infiltration of the plexus	43
Metastasis of the liver	9
Chronic pancreatitis	2

Requirements for Celiac Plexus Neurolysis

Requirements for a CT-guided celiac plexus neurolysis are [16, 18]:
- normal blood-clotting tests (PT, PTT, thrombocythes);
- intervenous line;
- no contra-indications to contrast medium (desirable, but not an absolute precondition);
- effective test-block with a local anesthetic (during the same session).

Technique

First a scanogram is made either in the supine or prone position followed by 8–10 mm thick CT scans from the lower end of the T12 vertebral body to the middle of the L2 vertebral body. The decision regarding from which side the puncture is to be made, or whether to puncture both sides, depends on the potential complications which could occur by the existing anatomic conditions such as puncturing liver, aorta, vena cava, kidney etc. After the CT identification of the celiac artery trunk, a puncture point is chosen on the skin. From this point a puncture of the area anterior to the aorta, immediately above the celiac artery trunk, can be performed. Normally, neurolysis is performed at the level of the L1 vertebral body. A fine needle with a maximum diameter of 0.7 mm is used. Many access routes are possible because of the low risk of injury with this fine needle. Furthermore, blockades have been performed transabdominally from an anterior, transhepatic and translumbar approach, the latter also involving a transaortic puncture (Figs 19.1.–19.7.).

The following procedure is normally independent of the approach (i.e. anterior, transhepatic or translumbar). After local anesthesia of the skin, the needle is introduced and local anesthetic is injected as the needle is advanced. When the needle tip is just anterior to the aorta, immediately above or – less desirable but in most cases also acceptable – immediately below the celiac artery trunk, an aspiration is performed. After a negative aspiration (if positive, the needle position must be corrected), the injection of 1–2 ml of diluted contrast medium (Ultravist 300, Schering; Solutrast 300, Byk-Gulden, diluted 1:5–7 with physiologic solution) is performed.

If the CT scan demonstrates that the injected contrast medium is distributed anterior to the aorta and on both sides, then a test blockade is performed with 5–10 ml 2% Lidocaine. If there are no complications and the patient has alleviation of his or her pain, a permanent blockade is performed. Many physicians use pure, high-proof alcohol for the neurolysis. However, 96% alcohol can cause severe pain and can also carry an increased risk of complications. For neurolysis of the celiac plexus the authors prefer an injection of 20–50 ml of the following: (see page 186).

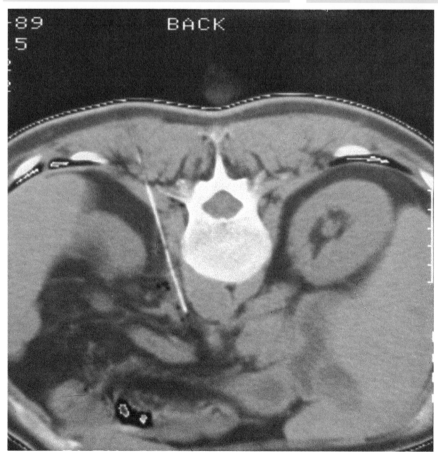

Fig. 19.1. This patient had a predominantly left-sided pain due to a pancreatic metastasis growing from the left side into the celiac plexus. Neurolysis of celiac plexus was performed after a fine-needle puncture from a posterolateral approach. The needle tip was advanced between left adrenal gland and aorta.

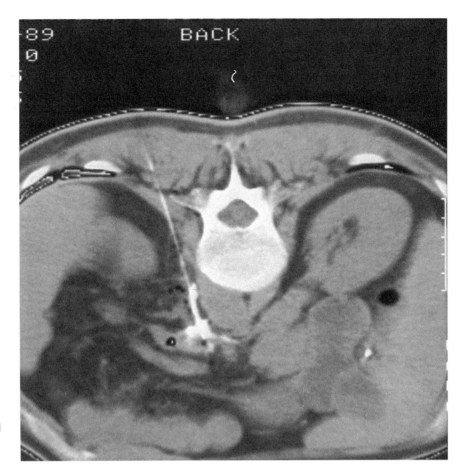

Fig. 19.2. Same patient as in Fig. 19.1. After contrast injection, a good distribution of contrast is visualized in the region of the celiac plexus.

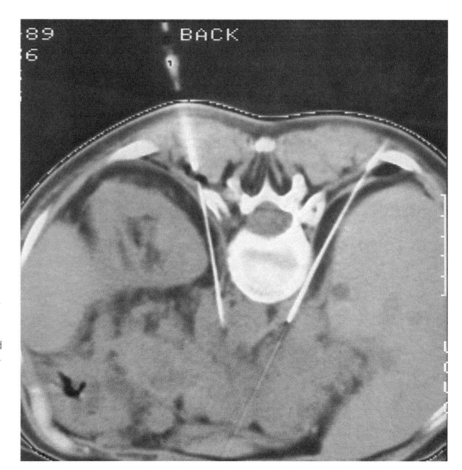

Fig. 19.3. Simultaneous bilateral neurolysis of the celiac plexus. On each side the needles were advanced alongside the diaphragmatic crura, up to the celiac plexus. On the left, the needle was advanced between an adrenal gland metastasis and the aorta, to the origin of the celiac artery trunk.

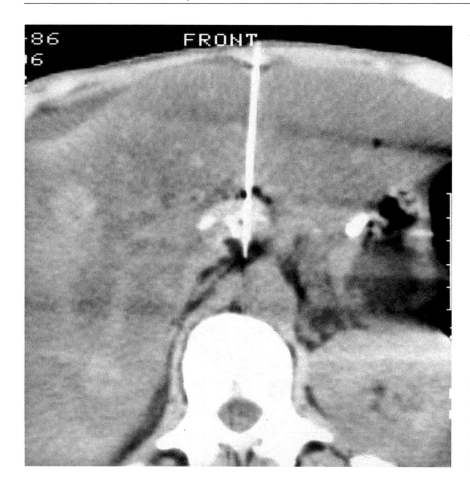

Fig. 19.4. For puncturing the celiac plexus, several access routes are possible. Here the puncture was performed transhepatically from an anterior approach. The needle tip is immediately adjacent to the celiac artery trunk. The alcohol solution was well distributed in the celiac plexus.

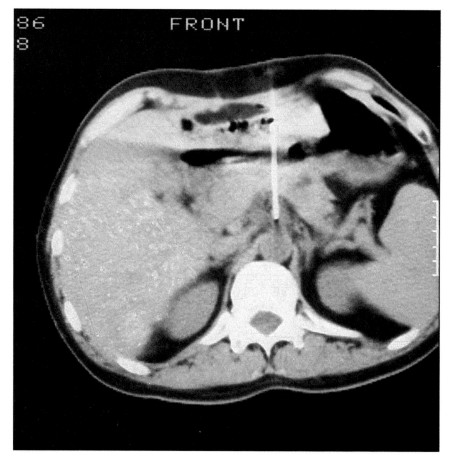

Figs. 19.5.–19.7. A patient with carcinoma of the pancreatic head with metastasis to the celiac plexus. An anterior approach is used, with the needle immediately above the transverse colon and below the stomach.

Fig. 19.5. The needle is superior to the pancreas and superior the origin to the superior mesenteric artery. The needle tip is close to the aorta in this patient.

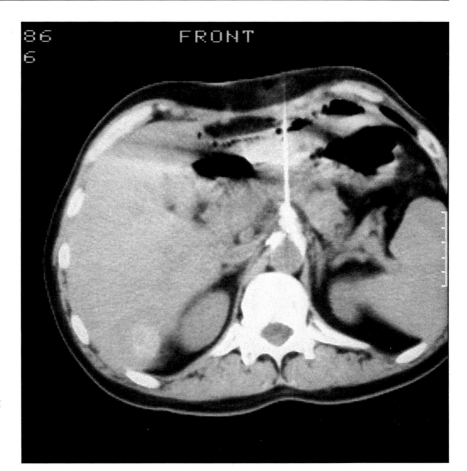

Fig. 19.6. After contrast-medium injection, the exact distribution at the level of the celiac plexus is visualized. The contrast medium remains extravascular.

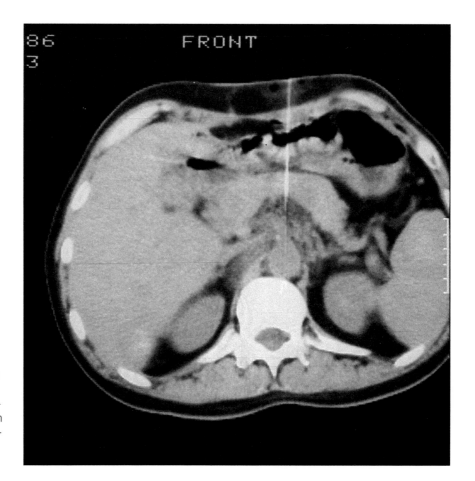

Fig. 19.7. After alcohol injection there is an increase in distance between vena cava and the aorta. The alcohol is distributed on both sides of the crura of the diaphragm and up into the retropancreatic region.

- 6–7 parts absolute ethanol (Caution: alcohol must be suitable for parenteral application!)
- 3–4 parts of a long-acting local anesthetic, i.e. 0.5% bupivacaine (Carbostesin).
- approximately 1 part contrast medium (compatible with the mixture) for which Iopamidol is used (Ultravist 300, Schering; Solutrast 300, Byk-Gulden).

Due to the local anesthetic, the injection is almost painless. The addition of the contrast medium allows observation of the distribution of the solution. A CT scan is used to monitor the injection after the first half of the injection and at the end.

Alternatively, a 1:1 mixture of 96% ethanol with Bupivacaine 1% without the addition of contrast medium is often used. The distribution of this mixture can also be documented with CT due to the negative contrast of the solution (Fig. 19.8.). If the CT scan shows that the neurolytic solution is not distributed equilaterally about the celiac artery trunk region or the aorta, then in the same session, a second puncture can be performed. However, the positioning of the second needle tip can be difficult due to the contrast medium already being injected (Figs. 19.9.–19.12.). The total amount of injected solution

should not exceed 60–70 ml. Alternatively, the authors believe that a more logical approach is to wait for the clinical results of the original injection and then a decision can be made about a second injection. Additionally, because of the possibility of hypertension or other cardiovascular problems, after the neurolysis the patient remains in hospital for 24 hours [3, 6, 9, 10, 13, 16–18].

Side-effects

Pain during and after the injection caused by irritation of abdominal structures occurs in a considerable number of patients only after the use of a pure alcohol solution. This can be avoided to a large extent by adding a local anesthetic to the neurolytic solution. Pain persisting for more than two to three hours after the procedure and/or peritonitis requires further investigation as to the clinical cause.

A significant drop in blood pressure has been described in the literature in up to 20% of cases; however, this has rarely been observed with the use of the above procedure. Often observed is an improvement in the patients' impaired bowel function after neurolysis, often to the delight of the patients.

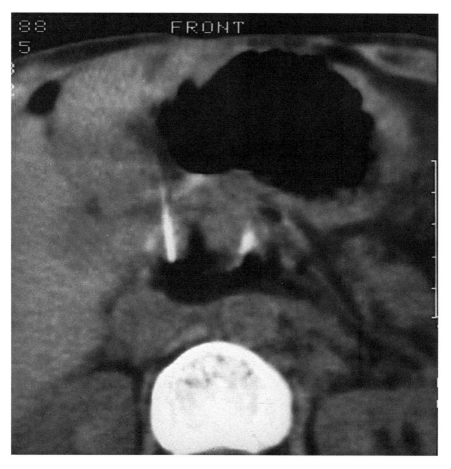

Fig. 19.8. For this celiac plexus neurolysis, the fine needle was advanced from an anterior oblique paragastric approach past the left lobe of the liver. In front of the needle tip, the 50% alcohol solution is seen as a hyperdense structure which outlines the front of the vena cava and aorta. Using this technique, the distribution can be checked without adding contrast medium. The previously injected contrast medium used for documenting the extravascular needle position is still recognized at the outer edge of the alcohol distribution.

Figs. 19.9.–19.12. 53-old patient with a recurrence of carcinoma in the pancreatic tail. The left-sided tumor has grown para-aortic into the celiac plexus and has caused severe pain. The neurolysis puncture was performed through the left lobe of the liver.

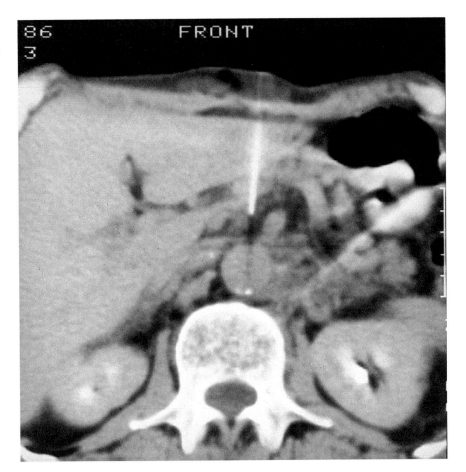

Fig. 19.9. The needle tip is just to the right of the superior mesenteric artery.

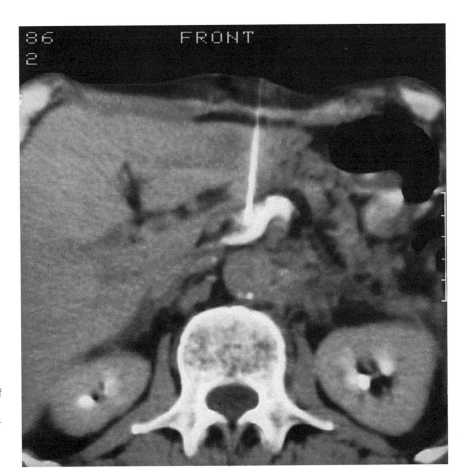

Fig. 19.10. After the contrast medium injection, there is good distribution of the solution on the right side. However, the neurolysis did not lead to a complete resolution of the patient's pain.

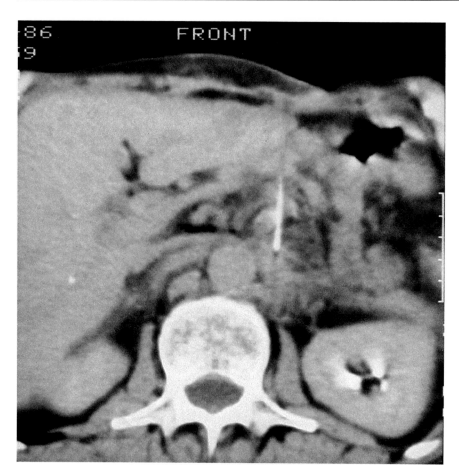

Fig 19.11. Because of the continued pain, during the same session a second puncture was performed on the left, past the superior mesenteric artery, into the tumor.

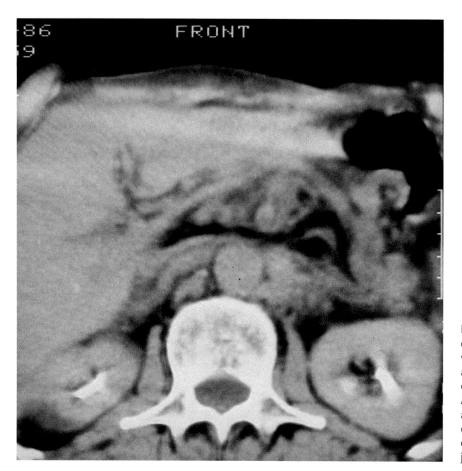

Fig. 19.12. After this second injection the patient was pain-free. The injected alcohol is seen as a hyperdensity in front of the aorta. Also seen between tumor and aorta is a small hyperdense border which is caused by the alcohol injection in this area.

Severe diarrhea can be observed in up to 60% of patients treated with celiac plexus neurolysis but this generally stops after two days. So far the clinic has observed only one case of long-lasting diarrhea which occurred for several days.

Complications

Complications such as infection or bleeding, and in the case of a pancreas puncture the possibility of pancreatitis, are associated with any kind of fine-needle puncture. The authors did not, however, observe any of these complications with the transabdominal procedure from an anterior approach.

Complications of a CT-guided plexus blockade from a posterior approach reported in the literature are:
- temporary hematuria from kidney puncture;
- spinal canal puncture without consequences;
- disk puncture without consequences.

In the literature, there are reports of grave consequences of fluoroscopy-guided plexus blockades such as:
- paraplegia (spinal ischemia can be caused by an injection intramurally or at/into a lumbar artery supplying the spinal cord);
- partial leg paralysis from the influence of the neurolytic solution on the lumbar plexus.

There are further reports about sexual dysfunction and urination disorders. However, the fear that a plexus blockade could mask the symptoms of an acute abdomen has not been verified in the literature [2-4, 7, 10, 12, 13, 16-19].

Results and Discussion

In the literature, between 33% and 94% of patients experience an improvement of their pain symptoms after celiac plexus blockade. 80% of the patients at MKI showed a diminution of pain, half of them became pain-free. However, with progression of the basic disease process, especially a pancreatic carcinoma, this pain may recur or intensify. In these cases, nerves can be irritated which do not run through the celiac plexus, such as intercostal nerves or the thoracic sympathetic trunk.

Under CT guidance these nerves can also be destroyed in a combined procedure (see Chapter 21) (Figs. 19.13. and 19.14.). As a rule, this combined approach can be performed in one or two sessions. Patients with diffusely growing epigastric tumors can become free of pain for the rest of their lives with this procedure. In the authors' study the duration of the plexus neurolysis effect is between four weeks and seven months. This time span is simular to that reported in the literature.

The success rate of plexus block in chronic pancreatitis is less than in pancreatic carcinoma. This is perhaps because of the partially different origin of the pain in these patients which is perineural edema. With injection of steroids in lieu of neurolytic therapy the authors achieved a better result in chronic pancreatitis which supports this thesis [2, 3, 5, 9, 11, 16–20].

Instrumentation and Medication	
Needle	10-15 cm 22-G needle DCHN 22-5.0 SI (Cook)
Local anesthetic	15-30 ml Bupivacaine 1%
Alcohol for injection 50%	20-50 ml (mixture with the local anesthetic)
Contrast medium	3-5 ml Iopromid/Iopamidol (diluted)

Causes of Insufficient Effectiveness of a Celiac Plexus Neurolysis

There are several reasons for only partial success or a complete failure of celiac plexus blockades:
- inaccurate positioning of needle;
- insufficient retroperitoneal diffusion or too little neurolytic solution injected;
- anatomic variations of the celiac plexus;
- pain transmitted through nerves which do not go through the celiac plexus and therefore would not be blocked, such as the intercostal nerves. This situation is present in many cases of extensive tumor diseases and/or is observed during the progress of the disease;
- narcotic abuse.

If the effect is only temporary, an alcohol neurolysis of the celiac plexus should be repeated. This can be because of a regeneration of nerves or the extension of the basic disease and/or a possible metastasis [3, 6, 9-11, 15-19].

References

1. Bonica J.J.: Autonomic innervation of viscera in relation to nerve block. Anesthesiology 29 (1968) 793
2. Bridenbaugh L.D., Moore D.C., Campbell D.D.: Management of upper abdominal cancer pain. J. Amer. med. Ass. 190 (1964) 877
3. Buy J.-N., Moss A.A., Singler R.C.: CT-guided celiac plexus and splanchnic nerve neurolysis. J. Comput. assist. Tomogr. 6 (1982) 315
4. Cherry D., Lamberty J.: Paraplegia following celiac plexus block. Anaesth. Intensive Care 12 (1984) 59

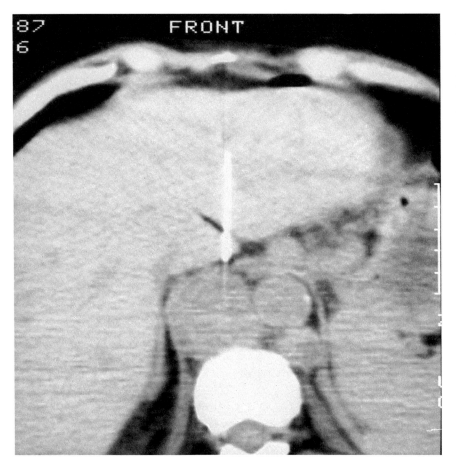

Figs. 19.13. and **19.14.**
CT scan in a patient with a renal cell carcinoma. Extensive metastases into the celiac plexus (are seen prevertebral and dorsal to the crura of the diaphragm). The aorta is lifted off the spinal column and displaced to the left. Because of the complex pain symptoms a combination treatment was performed. First, a transhepatic puncture of the celiac plexus, followed by a neurolysis in typical manner, was performed. (Fig. 19.13.).

Fig. 19.13

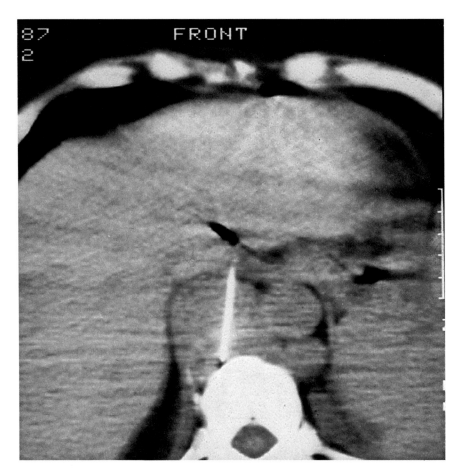

Fig. 19.14. Following this, the needle was advanced to the prevertebral region through the metastatic lymph node to the thoracic sympathetic plexus. Immediately after this neurolysis the patient was pain-free.

5. De Takats J.R.: Splanchnic anaesthesia: a critical review of the theory and practice of this method. Surg. Gynec. Obstet. 44 (1972) 501

6. Filshie J., Golding S., Robbie D.S., Husband J.: Unilateral computerised tomography guided celiac plexus block: a technique for pain relief. Anaesthesia 38 (1983) 498

7. Galizia E.J., Lahiri S.K.: Paraplegia following celiac plexus block with phenol. Brit. J Anaesth. 46 (1974) 539

8. Gorbitz C., Leavens M.E.: Alcohol block of the celiac plexus for control of upper abdominal pain caused by cancer and pancreatitis. J. Neurosurg. 34 (1971) 575

9. Greiner L., Ulatowski L., Prohm P.: Sonographisch gezielte und intraoperative Alkoholblockade der Zöliakalganglien bei konservativ nicht beherrschbaren malignombedingten Oberbauchschmerzen. Ultraschall in Med. 4 (1983) 57

10. Haaga J.R., Kori S.H. Eastwood D., Borkowski, G.: Improved technique for CT-guided celiac ganglia block. Amer. J. Roentgenol. 142 (1984) 1201

11. Hanowell S., Kennedy S., Macnamara T., Lees D.: Celiac plexus block: Diagnostic and therapeutic applications in abdominal pain. South Med J 33 (1980) 1330

12. Hegedues V., Relief of pancreatic pain by radiography-guided block. Amer J Roentgenol 133 (1979) 1101

13. Ischia S., Luzzani A., Ischia A., Faggion S.: A new approach to the neutolytic block of the celiac plexus: the transaortic technique. Pain 16 (1983) 333

14. Kappis M.: Sensibilität und lokale Anästhesie im chirurgischen Gebiet der Bauchhöhle mit besonderer Berücksichtigung der Splanchnicus Anästhesie. Beitr. Klin. Chir. 115 (1919) 161

15. Mandl F.: Blockade und Chirurgie des Sympathikus. Heidelberg 1953

16. Moore, D.C.: Regional Block, 4th ed. Springfield, III, 1978

17. Moore D.C., Bush W.H., Burnett L.L.: Celiac plexus block: A roentgenographic anatomic study of technique and spread of solution in patients and corpses. Anaesth Analg 60 (1981) 369

18. Muehle C., van Sonnenberg E., Casola G., Wittich G.R., Polansky A.M.: Radiographically guided alcohol block of the celiac ganglia. Semin. Intervent. Radiol. 4 (1987) 195

19. Schild H.: Perkutane Neurolyse des Plexus coeliacus. In: Günther R.W., Thelen M. Interventionelle Radiologie. Stuttgart 1988.

20. Schild H., Günther G., Hoffmann G., Goedecke R.: CT-gesteuerte Blockade des Plexus coeliacus mit ventralem Zugang. Fortschr. Röntgenstr. 139 (1983) 202

21. Thompson G.E., Moore D.C., Bridenbaugh L.D., Artin R.Y.: Abdominal pain and alcohol celiac plexus nerve block. Anaesth. Analg. 56 (1977) 1

22. Wall P., Melzack R.: Textbook of pain. New York 1984

23. Ward E.M., Rorie D.K., Nauss L.A., Bahn R.C.: The celiac ganglia in man: normal variations. Anaesth. Analg. 58 (1979) 461

Chapter 20
CT-Guided Neurolysis of the Presacral and Precoccygeal Sympathetic Trunk

R.M.M. Seibel, D.H.W. Grönemeyer

CT-guided neurolysis of the presacral and precoccygeal sympathetic trunk is another important method for local pain therapy. In patients with tumor infiltration of the pelvis (mostly from colorectal and gynecologic carcinomas), the authors were able to achieve very good results with neurolysis of the presacral and precoccygeal sympathetic trunk.

Anatomy

The bilateral sacral sympathetic trunks are located medial to the sacral foramina and merge inferiorly as the coccygeal (impar) ganglion which is located anterior to the coccyx. The presacral portions consist of three to four paired ganglia, covered by parietal peritoneum. Gray

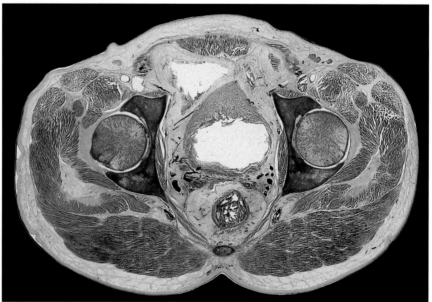

Fig. 20.1

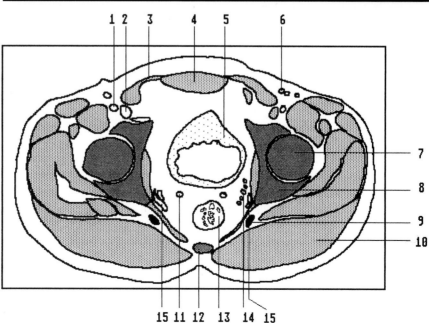

Figs. 20.1. and **20.2.** Neurolysis of the precoccygeal sympathetic trunk (anatomy and illustration). *1* Femoral artery; *2* femoral vein; *3* internal oblique muscle; *4* rectus abdominis muscle; *5* urinary bladder; *6* lymph node; *7* femoral head; *8* ischium; *9* inferior gluteal vein and sciatic nerve; *10* gluteus maximus muscle; *11* ureter; *12* coccyx; *13* rectum; *14* internal iliac artery and vein; *15* sacral plexus.

communicating branches connect the ganglia with the segmental spinal nerves. Only post-ganglionic fibers run inside these branches. The sympathetic innervation of the pelvic organs occurs predominantly through the left and right hypogastric nerves which extend over the prom-ontory of the sacrum (Anatomy, see Figs. 20.1. and 20.2.).

Indications

Pelvic pain caused by tumor infiltration of the pelvis

Pelvic-leg pain caused by tumor infiltration of the pelvis

Patients

25 patients with colorectal or gynecologic carci-nomas, which had infiltrated the presacral or precoccygeal sympathetic trunk, were treated. These were either primary tumors (including local recurrent carcinomas) which had grown directly into the plexus, or metastases to the plexus. The clinic performed 112 treatments in the 25 patients.

Technique

Contrary to lumbar sympathetic trunk and celiac plexus neurolysis, presacral and precoccy-geal neurolysis normally requires multiple ther-apies for complete neurolysis. Generally, these treatments are conducted in four separate ther-apies. At each treatment between 5 and 8 ml alcohol are injected into the plexus. The punc-ture is most often performed from a lateral approach, but can sometimes also be made from

an anterior approach. The needle tip is posi-tioned in a presacral or precoccygeal position. However, in the presacral puncture an anterior access is sometimes required. This is necessary for the superior parts of the plexus. In the pre-coccygeal neurolysis, a puncture from a lateral or posterolateral position is the most convenient approach. In each neurolysis, an assessment of the potential alcohol distribution has to be per-formed prior to the injection of alcohol. There-fore, dilute contrast medium is injected after the placement of the needle tip. Additionally, after two to three weeks, the procedure is repeated (Figs. 20.1.–20.10.).

Instrumentation and medication	
Needle	20–15 cm 22-G needle DCHN 22–20–0–S1 or DCHN 22–15–0–S1 (Cook, Inc.)
Local anesthetic	10–20 ml Mepivacaine 1%
Ethanol for injection 96%	5–8 ml

Results

In approximately 75% of cases, the therapy resulted in a significant reduction in pain. Pa-tients with bladder and rectal disorders (the ma-jority of the patients) had partial improvement in these disorders after therapy. A progression of these symptoms after neurolysis was not observed in any of the patients.

By the combination of a lumbar with a presacral and precoccygeal neurolysis of the sympathetic trunk, the patients with typical pelvic-leg pain caused by a diffusely infiltrating tumor in the iliac region could be saved a chordotomy.

Figs. 20.3.–20.7. Technique for neurolysis of the precoccygeal sympathetic trunk. 48-year old patient with a recurrence of rectal carcinoma in the anastomosis. The tumor extends from the clips into the right pararectal fat. Additionally, a metastasis to the precoccygeal plexus is seen in the presacral area.

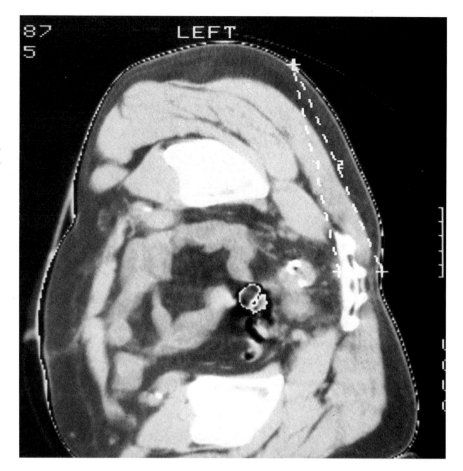

Fig. 20.3. With the patient in the lateral position, the best access route to the precoccygeal sympathetic trunk is determined and measured.

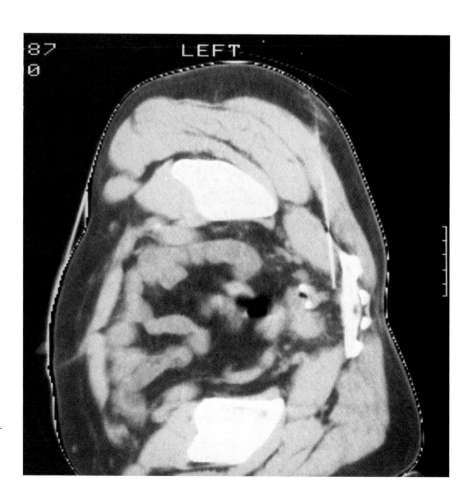

Fig. 20.4. A 22-G fine needle is positioned directly in front of the presacral metastasis.

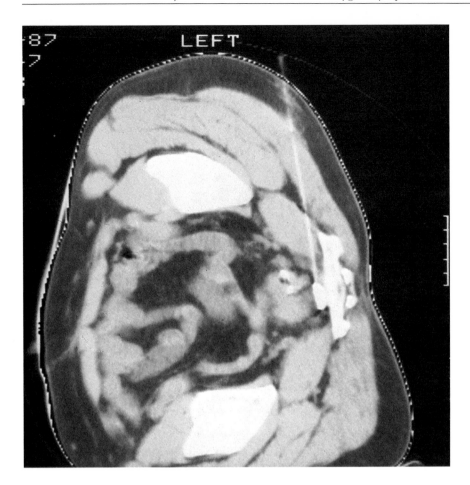

Fig. 20.5. After correcting the position of the needle tip over the mid-line, contrast medium is then injected which is seen distributed in the presacral area.

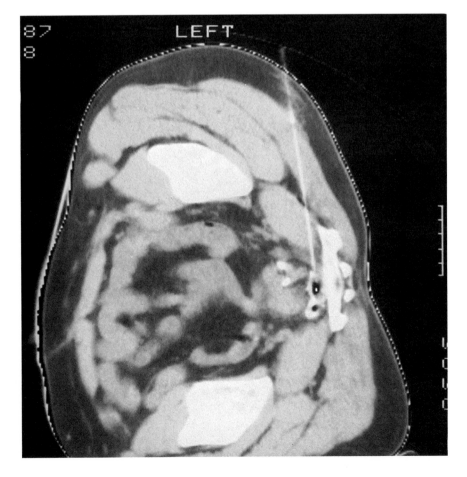

Fig. 20.6. Injection of a total of 8 ml 96% alcohol is performed. CT scan during the injection to check the distribution. The alcohol is seen as a hypodense area presacrally.

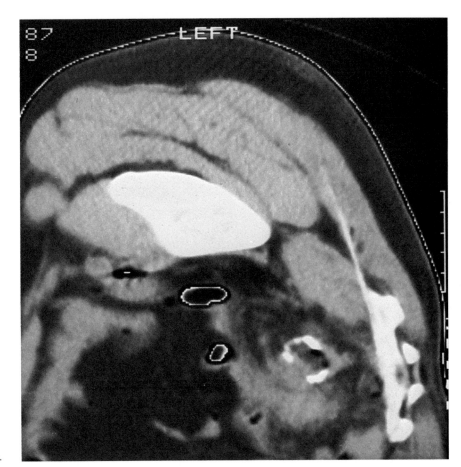

Fig. 20.7. Second treatment of this patient. The needle tip is between metastasis and anterior coccyx. In most cases, the therapy has to be performed four separate times.

Figs. 20.8.–20.10. 54-year old female patient with severe burning pain after colon resection and anastomosis for a rectal carcinoma. During rectoscopic follow-up, there was no evidence of local recurrence. After CT-guided fine needle biopsy, no evidence of tumor recurrence was found in the region of the precoccygeal scar. Due to the severe pain, a precoccygeal sympathetic trunk neurolysis was performed.

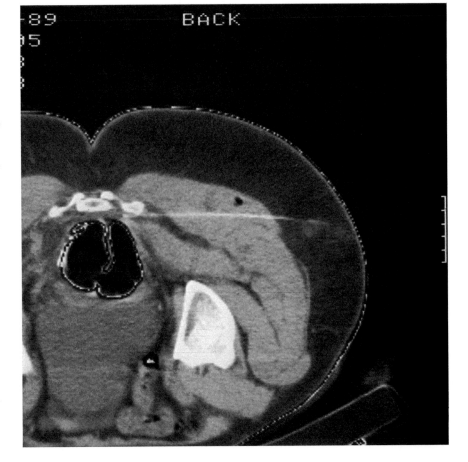

Fig. 20.8. With the patient in the prone position, a 22-G fine needle is advanced step by step into the precoccygeal scar tissue.

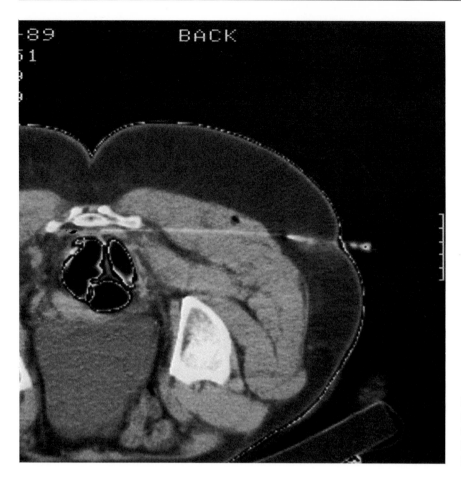

Fig. 20.9. The needle tip is now directly in front of the coccyx. The distance from the needle tip to the skin measures 19 cm.

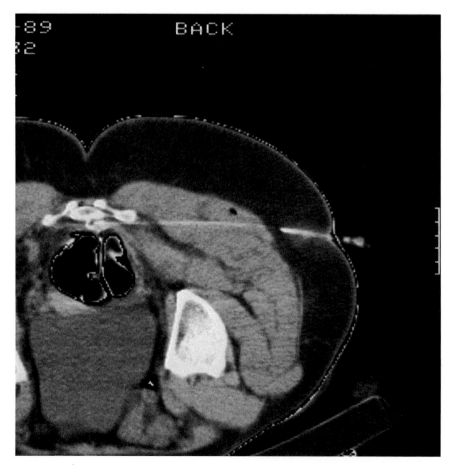

Fig. 20.10. After the precise dissemination of the contrast medium is seen, the alcohol is injected. Only 3 ml of 50% ethanol was injected in this case because there was no evidence of tumor found at FNA. After two treatments the patient was pain-free.

Figs. 20.11. and **20.12.**
64-year old patient with an extensive recurrence of cervix carcinoma. The tumor had encroached on the rectum and resulted in wide infiltration of the right pelvic wall. The patient had severe pelvic-leg pain on the right.

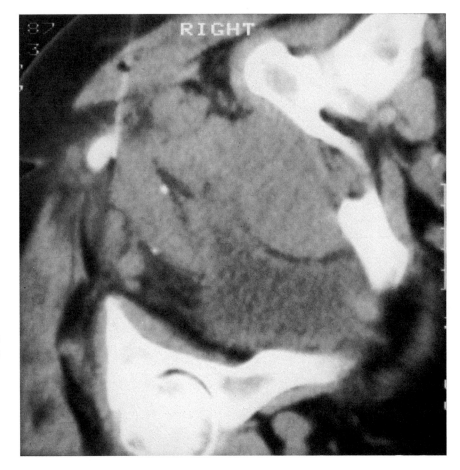

Fig. 20.11. Documentation of the needle-tip position in the precoccygeal area. The needle is advanced from a posterolateral approach through the gluteal musculature to the precoccygeal area. With this technique, the danger of injuring the sciatic nerve is minimized.

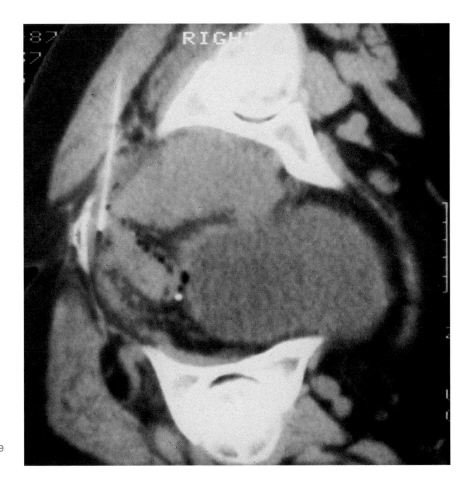

Fig. 20.12. In a second session, the cranial segments of the precoccygeal plexus are destroyed. Due to the configuration of the coccyx, a lateral puncture approach has to be selected in order to reach the precoccygeal plexus.

Percutaneous Lysis of Nerval Structures in Vascular Disorders

Chapter 21
CT-Guided Thoracic Sympathectomy

R.M.M. Seibel, D.H.W. Grönemeyer

Introduction

The first use of surgery in the sympathetic nervous system was by Alexander [2], who in 1889 unsuccessfully attempted to cure epileptics by removing the superior sympathetic trunk ganglia. After this, thoracic sympathectomy was used for a number of indications. Following an attempt to treat spastic paralysis, Royle [14, 15] discovered in 1924 that after sympathectomy there was an elimination of vasoconstriction. Thoracic sympathectomy was also used for the treatment of angina pectoris, bronchial asthma, hemoptysis, lung embolysis, hypertension, and in esophageial and aortic pain [17]. Today these indications have been abandoned. Circulatory disturbances of the upper extremities and chronic pain in the thorax region can, however, be effectively treated with thoracic sympathectomy.

Anatomy

The thoracic sympathetic trunk (Figs. 21.1. and 21.2.) consists of ten to twelve pairs of ganglia, which are located lateral to the vertebral body. The communicating branches are relatively short when compared with the lumbar sympathetic trunk. Connections of two ganglia with a

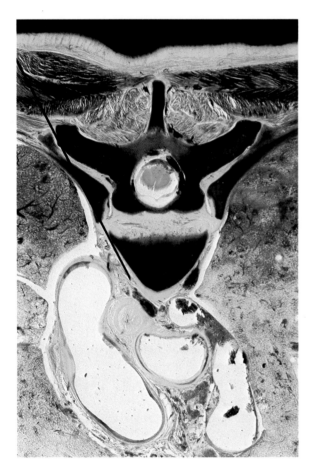
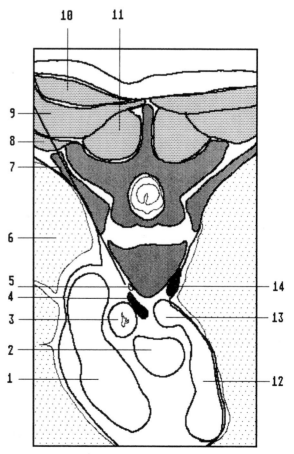

Fig. 21.1. and **21.2.** Thoracic sympathetic neurolysis (anatomy and illustration). *1* Aortic arch; *2* trachea; *3* esophagus; *4* hemiazygos vein; *5* thoracic ganglia; *6* lung; *7* rib; *8* intercostal muscle; *9* iliocostal muscle; *10* trapezius muscle; *11* erector spinae muscle; *12* superior vena cava; *13* azygos vein; *14* intercostal vein.

single segmental nerve or two segmental nerves connecting with one ganglion are possible. The majority of preganglionic fibers originate in the anterior roots of the spinal nerves and travel via the white rami communicantes into the ganglion. After synapsing in the ganglion, the postganglionic fibers run either directly alongside the nerves or vessels or over the gray rami communicantes with the intercostal nerves to their target organ. Preganglionic fibers can also directly synapse in other ganglia [12, 13].

Indications

Raynaud's phenomenon of the arms and hands is the most frequent indication for thoracic sympathectomy (TS). Also, in the same way as lumbar sympathetic neurolysis, peripheral occlusions can be treated with a high degree of success. Occlusions in the region of the axillery and of the brachial artery can be successfully treated just by TS when an operation or a lysis therapy is impossible. Peripheral necrosis due to poor blood supply can also be improved with TS therapy.

TS is an important treatment method for pain by brachial plexus infiltration or phantom type pain. For these two indications, often the TS is combined with therapy in the cervical region. Pain from infiltration by metastases or a primary tumor of the sympathetic trunk, vertebra or rib can be treated successfully with TS at the level of the tumor infiltration. TS can also prove helpful in a post-herpetic neuralgia (Table 21.1.).

Contraindications

TS is contra-indicated in cases of coagulation disorder.

Table 21.1. Indications for CT-guided thoracic sympathectomy.

Circulatory disturbance in the upper extremity
  Raynaud's phenomenon in the upper extremity
  Non-operable arterial occlusion disease of upper extremity
  Contraindications for a local lysis therapy in the upper extremity
Hyperhydrosis
Tumor pain in thorax region
Tumor pain in lower brachial plexus
Brachial plexus damage after radiation therapy with trophic disorders of hand
Phantom pain
Post-herpetic neuralgia

Technique

The CT-guided thoracic sympathectomy is performed under local anesthesia. In the prone position the upper vertebral spinal column is identified. The TS is normally performed at the level of the second or third thoracic vertebra in order to achieve better blood circulation in the arm. The puncturing point, the puncturing angle, and the distance to the skin are determined from a localization CT scan. After local anesthetics have been injected in the skin and the thoracic iliocostal muscle, a coaxial two-needle system consisting of a 22-G fine needle with stylet is advanced along the pleura into the ganglion, or in the immediate vicinity of the ganglion, without injuring the lung. This procedure is performed by the technique described in Figs. 21.3.-21.6. Then, a second local anesthetic is given at the level of the ganglion. Following this an injection of a diluted contrast medium is performed so that the anticipated distribution of the injected alcohol can be seen. For the neurolysis of the thoracic sympathetic trunk as little as 2 ml 96% ethanol is necessary, when the needle tip is in the precise position. Prior to each step a CT scan is performed (Figs. 21.3.–21.6.). In the lower thoracic region the TS can also be performed from an anterior approach (Fig. 21.7.)

For neurolysis of the sympathetic trunk for treatment of tumor pain, the level at which the tumor has infiltrated the trunk is first determined with a diagnostic CT. Then, after identification of the pathologic anatomy the procedure is planned. Neurolysis of the sympathetic trunk is performed in the same manner as previously described (Figs. 21.8. and 21.9.). This procedure is normally combined with an intra- or peritumoral therapy (see Chapter Tumor Therapy). If there is no success, the treatment is repeated after four weeks or in a neighboring segment.

Patients

During the last three years the clinic performed a total of 108 CT-guided TS. In 26% of patients the TS was performed bilaterally. The youngest patient was 19 and the oldest 61 years old. The average age was 35 years. The indications in these patients are shown in Table 21.2.

Table 21.2. Indication for CT-guided neurolysis of the thoracic sympathetic trunk (n = 108).

Circulatory disturbances in the upper extremity	57
Tumor pain	49
Phantom pain	2

Figs. 21.3.-21.6. Technique for thoracic sympathic neurolysis: The puncture is made through the back musculature. The needle tip is located at the level of the synovial joint of the superior and inferior processes. Note the approximately 1mm wide space between the vertebral body and the pleura. The needle is advanced alongside the intervertebral foramen but relatively far away from the foramen in order not to injure the segmental nerve.

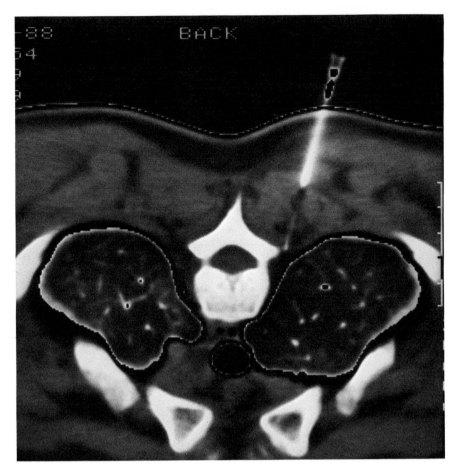

Fig. 21.3

Fig. 21.4. The needle tip has been advanced past the intervertebral foramen. The space between vertebral body and pleura has been widened by 4 to 5 mm by an injection of air and local anesthetic. With this technique an injury to the lung is avoided. The interventional needle must be advanced in contact with the vertebral body.

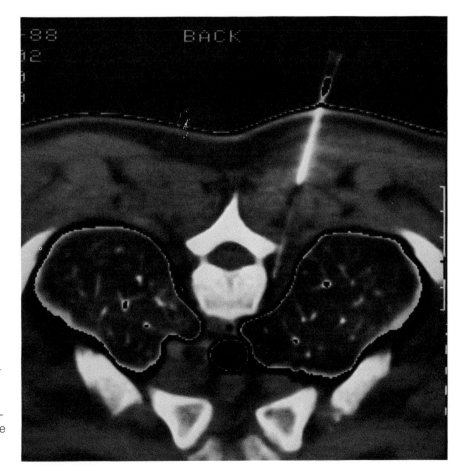

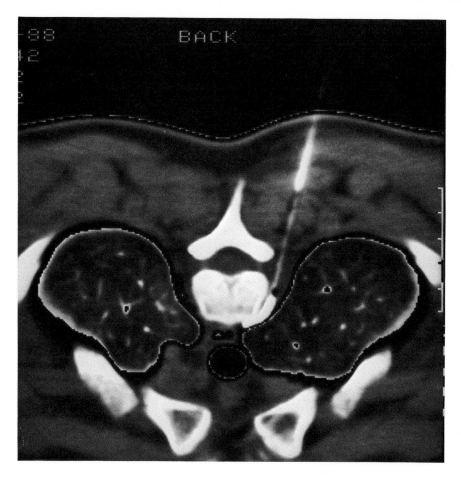

Fig. 21.5. Prior to injection of 96% ethanol a contrast injection is performed to outline the area where the alcohol will be distributed. In this scan the half-moon shaped distribution of contrast medium around the thoracic ganglion and paravertebral sympathic fibers is demonstrated. In a case where the pleura is injured or the puncture needle tip is intravascular, no contrast-medium enhancement will be seen on CT. In this case the needle is moved back and the procedure is repeated.

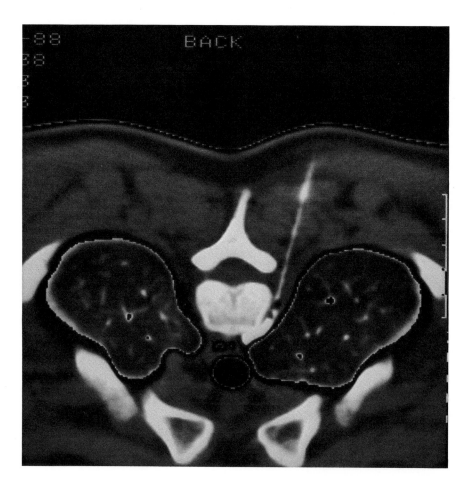

Fig. 21.6. Scan immediately after injection of ethanol. The distribution of the alcohol within the contrast medium must be documented: The alcohol is shown as a pearl-shaped hypodense (black) area anterior to the needle tip within the half-moon shaped area of contrast medium.

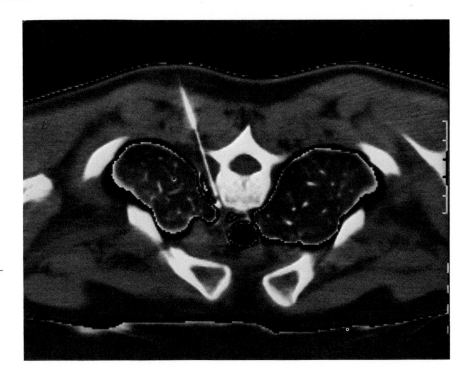

Fig. 21.7. Thoracic sympathetic neurolysis for Raynaud's disease at the T2/3 level. The needle tip and the contrast medium are documented in the region of the thoracic ganglion.

Complications

Complications did not occur after TS.

Side-effects

After TS three patients experienced symptoms in the upper thoracic region comparable to Horner's syndrome with miosis and ptosis. These symptoms resolved within one day. Irritations of the optic conjunctiva were seen in ten cases. These side-effects also lasted only a few hours. One patient showed a decrease in blood pressure which resolved with plasma volume expanders. Therefore, a cardiac cause for this decrease in blood pressure could be excluded.

Results of the CT-Guided TS

Approximately 70% of patients with circulatory disturbances (39 out of 57) had a prolonged rise of circulation in hand and arm after CT-guided TS. In 90% of the patients a warming-up of the affected extremity was felt during the neurolysis. Eight out of the eleven patients with occlusion diseases and necroses of the fingers had complete healing of the necrosis. In dry gangrene, a peripheral border-line amputation can be achieved after TS, as discussed in the Chapter Lumbar Sympathetic Neurolysis [16]. Phantom pain requires a segmental treatment, mostly in the form of periradicular therapy (see Chapter PRT), in addition to the thoracic sym-

pathetic neurolysis. In cases of tumor pain, a good reduction in pain could be achieved in 85% of patients (Table 21.3).

Table 21.3. Results after CT-guided neurolysis of the thoracic sympathetic trunk.

Prolonged rise in blood circulation of the upper extremity (n = 57)	75%
Healing of necroses (n = 11)	72%
Immediate warming-up (n = 57)	90%
Alleviation of tumor pain (n = 49)	85%

Discussion

Although current operative methods for sympathectomy do not put an excessive strain on the patient, a general anesthetic and a stay in hospital are still necessary [1, 3, 4, 5, 10]. CT-guided TS offers an alternative to operative thoracic sympathectomy in the therapy of circulatory disturbances of the upper extremity. With low-risk and only short-lasting side-effects the CT-guided TS should be performed before an operative TS. In a step-by-step concept the authors first recommend in their clinic the peripheric guanethidine blockade for elimination of peripheric sympathetic synapses. If there is no success with this method, the CT-guided TS is performed. Only in the case of an insufficient effect of CT-guided TS, will indication be given for an operation. Since the guanethidine blockade is performed in ischemia, it cannot be performed in many patients with a distinct arterial occlusion disease because ischemic damages and

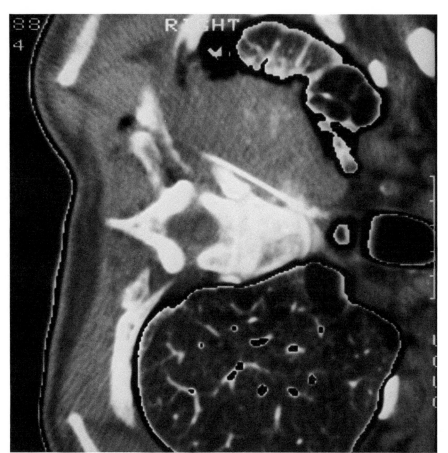

Figs. 21.8. and **21.9.** Thoracic sympathetic neurolysis in a patient with a pleura mesothelioma and severe pain.

Fig. 21.8. This scan shows the needle tip in the region of the thoracic ganglion and the paraganglionic sympathetic fibers. The contrast medium spreads out in half-moon shape configuration, posterior to the esophagus and around the vertebral body. After undergoing two treatments, the patient's pain perception was reduced by 85%.

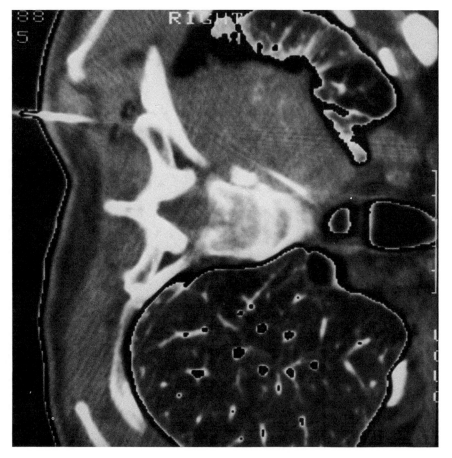

Fig. 21.9. Same patient as in Fig. 21.8. Note the arch-like pattern of the puncture needle and that it leaves the CT scan plain. The larger guiding needle is identified posterior to the spine, leaving the plain, with the intervention needle extending anteriorly, coming back into the same plain. Using this archlike technique the curvature of the needle allows the tip to be positioned anterior to the vertebral body. This three-dimensional procedure is a special puncture technique using a highly flexible needle.

occlusion would have to be expected during the procedure. In the case of an incompletely achieved ischemia there are also considerable circulatory reactions possible after a guanethidine dose. A fluoro-guided sympathetic blockade is contra-indicated due to the high rate of side-effects. For this reason several authors [6] consider a thoracic sympathetic treatment as obsolete. This recommendation has to be contrasted with the fact that, for the first time, with the utilization of CT an elegant method is available with low risk and with a high morphologic possibility of differentiation. Operative methods [7] and endoscopic operations according to Kux with installation of a pneumothorax [11] can be replaced in many cases by considerate use of the CT-guided sympathetic trunk disconnection even in cases of pathological findings.

Non-success of CT-guided TS for therapy of circulatory disturbances is explained by the presence of anomalies in sympathetic innervation in the upper thoracic region. Often these patients have a Kuntz's nerve [8, 9] which is a direct connection of the thoracic ganglion II or III with the plexus brachialis.

Undesirable side-effects of CT-guided TS occurred in the clinic at a low rate only and were merely temporary. Horner's syndrome can be avoided if during the injection the dissemination of alcohol is controlled and the thoracic ganglion I is taken care of.

CT-guided TS can also be performed after an unsuccessful operative thoracic sympathectomy. This may be explained by the possibility of elimination of regeneration fibers after operation by TS.

In cases of tumor infiltration of the lower cervical plexus or of the thoracic sympathetic trunk, and in metastases in the thoracic vertebral column with radicular pain, with the segmental sympathetic neurolysis very good pain reduction can be achieved, up to complete painlessness. To some extent an additional cervical or thoracic periradicular therapy is advisable (see Chapters on Tumor Therapy and Lumbar Sympathectomy). Neurolysis of the sympathetic trunk should always be performed at the level of tumor localization. A neurolysis of several sympathetic segments may be necessary.

References

1. Adson A.W.: Cervicothoracic ganglionectomy, trune resection and ramisectomy by the posterior intrathoracic approach. Amer. J. Surg. 11 (1931) 227–232

2. Alexander W.: The Treatment of Epilepsy, Pentland, Edinburgh 1889. Nat. Libr. Cat. 1955–1959

3. Atkins H.J.B.: Peraxillary approach to the stellate and the upper thoracic sympathetic ganglia. Lancet 11 (1949) 1152–1153

4. Atkins H.J.B.: Sympathectomy by the axillary approach. Lancet 1 (1954) 538–539

5. Carstensen G.: Eingriffe am Sympathetikus bei peripheren Durchblutungsstörungen. In: Baumgartl F., Kremer K., Schreiber W. (Ed.): Spezielle Chirurgie für die Praxis. Stuttgart 1975, 628–652

6. Hankemeyer U., Krizanits F.: Schmerztherapie bei akutem Herpes zoster und bei der postherpetischen Neuralgie. In: Lücking Ch., Thoden U., Zimmermann M. (Hrsg.) Nervenschmerz. Stuttgart, New York, Schmerzstudien 7, 1988, 105–115

7. Kuhlendahl H.: Operation am sympathischen und parasympathischen Nervensystem, in: Bier A., Braun H., Kümmerle H. (Hrsg.), Chirurgische Operationslehre. Leipzig 1973, 445–447

8. Kuntz A.: Distribution of the sympathetic rami of the brachial plexus: Its relation to sympathectomy affecting the upper extremity. Arch. Surg. 15 (1927) 871–877

9. Kuntz A.: The autonomic nervous system. Philadelphia 1929

10. Kux E.: Der endoskopisch transpleurale Zugang zum vegetativen System in der Brusthöhle. Dtsch. Med. Wschr. 74 (1949) 753–754

11. Kux E.: Thorakoskopische Eingriffe am Nervensystem. Stuttgart, New York 1954

12. Netter F.H.: Autonomes Nervensystem. In: Nervensystem 1. Neuroanatomie und Physiologie. Stuttgart, New York 1987, 69–80

13. Rickenbacher J., Landolt A.M., Theiler K.: Rücken In: v. Lanz, Wachsmuth (Ed.): Praktische Anatomie 2, 7. Berlin, Heidelberg, New York 1982, 152–156

14. Royle N.D.: A new operative procedure in the treatment of spastic paralysis and its experimental basis. Med. J. Austral. 1 (1925) 77–86

15. Royle N.D.: The treatment of spastic paralysis by sympathetic ramisection. Experimental basis and clinical results. Surg. Gyn. Obstet. 39 (1924) 701–720

16. Seibel R.M.M., Balzer K., Grönemeyer D.H.W.: Erfahrungen mit der CT gesteuerten Sympathikusausschaltung bei der Behandlung der peripheren AVK. Angio Arch. (1989) 75–77

17. Stiller H.: Indikation und Erfolg der Sympathikus-Chirurgie. Fortschr. Med. 78 (1960) 425–428

Instrumentation and Medication	
Needle	10-15 cm 22-G needle DCHN 22-15.0-S1 (Cook)
Local anesthetic	10-15 ml Mepivacaine 1%
Contrast medium	0.5 ml Iopromide (diluted)

Chapter 22
CT-Guided Lumbar Sympathetic Trunk Neurolysis for the Treatment of Occlusive Arterial Disease (OAD)

R.M.M. Seibel, D.H.W. Grönemeyer, K. Balzer, G. Carstensen, C. Sehnert

Introduction

The first peri-arterial sympathectomy was performed by Jaboulay in 1899 [7]. In 1913, this method was improved by Leriche [11]. In 1925, Adson and Brown [1] for the first time both removed the lumbar ganglia and severed the communicating branches. The first paravertebral chemical neurolysis of the sympathetic trunk with 85% ethanol was performed by Swetlow [21] in 1926. In 1949, Haxton [6] presented his results after lumbar sympathectomy with phenyl alcohol in 220 patients. After the introduction of CT guidance for sympathectomy, a puncture accuracy of 1 mm^3 could be achieved. Today, lumbar sympathectomy (LS) has an established place in the treatment of peripheral circulation disorders of the lower leg.

Anatomy

The lumbar sympathetic trunk consists of three to four pairs of ganglia, which lie on the anterior surface of the vertebral bodies. The communicating branches between the ganglia are relatively long. White communicating branches are found only in the upper one or two ganglia, whereas the gray communicating branches are in all of the lumbar ganglia. The preganglionic fibers in the lower lumbar sympathetic trunk run in the interganglionic branches. Furthermore, it is possible to have communication between two ganglia and one segment nerve or two segment nerves and one ganglion. After synapsing in the ganglion, the postganglionic fibers traverse with the lumbar spinal nerve. These fibers contain the vasomotor nerves [13, 15] (Figs. 22.1.–22.7.).

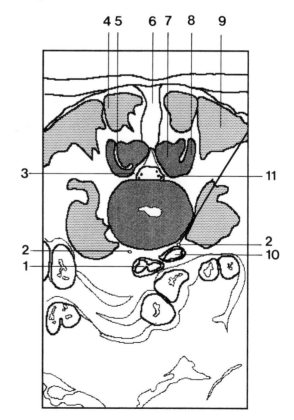

Figs. 22.1. and **22.2.** Lumbar sympathectomy (anatomy and drawing). *1* Aorta; *2* sympathetic-lumbar ganglion; *3* epidural space; *4* medial part of the back musculature; *5* synovial joint; *6* interspinous ligament; *7* superior articular process of L4; *8* inferior articular process of L3; *9* lateral part of the back musculature; *10* vena cava; *11* cauda equina.

Indications

Generally, a high rate of success is achieved in the therapy of localized peripheral occlusions by lumbar sympathectomy. The main indications for this therapy are occlusions of arteries in the lower leg and foot, as well as simultaneous femoral occlusions. Trophic peripheral ulcers and necrotic areas within the region of the toes can often be successfully treated with LS. The authors perform LS in many patients, as an additional therapy after revascularization of the femoral or popliteal arteries. In most cases, the indications are determined after an examination, including Doppler ultrasound and angiography, by a vascular surgeon or angiologist in accordance with criteria after Carstensen [2] (Table 22.1.).

Table 22.1. Indications for LS.

Occlusion of the arteries in the lower legs and feet
Combined thigh and lower leg occlusion
Trophic ulcers of the lower legs and feet
Necrosis of the toes
In addition to profunda prosthesis or femoro-popliteal bypass
Endarteries obliterans (Winiwarter-Buerger)
Functional circulation disorders

Contraindications

In older patients with generalized arteriosclerosis, the operative lumbar sympathectomy is contra-indicated. The main danger here is that a reduction in blood pressure from anesthesia and neurolysis can aggravate a patient's existing circulation disorders. Also, in isolated aortoiliac occlusions, advanced gangrene, and chronic edema of the lower leg, surgical LS is not performed. Additionally, a paradoxical decrease in circulation in the lower leg after vascular manipulation (mostly by calcium or thrombotic embolism) is often seen in these cases. Above all, a contraindication to general anesthesia makes surgical LS impossible, since it is performed only under general anesthesia [2] (Table 22.2.). Contraindications for CT-guided LS are isolated aortiliac stenosis and/or occlusion.

Table 22.2. Contraindications for surgical LSE.

Older patients with generalized arteriosclerosis
Isolated aortoiliac occlusions
Advanced gangrene
Treatment-resistant edema of lower legs and feet

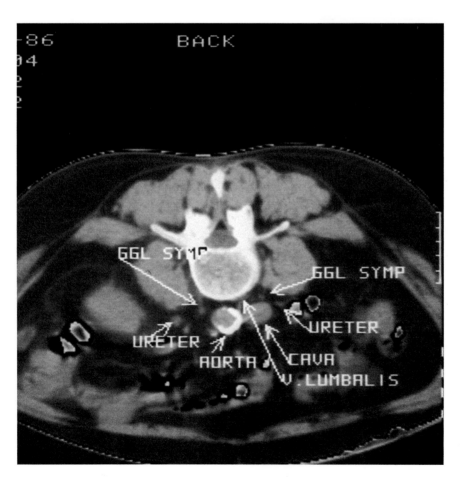

Fig. 22.3. CT scan in the middle of the L4 vertebral body. The sympathetic ganglia can be well demarcated bilaterally from the fat. Also, the neighboring structures such as blood vessels and ureters can be differentiated.

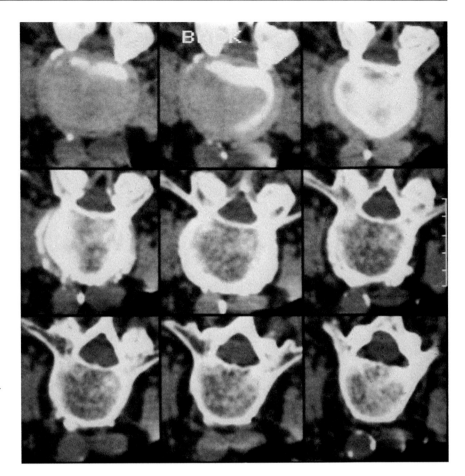

Fig. 22.4. In 2 mm contiguous scans, the left 4th lumbar ganglion can be observed at the anterior edge of the vertebral body between aorta and psoas muscle (bottom row, left picture).

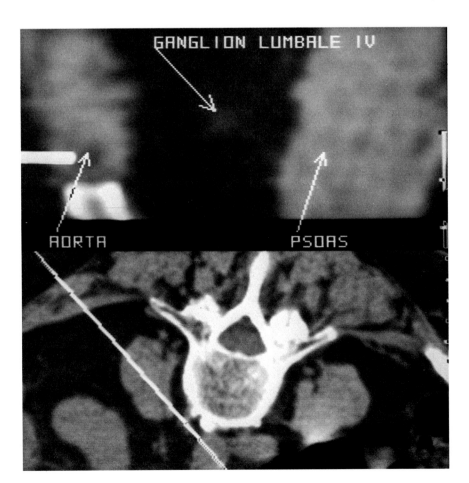

Fig. 22.5. In an oblique reconstruction, the 4th lumbar ganglion is seen between aorta and psoas muscle.

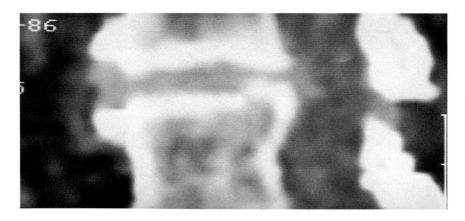

Fig. 22.6. Same patient as in Fig. 22.5. Sagittal reconstruction. The 4th lumbar ganglion is seen at the anterior edge of the vertebral body and extends cranially to the intervertebral disc level.

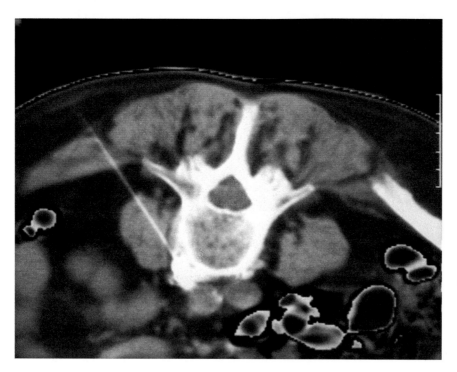

Fig. 22.7. Lumbar sympathectomy (cases Figs. 22.3.–22.7.). An optimal distribution of the contrast medium is seen at the anterior edge of the vertebral body.

The more peripheral and localized the occlusion, the greater the probability of a successful lumbar sympathectomy.

Technique

CT-guided LS requires only local anesthesia. After I.V. contrast medium injection, with the patient in the prone position, the sympathetic ganglia and ureters are visualized. Then, a determination of the puncture point, puncture angle, and distance to the skin is made. After local anesthesia of the skin and ileocostal muscle, using the guide needle from a coaxial fine needle system, a 22-G fine needle with a mandril is advanced through this guide needle. The fine needle is then advanced through the psoas muscle into the ganglion or its immediate vicinity. Local anesthesia is again injected, especially to demonstrate the effect on the sympathetic tone. By injection of diluted contrast medium, the anticipated distribution of the alcohol in the region of the sympathetic trunk can be checked. For neurolysis of the sympathetic trunk only 3 ml of 96% ethanol is used, when the needle tip is correctly positioned. CT-scans are performed prior to each step (Figs. 22.8.–22.11.). The access route used for the CT-guided procedure can be considerably simpler and in most cases shorter than the route needed in surgical LS (Figs. 22.12. and 22.13.).

Figs. 22.8.–22.11. Technique of the lumbar sympathectomy.

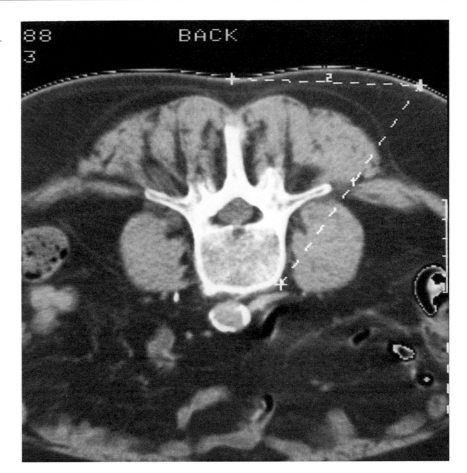

Fig. 22.8. After I.V. contrast-medium injection and documentation of the ureters which are located anterior to each psoas muscle, measurement of the best access route is performed, normally in the prone position.

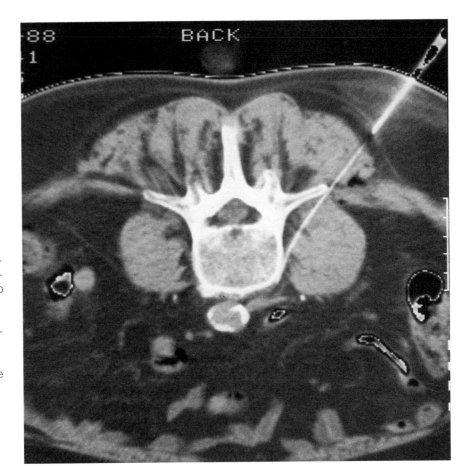

Fig. 22.9. With a coaxial needle system, from a posterolateral approach, the interior needle is advanced to the lumbar ganglion or to its immediate vicinity. During the advancing, local anesthetic is injected. Additionally, it can be useful, as in this case, to advance the interior needle at a slight arch along the vertebral body to the ganglion. The puncture tract is through the iliocostalis and psoas muscle.

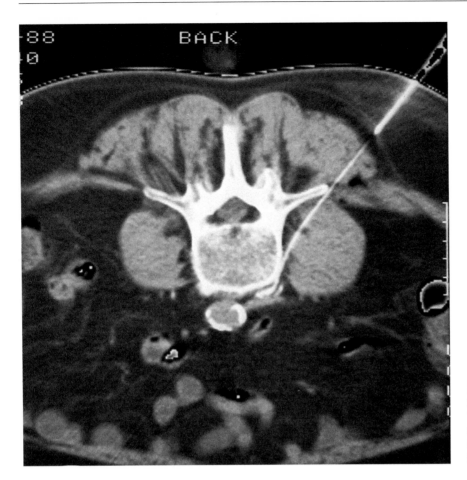

Fig. 22.10. After injection of 3 ml local anesthetic, 1 ml diluted contrast medium was also injected, which extends retrocavally in this case.

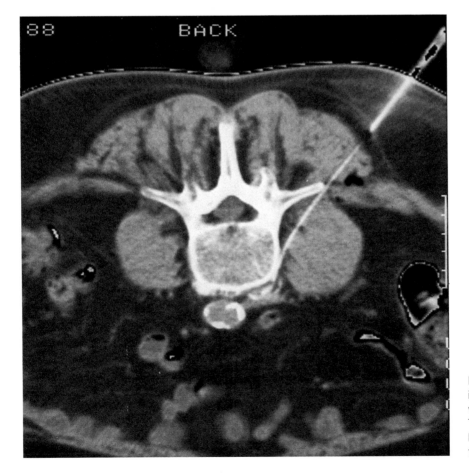

Fig. 22.11. The sympathetic trunk is then destroyed with 2 ml of 96% ethanol. The ethanol injection can be recognized by the dilution of the contrast.

Figs. 22.12. and **22.13.**
With this female patient the operative lumbar sympathectomy would be difficult to perform due to an extensive herniation through the anterior abdominal wall (Fig. 22.12.). The anteroposterior radius of the patient is 44.3 cm. The distance of the access route to the sympathetic ganglion is only 11 cm for the CT-guided lumbar sympathectomy (Fig. 22.13.).

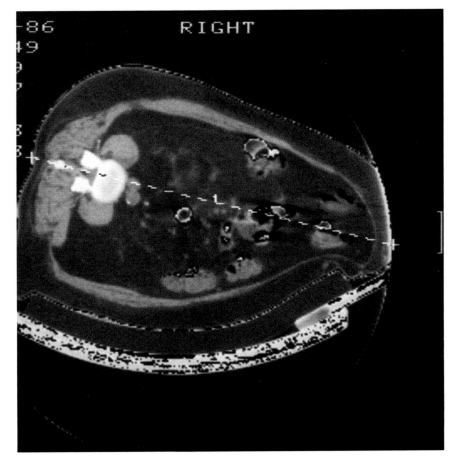

Fig. 22.12

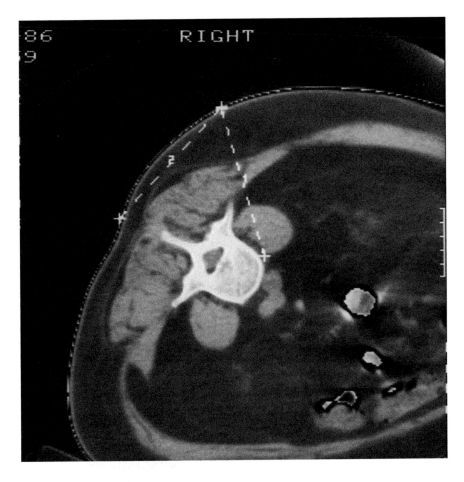

Fig. 22.13

Patients

During the past 3 years the authors performed a total of 510 CT-guided LS. In 26% of the patients, the intervention was performed bilaterally. Normally, bilateral treatment is performed in two separate sessions. However, in some cases, the bilateral treatment was performed in a single session (Figs. 22.14.–22.17.). The patients were between 14 and 94 years old with an average age of approximately 65 years. Furthermore, 20% of the patients had diabetes and 72% were either in stage III or IV on the Fontaine scale of occlusive diseases (Table 22.3.).

Table 22.3. Scale of occlusive arterial diseases (OAD).

OAD Stage II	28%
OAD Stage III	33%
OAD Stage IV	39%
Diabetes mellitus (in all stages)	20%

Side-effects and Complications of Surgical and CT-Guided LS

Despite excellent anesthesia techniques, post-operative mortality of 0.5-7% occurred in extensive operative studies which had between 150 and 830 patients each. Post-operative hyperesthesia in the region of the genitofemoral or lateral cutaneous nerve of the thigh occurred in 5-18% of cases. These hyperesthesias were observed in only 2% of the patients. Furthermore, with CT-guided perineural infiltration of the genitofemoral nerve these symptoms disappear after one week at the most. Especially with the surgical removal of the 1st lumbar ganglia bilaterally, sexual disorders appeared in 2-9% of the patients [9]. The authors did not observe these side-effects with CT-guided LS, which is normally performed at the L3 and L4 level. The paradoxial effect of operative LS was not observed after CT-guided LS. In 1% of the surgical LS cases, the ureter was severed or removed. In their group of patients the authors had one patient (0.2%) who developed a ureter fistula. For this reason they determine the location of the ureters with an I.V. contrast-medium injection prior to the procedure.

Results of CT-Guided LS

75% of the patients after CT-guided LS had an observable increase in blood circulation to the skin. In 85% "warming-up" was noticed during the procedure. This immediate therapeutic effect had a beneficial effect on patients. In 66% of the patients, there was a notable increase in walking distance. The maximum beneficial effect from LS is obtained after approximately 6-8 weeks of intensive walking exercise. In 45% of the patients with OAD at stage IV, there was complete healing of the area of necrosis. The subjective effect of the CT-guided LS is also important. 82% of the patients had a subjective improvement (Table 22.5.). In 135 patients, there was a follow-up observation period of two years. In many of these patients an improvement of the OAD stage occurred after the lumbar sympathectomy. The patients at stage III showed the greatest improvement (Table 22.6.).

Table 22.4. Complications after lumbar sympathectomy.

	Surgical LS	CT-guided LS
Mortality	0.5%-7.0%	0%
Hyperesthesia of the genitofemoral nerve	5.0%-18.0%	2.0%
Sexual disorders	2.0%- 9.0%	0%
Paradoxic gangrene	1.0%- 4.0%	0%
Ureteral damage	1.0%	0.2%

Table 22.5. Results after CT-guided lumbar sympathectomy (n = 510).

Blood circulation increase	75%
Immediate feeling of warmth	85%
Increased walking distance	66%
Subjective improvement	82%
Healing of necrosis	45%

Table 22.6. Change in stages of OAD after CT-guided LS (results after two years) (n = 135).

Stage II	unchanged	55%
Stage II	to stage I	39%
Stage II	to stage III	6%
Stage III	unchanged	4%
Stage III	to stage I	4%
Stage III	to stage II	85%
Stage III	to stage IV	7%
Stage IV	unchanged	66%
Stage IV	to stage I	3%
Stage IV	to stage II	31%

In 18.5% of the patients, amputation had to be performed after LS, but in many of these patients, the authors were able to achieve a border-line amputation. The frequency of amputations showed a distinct correlation with the stage of occlusion (Table 22.7.).

Figs. 22.14.–22.17.
Simultaneous lumbar
sympathectomy performed
bilaterally.

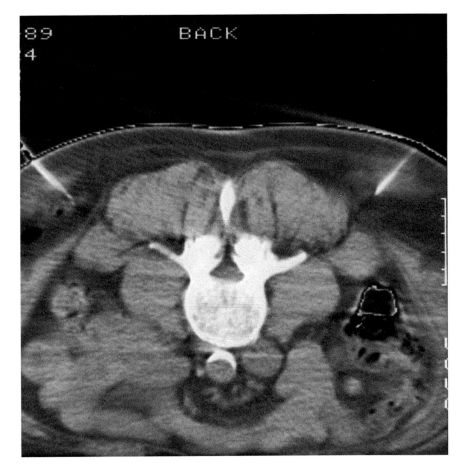

Fig. 22.14. CT-scan at the
level of the middle of the
4th lumbar vertebra. After
subcutaneous injection of
local anesthesia, both
guide needles are now in
the correct position for advancement of the therapy
needles.

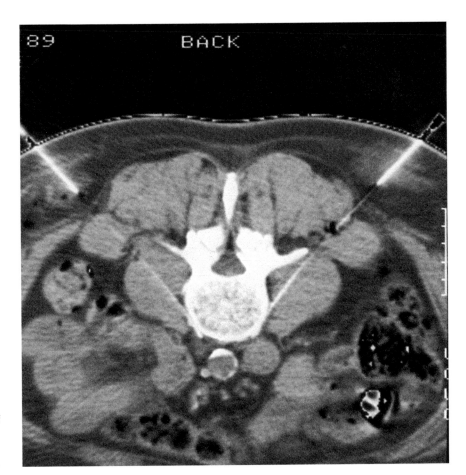

Fig. 22.15 CT-scan show-
ing the exact positioning of
the therapy needles which
have been advanced
through the guide needles.

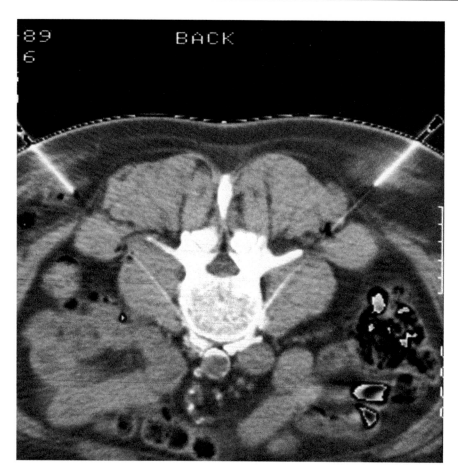

Fig. 22.16. Good distribution of the contrast medium in the retrocaval area, retroaortal area and bilaterally around the ganglia.

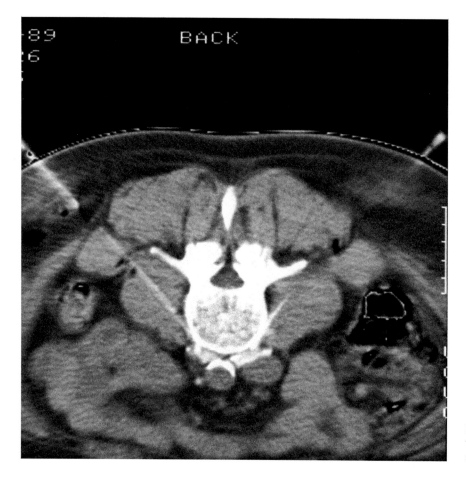

Fig. 22.17. Bilateral injection of 3 ml ethanol for the sympathectomy.

Table 22.7. Amputations versus stages of OAD after CT-guided lumbar sympathectomy.

Total	18.5%
Stage IV	40.8%
Stage III	9.7%
Stage II	2.9%

Discussion

A quantitative appraisal of the success of lumbar sympathectomy has been difficult to evaluate since the effects of both the therapy and the walking exercise cannot be differentiated with respect to the increase in walking distance. After intensive walking exercise, the patients are able to improve circulation considerably following lumbar sympathectomy. Undisputed, however, are the effects of LS in Fontaine stage III. This was not only seen at MKI, but was also proven in a randomised prospective study by Cross and Cotton [3]. In the authors' patients with rest pain, there was an improvement with a change from stage III to stage II in 85% of the cases [20]. Even at stage IV (associated necroses), patients can have favorable results after LS. Also, the rate of success increases when the necrosis is located more distally. Lee et al. were able to preserve the toes in 51% of their patients with distal necrosis and the leg in 71% by LS alone [10]. In clinic patients with extensive necroses, a border-line amputation could be performed after an LS in most cases. In 45% of the patients with necrosis, there was complete healing.

The combination of LS with a vascular operation or angioplasty for improvement of the peripheral circulation has been a successful therapy. The most common types of vascular operations performed with LS are profunda prosthesis, femoropopliteal bypass, and bifurcation prosthesis. The indication for a combination of LS and vascular surgery is the case of diffuse small vessels disease. Also, after dilation or percutaneous aspiration thrombo-embolectomy in the pelvis-leg region, an LS should be performed if insufficient circulation of the lower leg and foot arteries is still present.

If LS only is performed, a check of the sympathetic tone before the procedure should be made in order to assess the beneficial effect of LS. To estimate the potential success of LS, a predictive test using local anesthetics for a temporary sympathetic trunk blockade can be helpful [8]. Also, circulation measurements with an infra-red camera after blockade of the sympathetic trunk can be useful [12]. Therefore, a diagnostic blockade of the lumbar sympathetic trunk with local anesthetic is conducted prior to the LS. If the desired effect is achieved, then a neurolysis using an alcohol injection is performed in the same session.

Contrary to the phenol injection, where a dose of up to 15 ml of liquid may be required [4, 16], the ethanol injection is performed with a volume of only 2-5 ml. This leads to a more accurate distribution of the alcohol in the region of the sympathetic trunk (Figs. 22.18.–22.23.). Another interesting finding is that the neurolysis of two segments compared with that of one segment does not show any advantages [5].

In all patients with OAD, the basic disease is not treated by lumbar sympathectomy. Nevertheless, in 82% of the authors' patients, there was a subjective improvement after lumbar sympathectomy. Furthermore, 85% of the patients noticed a warming-up of the treated leg during the interventional procedure.

The authors found no significant difference in response to LS in diabetics, when compared with other patients. This has been verified by other authors [10, 17]. CT-guided LS can be repeated if the sympathetic tone reappears [19]. The cause for this return of sympathetic tone may be incomplete denervation or partial regeneration of the sympathetic trunk.

Instruments and Medication	
Needle	10-15 cm 22-G needle DCHN 22-15.0 S1 (Cook, Inc.)
Local anesthetic	10-15 ml Mepivacaine 1%
96% ethanol for injection	3-5 ml
Contrast medium	0.5 ml Iopromide (diluted 1:5 with local anesthetic)

In conclusion, for the lumbar sympathectomy, CT-guided neurolysis is an effective method which is less traumatic for the patient and has a lower complication rate than surgical LSE. Due to the high tissue differentiation and three-dimensional control of the distribution of the alcohol, LS (and other nerve neurolyses) should only be performed with the use of CT guidance. Contrary to fluoroscopy guidance only, the danger of inaccurate injections, e.g. into the psoas muscle, and complications such as ureter lesions and injuries of large vessels are minimized [18].

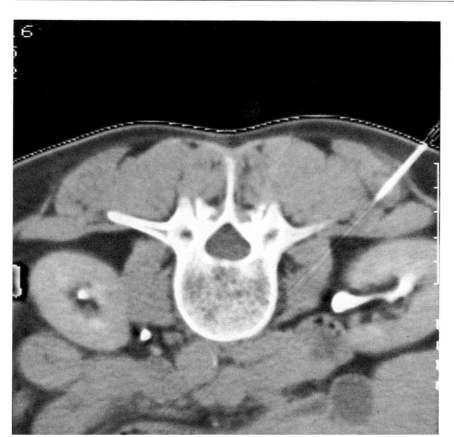

Figs. 22.18.–22.23. Female patient with OAD stage III.

Fig. 22.18. Adjacent to the 3rd lumbar vertebra, the guide needle has been inserted and local anesthesia is injected in the previously described manner. The "target artifact", a line-like artifact, points in the direction of the lumbar ganglion. The ganglion can be identified retrocavally at the anterior edge of the vertebral body.

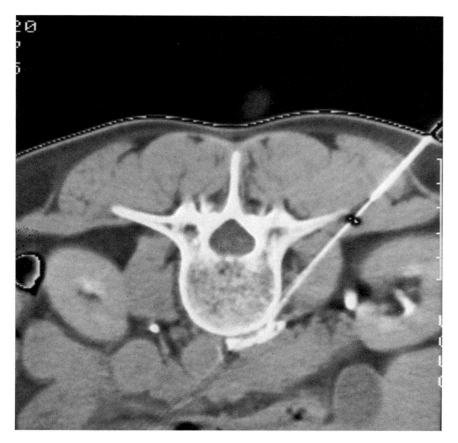

Fig. 22.19. After positioning the 22-G fine needle through the guide cannula, injection of diluted contrast medium is performed. The contrast extends retrocavally and retroaortically to the opposite side. The vena cava lies on the spinal column prior to injection of the contrast medium (Fig. 22.18). The needle tip is exactly 1 mm posterior to the vena cava. This is a very difficult procedure which requires an acute puncture angle. After injection of contrast medium and local anesthetic, the vena cava has shifted several millimeters.

Figs. 22.20. and **22.21.** CT documentation of the exact distribution of the alcohol along the anterior edge of the vertebral body.

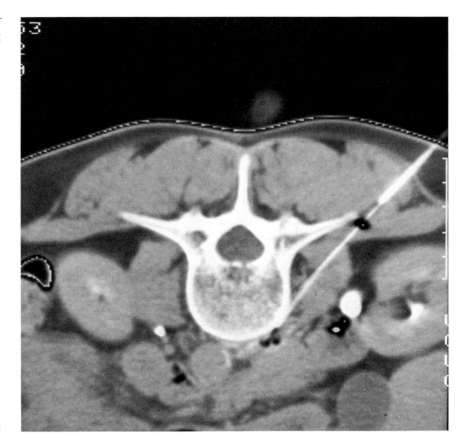

Fig. 22.20

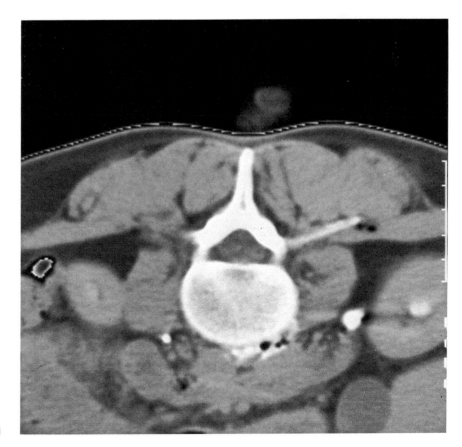

Fig. 22.21

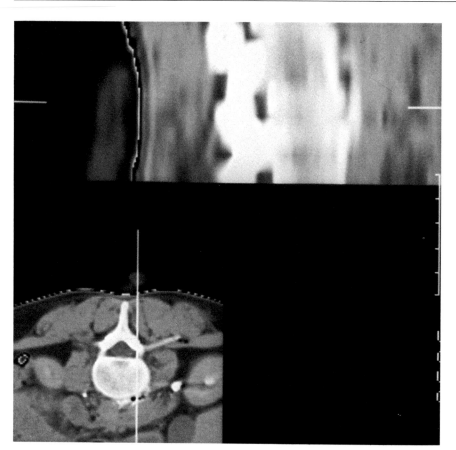

Figs. 22.22. and **22.23.**
Documentation of the cranio-cardinal extension of the alcohol. Sagittal reconstructions of the axial control scans. On both images, the distribution of the contrast medium and alcohol is recognized at the anterior edge of the vertebral body and has a maximum extension of 3 cm.

Fig. 22.22

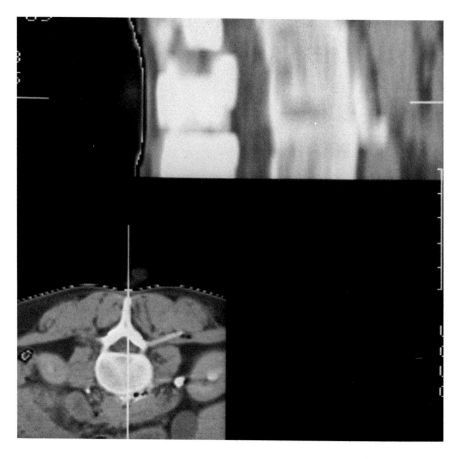

Fig. 22.23

Summary

CT-guided lumbar sympathectomy has important advantages compared with the operative method:

1. Only local anesthesia is necessary for the procedure.
2. Treatment can be performed in older patients with whom it is more frequently indicated.
3. Immediately following LS, walking exercise therapy is possible. This increases the effectiveness of the LS therapy.
4. The CT-guided method has few side-effects and complications.
5. More than 80% of the patients notice a warming-up in the cold leg during the procedure and later on a relief of pain.
6. The CT procedure can be performed on an out-patient basis.

References

1. Adson A.W., Brown G.E.: Treatment of Raynaud's disease by lumbar ramisection ganglionectomy and perivascular sympathetic neurectomy of the common iliacs. J. Amer. med. Ass. 84 (1925) 1908–1910
2. Carstensen G.: Eingriffe am Sympathikus bei peripheren Durchblutungsstörungen. In: Baumgartl F., Kremer K., Schreiber W. (Hrsg.) Spezielle Chirurgie für die Praxis. Stuttgart 1975, 628–652
3. Cross F.W., Cotton L.T.: Chemical lumbar sympathectomy for ischemic rest pain. A randomized, prospective controlled clinical trial. Amer. J. Surg. 150 (1985) 341–345
4. Dondelinger R., Kurdziel J.C.: Percutaneous phenol neurolysis of the lumbar sympathetic chain with computed tomography control. Ann. Radiol. 27, 4 (1984) 376–379
5. Hatangi V.S., Boas R.A.: Lumbar sympathectomy: A single needle technique. Br. J. Anaesth. 57 (1985) 285–289
6. Haxton H.A.: Chemical Sympathectomy. Br. Med. J. (1949) 1026–1028
7. Jaboulay M.: Le traitement de quelques troubles trophiques du pied et de la jambe par la dénudation de l'artère fémorale et la distension des nerfs vasculaires. Lyon méd. 91 (1899) 467–468
8. Kruse C.A.: Thirty years experience with predictive lumbar sympathectomy. Method for selection of patients. Amer. J. Surg. 150 (1985) 232–236
9. Lemmens H.A.J.: Sympathikus. In: Carstensen G. (Hrsg.) Intra- und postoperative Komplikationen. Berlin, Heidelberg, New York 1983, 101–106
10. Lee B.Y., Madden J.I., Thoden W.R., McCann W.J.: Lumbar sympathectomy for toe gangrene. Long-term follow-up. Amer. J. Surg. 145 (1983) 398–401
11. Leriche R.: De l'élongation et de la section des nerfs périvasculaires dans certains syndromes douloureux d'origine artérielle et dans quelques troubles trophiques. Lyon chir. 10 (1913) 378–382
12. McCollum P.T., Spence V.A., Macrae B., Walker W.F.: Quantitative assessment of the effectiveness of chemical lumbar sympathectomy. Br. J. Anaesth. 57 (1985) 1146–1149
13. Netter F.H.: Autonomes Nervensystem. In: Nervensystem 1. Neuroanatomie und Physiologie Stuttgart, New York 1987, 69–80
14. Rau G.: Sympathektomie. In: Heberer G., Rau G., Schoop W. (Hrsg.): Angiologie. Stuttgart 1974, 152–156
15. Rickenbacher J., Landolt A.M., Theiler K.: Rücken In: V. Lanz, Wachsmuth (Hrsg.) Praktische Anatomie 2, 7, Berlin, Heidelberg, New York 1982, 152–156
16. Redman D.R.O., Robinson P.N., Al-Kutoubi M.A.: Computerised tomography guided lumbar sympathectomy, Anaesth. 41 (1986) 39–41
17. Rosen R.J., Miller D.I., Imparato A.M., Riles T.S.: Percutaous phenol sympathectomy in advanced vascular disease. Amer. J. Roentgenol. 141 (1983) 597–600
18. Schild H., Grönninger J., Günther R., Thelen M., Schwab R.: Transabdominelle CT-gesteuerte Sympathektomie. Fortschr. Röntgenstr. 141 (1984) 504–508
19. Schild H.: Perkutane Neurolyse des lumbalen Sympathikus. In: Günther R.W., Thelen M. (Hrsg.): Interventionelle Radiologie. Stuttgart, New York 1988, 409–415
20. Seibel R.M.M., Balzer K., Grönemeyer D.H.W.: Erfahrungen mit der CT-gesteuerten Sympathikusausschaltung bei der Behandlung der peripheren AVK. Angio Arch. 17 (1989) 75–77
21. Swetlow G.I.: Alcoholic injections into nerve tissue for the relief of pain. Amer. J. med. Sci. 171 (1926) 397–407

Percutaneous Management of Fluid Collections and Urinary Diseases

Chapter 23
Percutaneous Decompression of the Urinary System

W.R. Werner, R.M.M. Seibel, D.H.W. Grönemeyer

The use of CT-guided puncture for a dilated renal pelvis makes surgical decompression rarely necessary. CT-guided procedures have a low complication rate and can be performed without general anesthesia. Furthermore, they do not require extensive pre-operative tests. The frequently observed anatomic variations of the renal pelvis do not present a contraindication for percutaneous nephrostomy; these variations can be documented non-invasively with CT, even without contrast medium. Therefore, patients that are allergic to contrast media or patients with a renal insufficiency may be candidates for CT-guided decompression.

Technique

Prior to puncture of the renal-caliceal system, a current blood-clotting status and renal function-status should be obtained. In patients with coagulation disorders, the puncture of the renal collecting system is contraindicated.
A CT of the retroperitoneum defines the anatomic conditions of the urinary tract. The puncture of the dilated collecting system is performed with the patient in the prone position. A 22-G fine needle is advanced through the guide needle from a posterior approach after local anesthesia with Mepivacaine 1%. The aspirated fluid is sent for microbiological and chemical tests. The appropriate antibiotic therapy in case of an inflammatory hydronephrosis is then possible.
After checking the needle position with CT, a controllable guide wire is placed into the collecting system, using the Seldinger-technique. This is followed by the introduction of a 7 F-kidney fistula catheter. The tip of the catheter should be positioned in the renal pelvis and not in the neck of a calix. Finally, the catheter is fixed with a skin suture.

Catheter Care and Follow-up Examinations

The most important factor for the success of the procedure and the anti-inflammatory therapy is the catheter care. Furthermore, sterile saline and Betadine flushes several times a day are important.
Often the patient can be treated as an outpatient. Periodical follow-up blood tests (CBC and SMA 20) and daily fluid balances are necessary. In cases of renal abscess drainage, the patients should be afebrile after 24–48 hours for the drainage to be successful.
Follow-up renal ultrasound is performed regularly to monitor the progress of the drainage. Additionally, a Dopplersonography of the punctured kidney is recommended in order to detect AV-fistulas at an early stage not invasively.
With adequate catheter care, the catheter can remain in place for several weeks.
Inflammatory lesions of the renal pelvis are normally completely healed after 14 days of drainage.

Indications and contraindications for
CT-guided percutaneous nephrostomy

Indications
Inflammatory hydronephrosis
Non-inflammatory hydronephrosis

Contraindication
Coagulation disorders

Chapter 24
CT-Guided Antegrade Ureter Stent

R.M.M. Seibel, D.H.W. Grönemeyer, W.R. Werner

If during decompression of the dilated collecting system a disorder of the urine flow occurs or a compression of the ureter is present, a percutaneous renal fistula can be transformed into an internal ureter stent. This is performed using the Seldinger technique. If the ureter is compressed by a tumor (i.e. at the true pelvis), then a guide wire is advanced past the ureteral stenosis. Over this guide wire, a ureter catheter is percutaneously introduced and then uncoupled from the introducer. It will then function as an internal ureteral stent.

In the case of a continuous drainage, the conversion of the percutaneous nephrostomy to a ureter stent should always be attempted in order to improve the patient's quality of life. If it is possible to correct the ureter compression with appropriate therapeutic measures (such as chemotherapy, radiation or operation), then the internal ureter stents can be easily removed using cystoscopy.

nique and insertion of a polyethylene catheter into the collecting system. This method has become the procedure of choice for the decompression treatment of hydronephrosis [2]. With time, the method was improved by better imaging modalities, i.e. ultrasound and CT, thereby decreasing the risk to the patient.

Shortly after the introduction of whole-body CT, Haaga and co-workers in 1977 [3] described the first CT-guided antegrade pyelography and percutaneous nephrostomy. With the better differentiation of tissue densities, structures which do not contain contrast can easily be punctured. The use of ultrasound also made percutaneous decompressions possible without radiation [4].

In a summary of the literature by Stables [6], there were already 516 percutaneous nephrostomies reported in 1978.

Otto [5] suggested in 1988 that, with further development, MRI may be an additional diagnostic instrument to perform invasive percutaneous procedures with only a few complications.

Indications and contraindication for the CT-guided antegrade ureter stent
Indications
Ureter compression from any cause
Ureter stent before extracorporeal shock-wave lithotripsy (ESWL)
Renal calix system obstruction of an inflammatory origin (abscess drainage)
Contraindication
Blood-clotting disorders

Literature Review

In 1948, Ferris [1] described the first percutaneous nephrostomy by means of a trocar tech-

References

1. Ferris D.O., Grindlay J.H.: Use of polyethylene and polyvinyl tubing in ureterostomy, nephrostomy and cystostomy. Proc. Staff Meet. Mayo Clin. 23 (1948) 385
2. Goodwin E.R., Casey W.C., Woolf W.: Percutaneous trocar (needle) nephrostomy. In: Hydronephrosis. J.A.M.A. (1955) 891
3. Haaga J.R., Zelch M.G., Alfidi R.J., Stewart B.H., Dougherty J.D.: CT-guided antegrade pyelography and percutaneous nephrostomy. Amer. J. Roentgenol. 128 (1977) 621–624
4. Harris R.D., McCullough D.L., Talner L.B.: Percutaneous nephrostomy. J. Urol. 115 (1976) 628–631
5. Otto R.Ch.: Interventionelle Maßnahmen unter sonographischer Kontrolle für Diagnostik und Therapie. Röntgen-Bl. 41 (1988) 419–425
6. Stables D.P., Ginsberg N.J., Johnson M.L.: Percutaneous nephrostomy: a review of the literature. Amer. J. Roentgenol. 130 (1978) 75–82

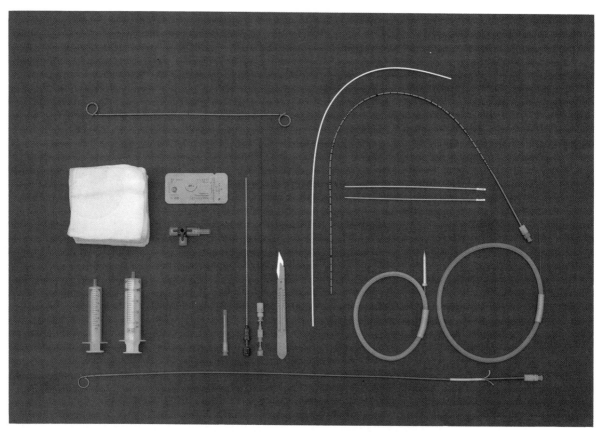

Fig. 24.1. Components of an interventional drainage/decompression set: *below:* pigtail catheter (7-F green); *from left to right: 1* syringes (5 ml, 10 ml); *2* guiding cannula; *3* interventional needle (22-G); *4* dilator; *5* scalpel; *6* pusher; *7* distance-marked stretched catheter; *8* guiding wires; *middle: 1* swabs; *2* suture material; *3* 3-way tap; *4* dilator; *at top:* double-pigtail.

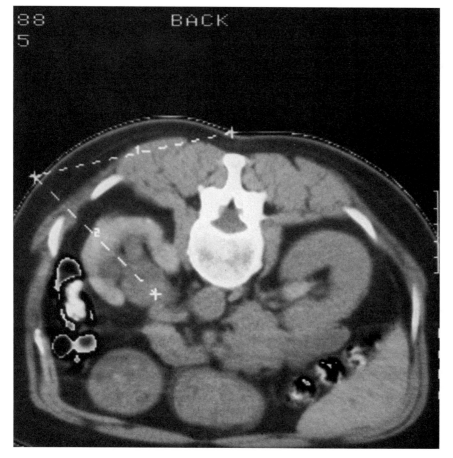

Figs. 24.2.–24.6. 58-year old patient with a recurrent carcinoma of the cervix which has resulted in hydronephrosis on the left. In the prone position, the correct puncture level is determined. Penetration depth and angle of puncture are determined using CT (Fig. 24.2).

Fig. 24.2

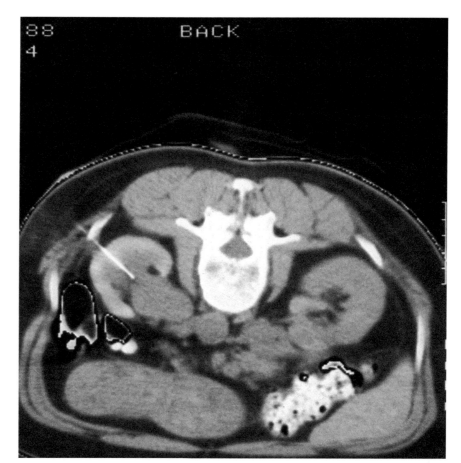

Fig. 24.3. In the prone position, the guide needle is introduced from a posterolateral approach. The injected local anesthetic is visible in the fatty tissue. Through the guide needle a 22-G fine needle is advanced into the renal pelvis with continued injection of local anesthetic.

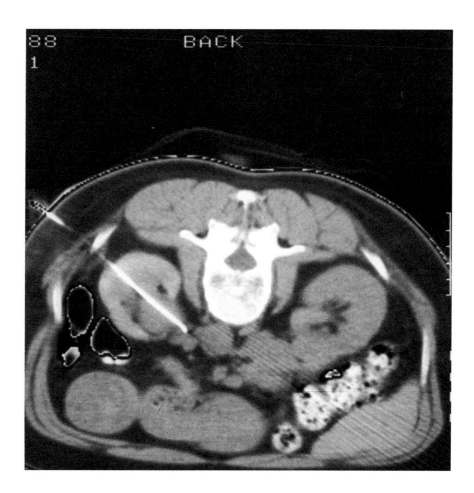

Fig. 24.4. A 18-G guide wire is introduced through the fine needle.

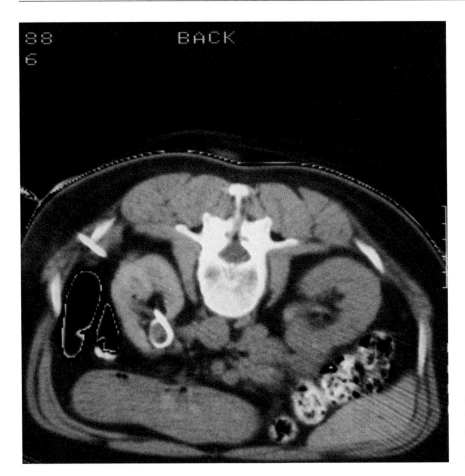

Fig. 24.5. After dilation of the puncture canal, a pigtail catheter is inserted into the renal pelvis and the pelvis drained.

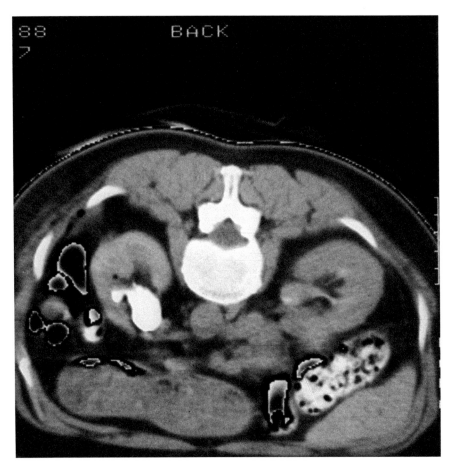

Fig. 24.6. The collecting system is then checked for leaks. Through the inserted catheter a diluted contrast medium is injected. No extravasation of the contrast is identified. Perforation of the collecting system can now be excluded.

Figs. 24.7.–24.10. 68-year old patient with a prostatic carcinoma and hydrone-phrosis on the right. After puncturing the massive enlarged renal pelvis with a 22-G fine needle (Fig. 24.7.), a pigtail catheter is inserted.

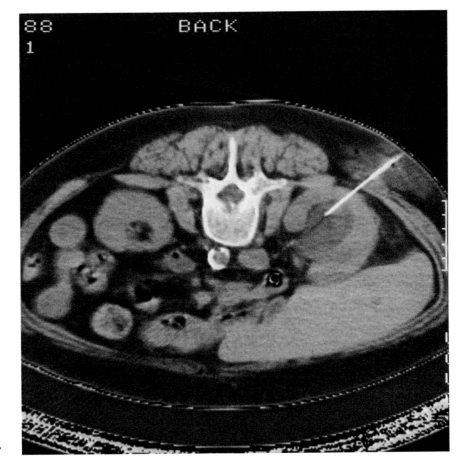

Fig. 24.7

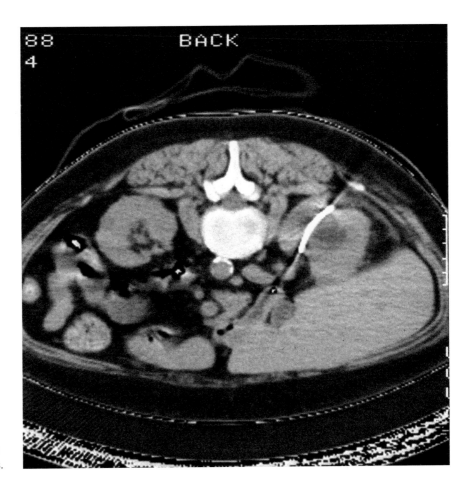

Fig. 24.8. The exact position of the catheter can be identified in the renal pelvis.

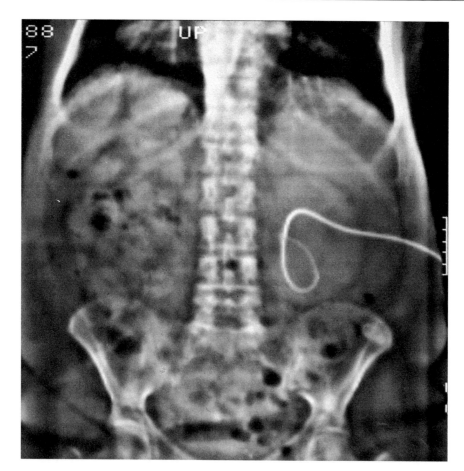

Fig. 24.9. CT-topogram for documentation of the correct position of the inserted 7-F pigtail catheter in the renal pelvis.

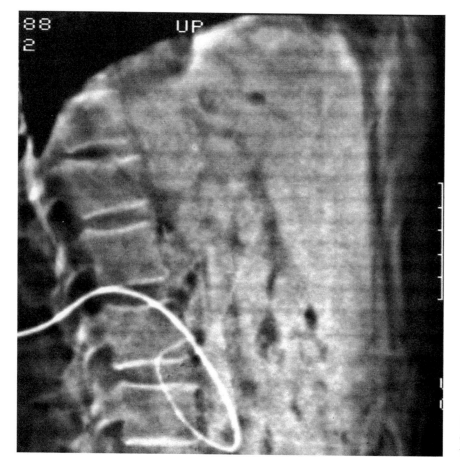

Fig. 24.10. Lateral topogram for documentation of the renal fistula catheter.

Figs. 24.11.–24.19. 60-year old patient with extensive recurrent cervical carcinoma which has resulted in bilateral hydronephrosis. At admission, a creatinine value of 7.6 mg% was found. After diagnostic CT, a percutaneous nephrostomy is performed. The planning of the puncture is carried out in the usual manner (Fig. 24.11.).

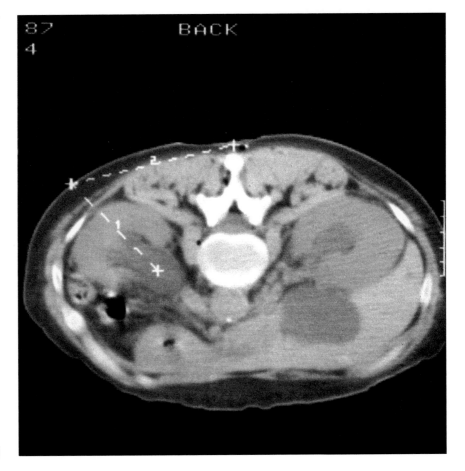

Fig. 24.11

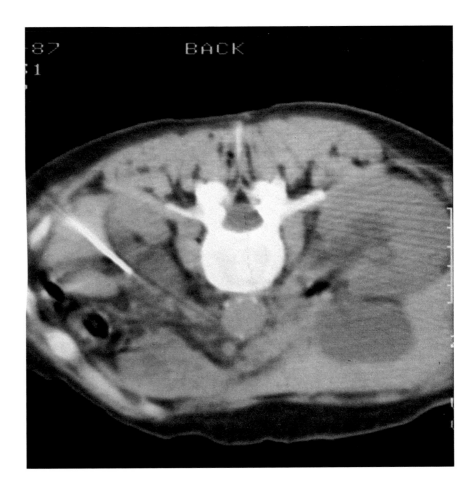

Fig. 24.12. A 22-G fine needle is in the massive enlarged left renal pelvis.

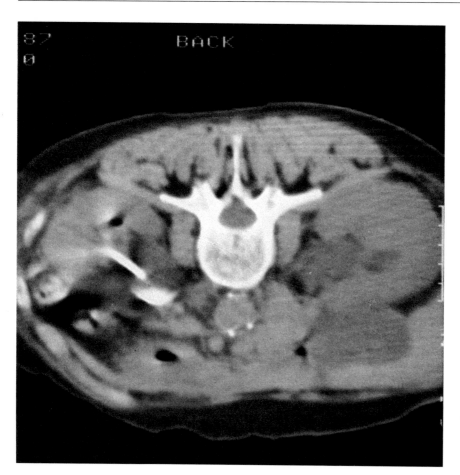

Fig. 24.13. After insertion of the pigtail catheter, a check for extravasation with diluted contrast medium is performed. A contrast-fluid level is identified at the transition area of the renal pelvis with the enlarged ureter.

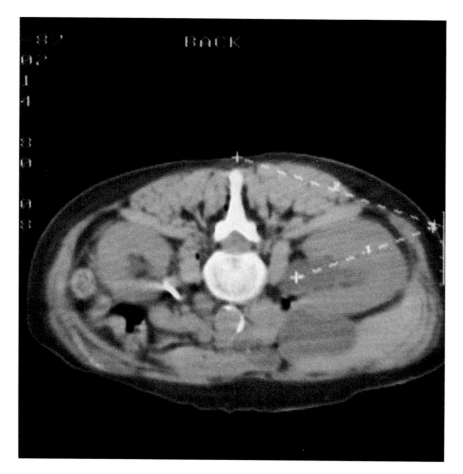

Fig. 24.14. Determination of the puncture angle for the right nephrostomy. After problem-free placement of the renal fistula catheter on the left, the right nephrostomy is then performed at the same session.

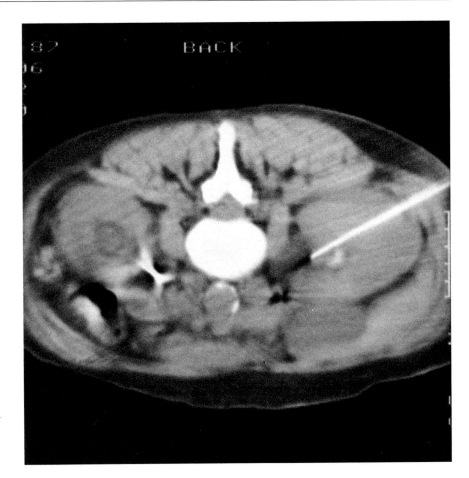

Fig. 24.15. Status post puncture of the enlarged right renal pelvis with a 22-G fine needle and introduction of a 18-G wire. Both can be seen in the renal pelvis.

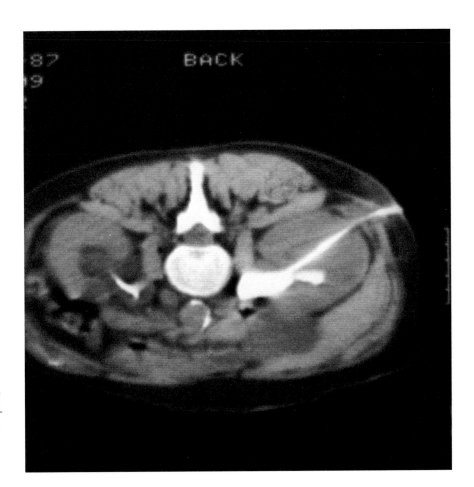

Fig. 24.16. After insertion of the catheter, a check of the contrast-medium distribution in the renal pelvis is performed. Extraluminar contrast medium is not detected.

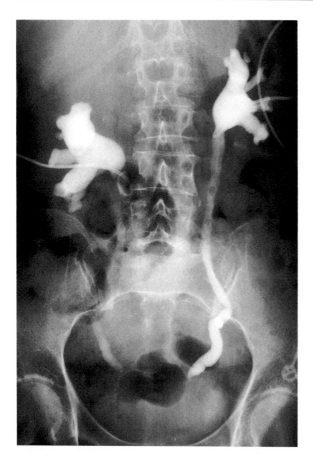

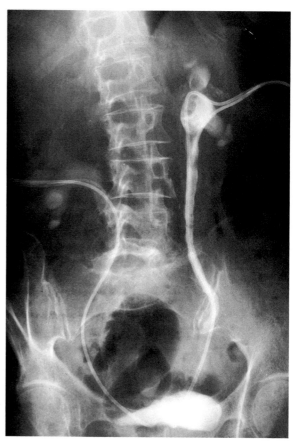

Fig. 24.17. After change in position of the patient to the supine, the fistula catheters and contrast are observed on a fluoro-image. The CT diagnosis of a subtotal bilateral occlusion, located directly in front of the ostia, is verified.

Fig. 24.18. On the same day, bilateral ureter stents were inserted. Additionally, bilateral nephrostomy flush catheters are in place and will remain for 72 hours. The contrast medium in the urinary bladder is a sign of ureter stent function.

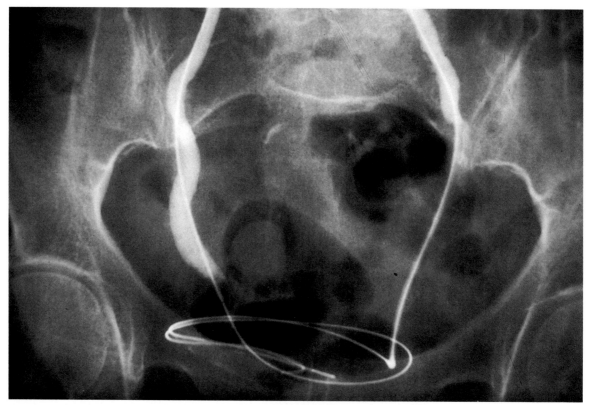

Fig. 24.19. With suitable catheters and wires the stenoses can be traversed bilaterally.

Figs. 24.20.–24.30.
71-year old patient with prostatic carcinoma and bilateral hydronephrosis. Massive renal parenchyma thinning is identified on the left. A fistula was installed in this kidney at another medical center. With sonographic guidance, a puncture of the right kidney was attempted. However, a fistula drain could not be installed. The nephrostomy procedure was halted because of bleeding into the renal pelvis.

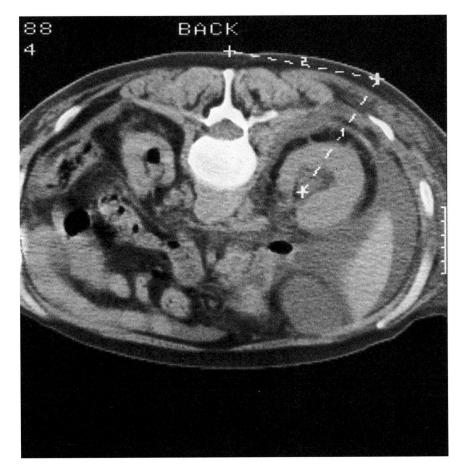

Fig. 24.20. Puncture angle for nephrostomy on the right. Ascites is observed.

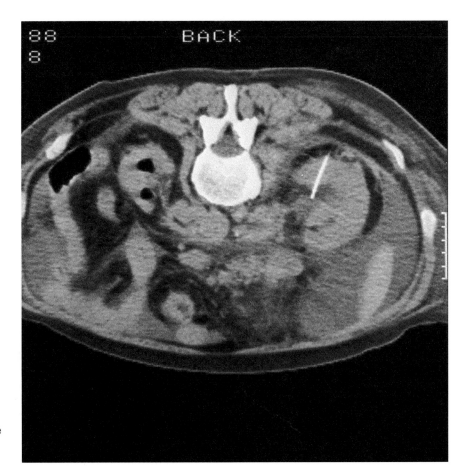

Fig. 24.21. Puncture of the renal pelvis with a 22-G fine needle.

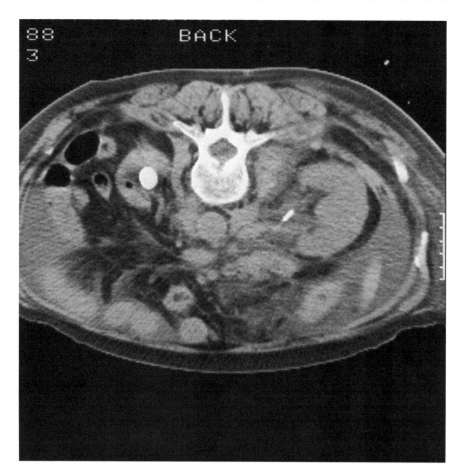

Fig. 24.22. Check of the 18-G wire in its inferior course.

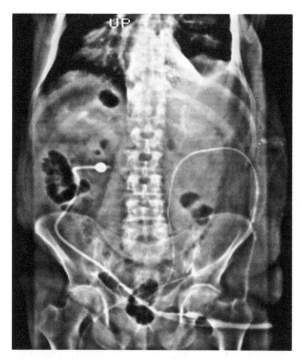

Fig. 24.23. CT topogram for evaluating the inserted renal fistula catheter. This catheter has been advanced into the urinary bladder.

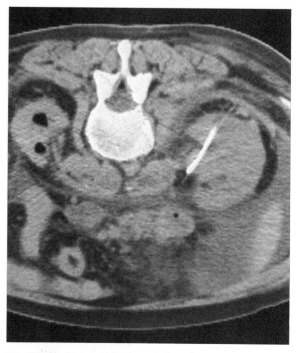

Fig. 24.24. Check of the inserted nephrostomy catheter.

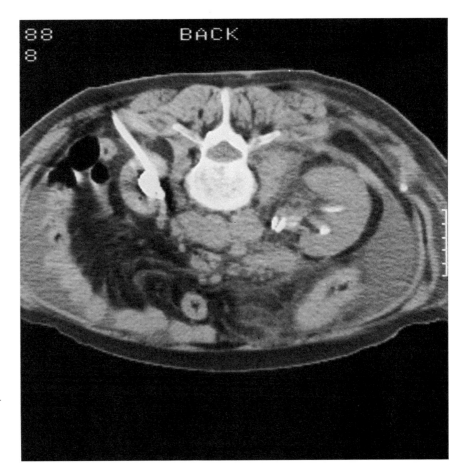

Fig. 24.25. After contrast-medium injection, coagulated blood is seen in the right renal pelvis from the previous nephrostomy attempt.

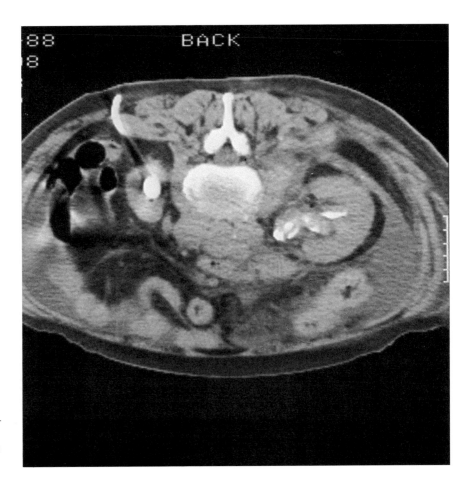

Fig. 24.26. The nephrostomy catheter is at the medial wall of the renal pelvis in the transition area of the ureter.

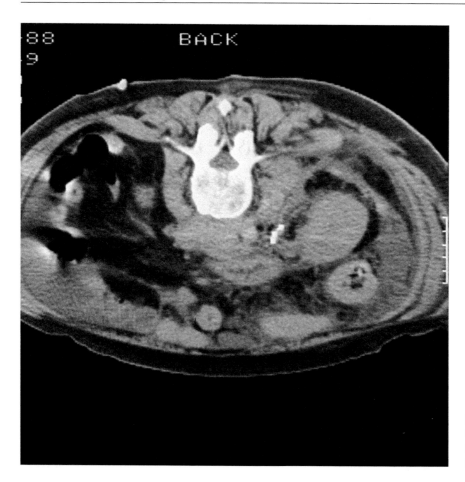

Fig. 24.27. Documentation of the fistula catheter in the ureter at the lower kidney pole.

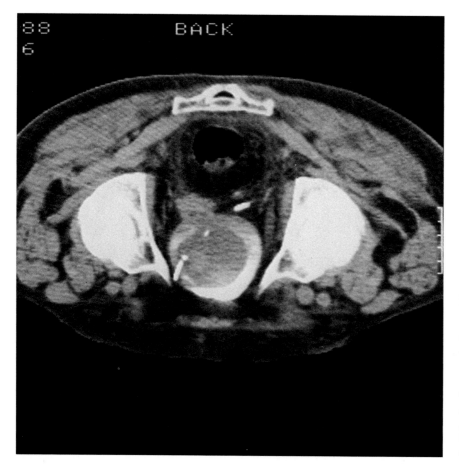

Fig. 24.28. The antegrade ureter stent, which is inserted from the right reaches the left base of the bladder. The impression on the bladder base from the prostatic carcinoma is readily visible. Also identified is an area of prostatic carcinoma infiltration in the posterior wall of the bladder at the region of the ostia.

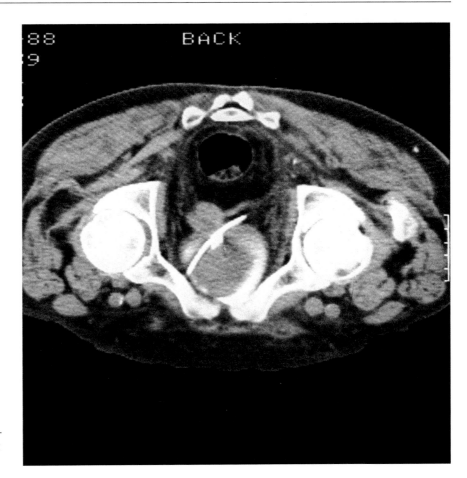

Fig. 24.29. CT scan at the level of the right ureteral ostium. The prostatic carcinoma extends from the left side to the right ostium.

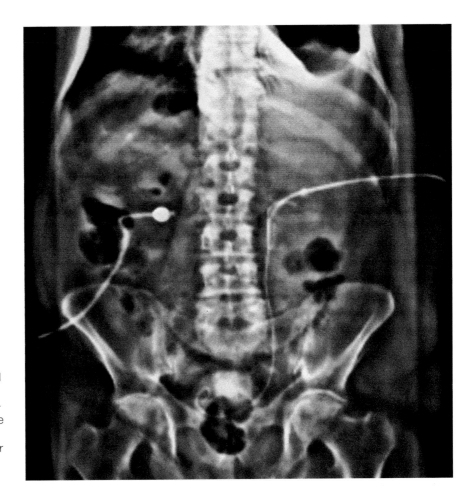

Fig. 24.30. During the final CT topogram, the exact position of the inserted antegrade ureter stent can be documented. For the next three days, a flush catheter will remain in the renal pelvis.

Chapter 25
CT-Guided Percutaneous Thoracic and Abdominal Abscess Drainage

R.M.M. Seibel, D.H.W. Grönemeyer, W.R. Werner, E. Starck, I.P. Arlart

Organ preserving therapy without surgical intervention is possible with the percutaneous abscess drainage (PAD). Also PAD can reduce the time the patient must be in hospital. Furthermore, surgical procedures are rarely indicated after PAD.

Technique

First a Bolus-CT (CT-angiogram) is performed for the abscess localization. With this technique, usually a hyperdense ring is identified which corresponds to the abscess wall. A further advantage of this method is the fact that the adjoining structures can be well differentiated. A precondition for PAD is an intact clotting system.

After abscess localization and local anesthesia, a 7 to 10F pigtail catheter is placed in the abscess cavity either by a Seldinger or trocar technique. In cases of larger abscess cavities (i.e. retroperitoneal abscesses) or pancreatitic necrosis, several pigtail catheters are placed into the cavity using a Seldinger technique. The contamination of healthy tissues (i.e. the pleura cavity) by abscess contents must be avoided. Placing a catheter in the diaphragmatic area (thoracic-abdominal passage) can be accomplished with the use of an externally controlled guide wire and additional fine needles to push away important structures. In case of complicated abscess cavities with fistulae into neighboring organs, the control of the catheter tip position can be accomplished three-dimensionally with a combination of CT and C-arm.

After PAD, a sinogram is most often performed by using an A-P and lateral CT-topogram without changing the patient's position. If a higher detailed image is necessary, especially for demonstrating fistula systems, the C-arm can simultaneously film the sinogram. The sinogram should be performed with antibiotics on board to avoid a sepsis.

Catheter Care

The success of PAD predominantly depends on catheter care. Immediately after placing the catheter, if possible, the entire abscess volume should be aspirated. The abscess cavity is then cleansed with a physiologic salt solution. In order to aspirate viscous and necrotic material through the pigtail catheter, acetylsteine (Mucomyst, Mead Johnson) is injected into the cavity via the catheter.

Biochemically, acetylcysteine breaks disulfate bridges and achieves a liquefaction of even the most viscous abscess contents. This acetylcysteine flushing should be performed at 3–4 hourly intervals.

Observation of the clinical and laboratory parameters is important for the evaluation of the PAD. Normalization of the body temperature and blood tests indicates a succesful PAD. As a rule , 24–28 hours after a PAD the patients should be afebrile.

The time for which the catheter remains in place is normally 14–21 days, but depends on the size and type of the abscess. After partial recovery, the patient can be treated on an out-patient basis with the catheter in place. With proper catheter care, operative revisions are rarely required. A systemic antibiotic therapy (after antibiogram) can shorten the time for which the catheter needs to be in place. An injection of antibiotics into the abscess cavity is rarely required. Sometimes the application of Betadine solution or other disinfectants is used to treat the abscess cavity.

Complications

Complications are rare when using CT guidance for PAD. Possible complications are injury to vessels, bleeding, bacterial contamination, pneumothorax, injuries to neighboring organs and fistula formation. In their patients the authors did not observe any major complications. Minor complications such as shivering attacks from bacteremia were observed and successfully treated.

Indication and contraindications for CT-guided PAD
Indication Abscesses at most locations Contraindications Coagulation disorders of any kind Echinococcus cysts

Literature Review

Van Waes et al. [9] describe 14 percutaneous abscess drainages in which they used acetylcysteine flushes. In their literature review of over 146 patients only 19% needed a surgical revision after PAD.

Knochel et al. [6] report a diagnostic accuracy of 96% for abdominal abscesses with whole-body CT. Van Waes [9] reports a mortality rate directly related to the percutaneous abscess drainage of only 4%. Other authors report that the operative mortality rate is between 30% and 80%, depending on the abscess localization [3, 5]. Berger et al. [1] describe successful percuteaneous liver abscess drainage in 24 patients. They also report of 9 cases where amebic abscesses were successfully treated with PAD, without an operative revision.

The major causes of early failure of percutaneous abscess treatment are too small catheterlumina and insufficient flushing procedures. Furthermore, local injection of antibiotics is not necessary for a successful PAD.

Berkman et al. [2] emphasize the advantages of the CT-guided puncture technique. Only CT is able to clearly define the abscess margins in relationhip to other viscera. For example, they describe a dangerous abscess localization in the area of esophagal varices.

An important paper by Gzozdanovic [4] reports of over 61 direct portograms which had been performed with a 16-G needle. Only one case of bleeding occured. Kumpan [7] describes postoperative compartments which can be a potential location of future abscesses. It is important to be aware of these compartments before a PAD is attempted.

What Ochsner and DeBakey [8] wrote in 1938 is still valid today: "The ideal method for a drainage is characterized by its directness, its simple application and, what is even more important, avoidance of an unnecessary contamination of healthy neighboring structures".

References

1. Berger H., Pratschke E., Berr F., Fink U.: Die perkutane Drainagebehandlung primärer Leberabszesse. Fortschr. Röntgenstr. 150, 2 (1989) 167–170
2. Berkman W.A., Harris W.A., Bernardino M.E.: Non surgical drainage of splenic abscess. Amer. J. Roentgenol. 141 (1983) 395–396
3. Bonfils-Roberts e.A., Barone J.E., Nealon T.F.: Treatment of subphrenic abscess. Surg. Clin. North Am. 55 (1975) 1361–1366
4. Gzozdanovic V., Hauptmann E.: Further experience with percutaneous lienoportal venography. Acta Radiol. 43 (1955) 177–200
5. Karlson K.B., Martin E.C., Frankuchen E.I., Mattern R.F., Schultz R.W., Casarella W.J.: Percutaneous drainage of pancreatic pseudocysts and abscesses. Radiology 142 (1982) 619–524
6. Knochel J.Q., Koehler P.R., Lee T.G., Welch D.M.: Diagnosis of abdominal abscesses with computed tomography, ultrasound, and In-111 leukocyte scans. Radiology 137 (1980) 425–432
7. Kumpan W.: Computertomographische Analyse postoperativer abdomineller Kompartimente und deren Bedeutung für die Abszeßausbreitung sowie Percutane Drainage unilokulärer Abszesse. 4. Workshop Interventionelle Radiologie, Bad Iburg; 7.-8. 11. 1987
8. Ochsner A., DeBakey M.: Subphrenic abscess: a collective review and an analysis of 3608 collected and personal cases. Int. Abstr. Surg. 66 (1938) 462–438
9. van Waes P.F.G.M., Feldberg M.A.M., Mali W.P.Th.M., et al.: Management of located abscesses that are difficult to drain; a new approach. Radiology 147 (1983) 57–63

Figs. 25.1. and **25.2.**
28-year old patient with
septic fever. CT shows evidence of a septated pleural
empyema in the left using
base with a small left he-
mithorax. After puncturing
the central fluid space,
contrast medium was
injected (Fig. 25.1.).

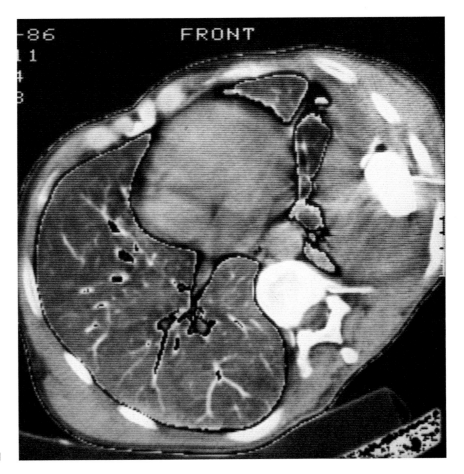

Fig. 25.1

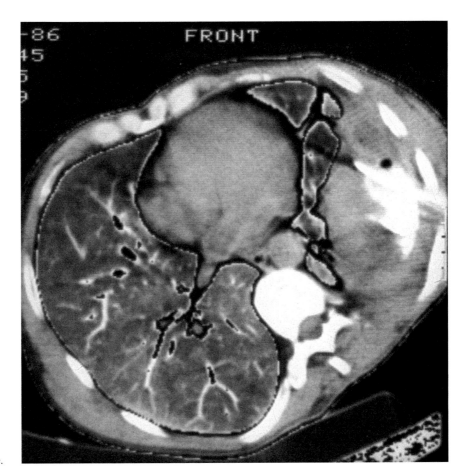

Fig. 25.2. Installation of a
van Sonnenberg drainage.
After the drain was placed
the patient became afebrile.

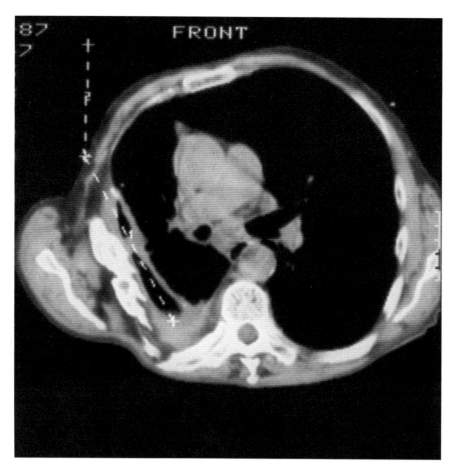

Figs. 25.3.–25.12. 69-year old patient with an old gunshot injury (from the 2nd World War) and pleura/empyema. Present status, post multiple operative revisions. When admitted, the patient was septic and had a high temperature. There was a strong suspicion of a tracheobronchial fistula. CT shows evidence of a large air-filled abscess cavity with an air-fluid level in the left posterolateral thoracic wall. On the right side deformed ribs from multiple thoracotomies are visible (Fig. 25.3.).

Fig. 25.3

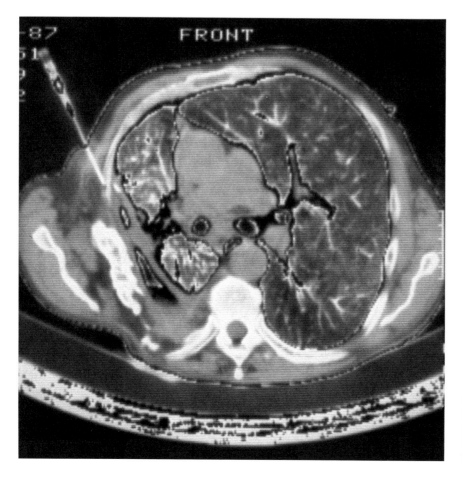

Fig. 25.4. From an anterolateral approach, a fine needle puncture is performed, in direct line with the abscess cavity.

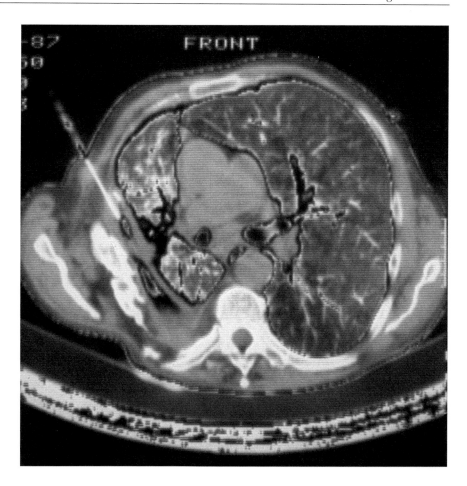

Fig. 25.5. The needle is inside the abscess.

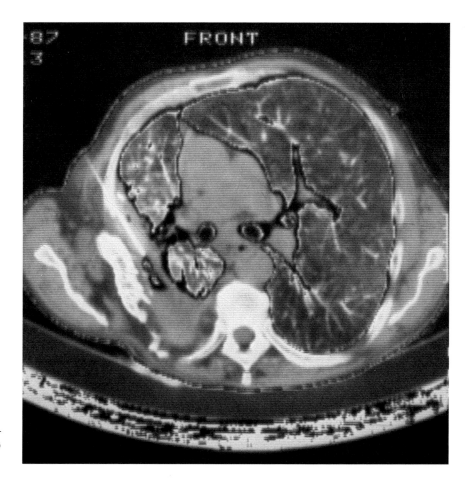

Fig. 25.6. Further advancement of the fine needle into the abscess cavity.

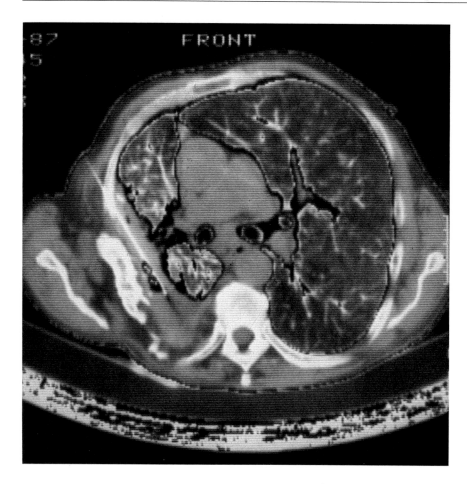

Fig. 25.7. Through the fine needle an 18-G wire is inserted.

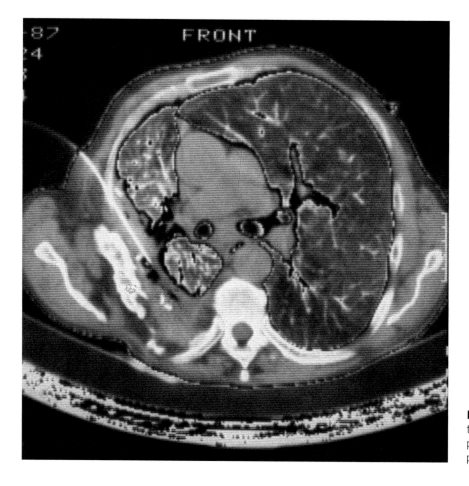

Fig. 25.8. After dilation of the puncture canal, a 7-F pigtail catheter can be placed.

Figs. 25.9. and **25.10.**
Level-by-level documentation of the pigtail catheter
position.

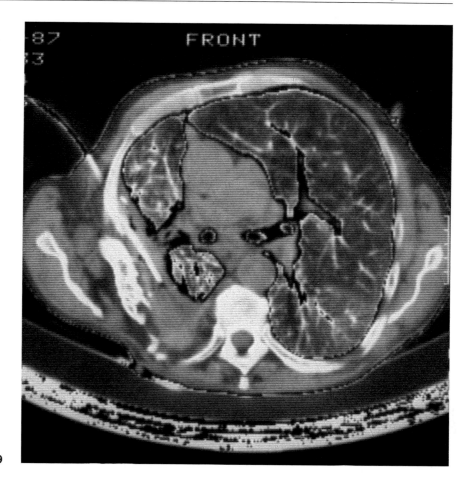

Fig. 25.9

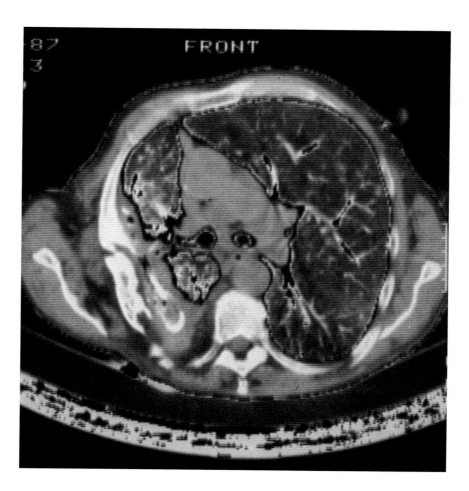

Fig. 25.10

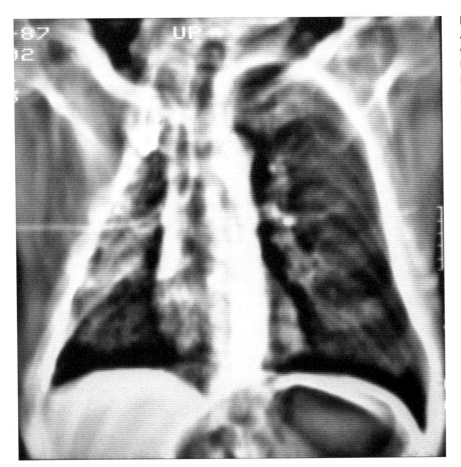

Figs. 25.11. and **25.12.**
A-P and lateral CT topogram after catheter placement. Following this the patient became afebrile. In a second therapy, the fistula was closed using a bronchoscope (Fig. 25.11.).

Fig. 25.11

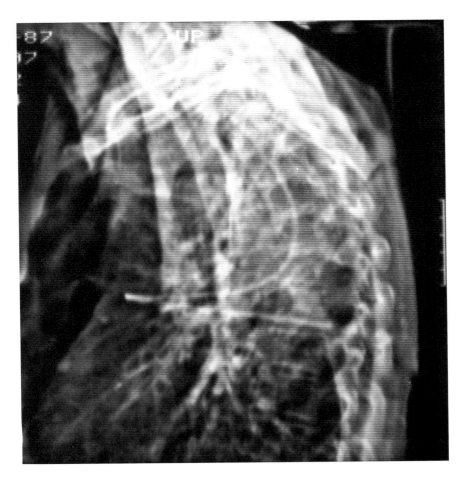

Fig. 25.12

Figs. 25.13.–25.18. Large left-sided psoas abscess. The abscess extends into the subcutaneous fat on the left. Initial focus for this graviation abscess is the pyelonephritic arteriosclerotic left kidney. After puncture, the needle is inside the abscess (Fig. 21.13.).

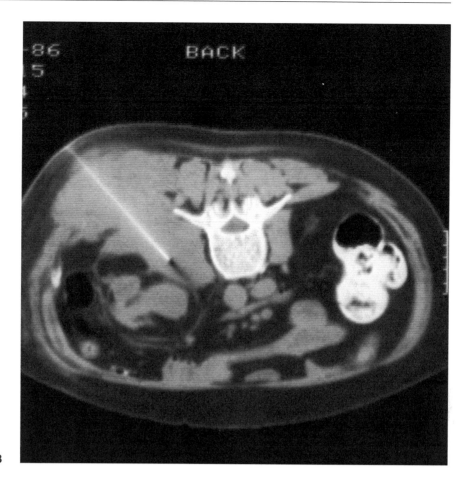

Fig. 25.13

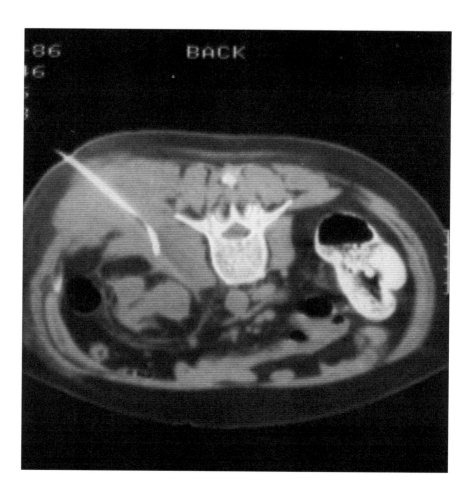

Fig. 25.14. The puncture canal is dilated.

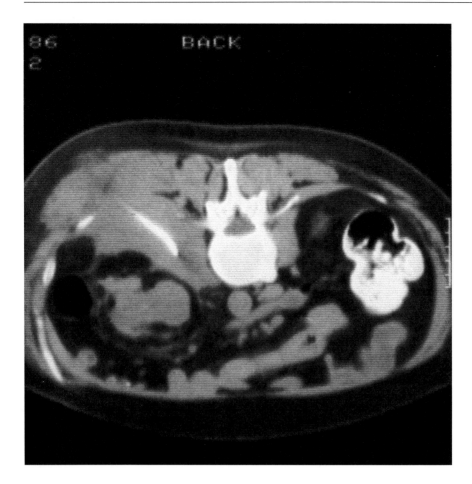

Fig. 25.15. Then a 10-F pigtail catheter is placed.

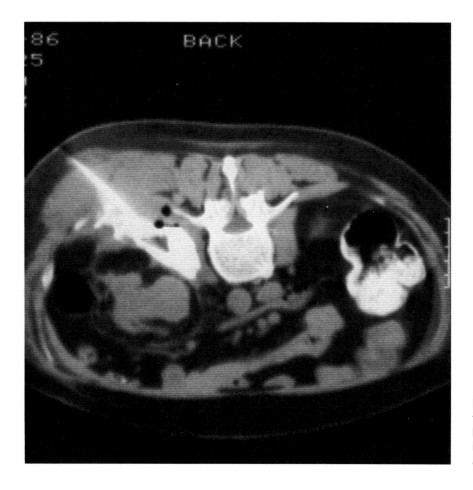

Fig. 25.16. After the contrast-medium injection, a homogeneous distribution is seen within the abscess area.

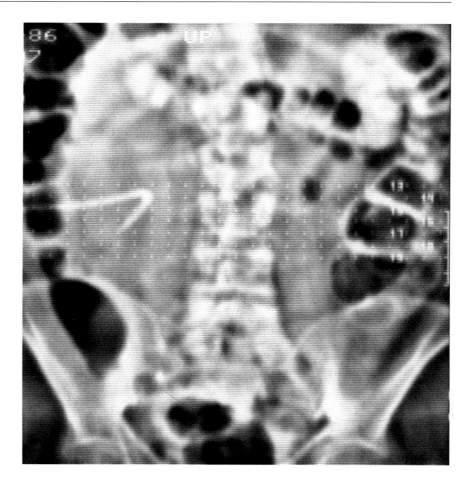

Fig. 25.17. A-P CT-topogram after positioning the drainage catheter. Following afebricity of the patient, the infected arteriosclerotic kidney was removed. An operative revision of the abscess was not required.

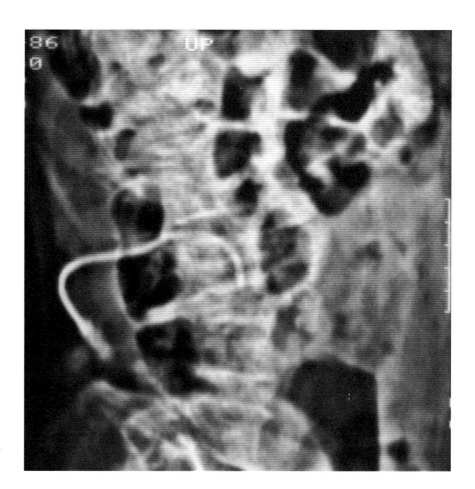

Fig. 25.18. Lateral topogram for documentation of the catheter position.

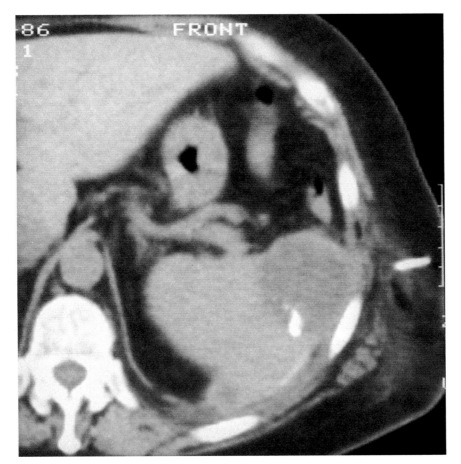

Figs. 25.19.–25.21.
76-year old female patient with septic fever. CT shows evidence of a purulent splenitis. Puncture of the largest abscess is performed from a left lateral approach (Fig. 25.19.).

Fig. 25.19

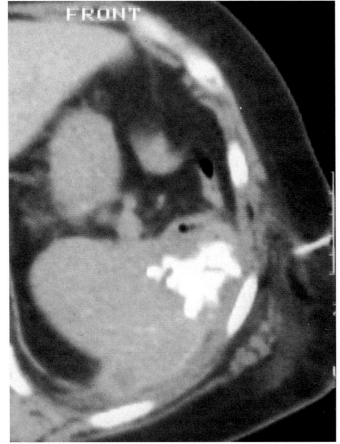

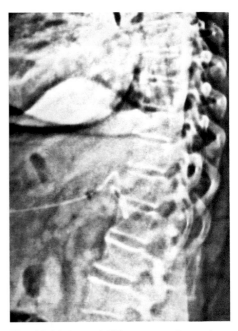

Fig. 25.20. Lateral CT-topogram for catheter position (7-F pigtail). Microbiologic evidence of Klebsiellas. Afebricity of the patient occurred after repeated flushing treatments.

Fig. 25.21. After injection of contrast medium, the distribution within the abscess is easily visible.

Figs. 25.22.–25.30.
66-year old female patient.
Because of choledochus
concrements, a papillotomy
was performed first. During
this therapy, bleeding and
an extensive pneumoretro-
peritoneum developed.
After three days, sepsis
also appeared.

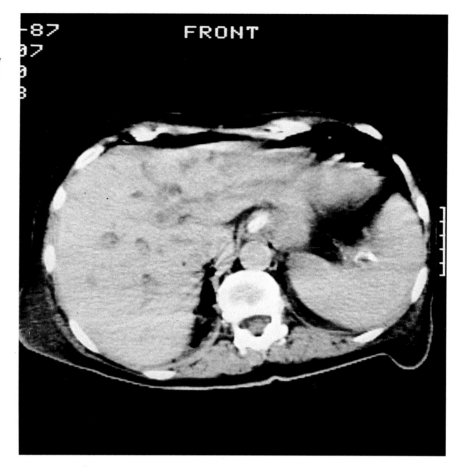

Fig. 25.22. CT scan at the
level of the renal hilus.
Pneumoretroperitoneum
with air below the dia-
phragm is identified on the
right.

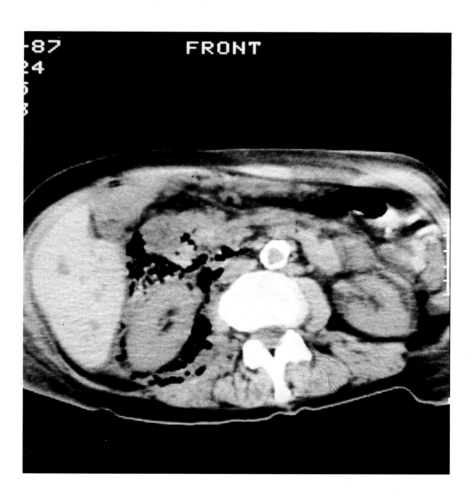

Fig. 25.23. Extensive air
accumulation around the
right kidney.

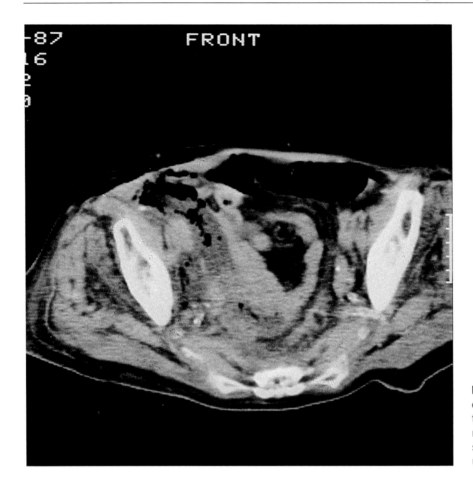

Fig. 25.24. Retroperitoneal extension of fluid around the iliac vessels from the right side. Additionally, air is seen in the retroperitoneum.

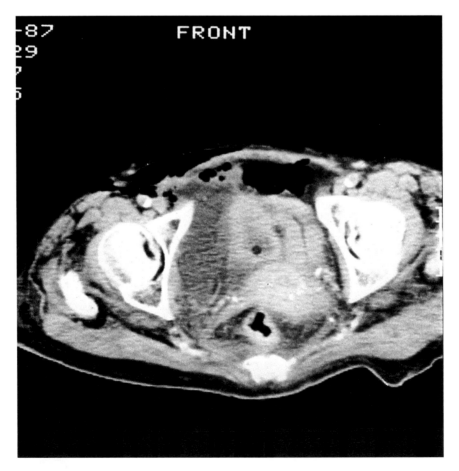

Fig. 25.25. Large fluid accumulation in the right pelvis with displacement of the small intestine. Air is entering the subcutaneous fat under the right inguinal ligament.

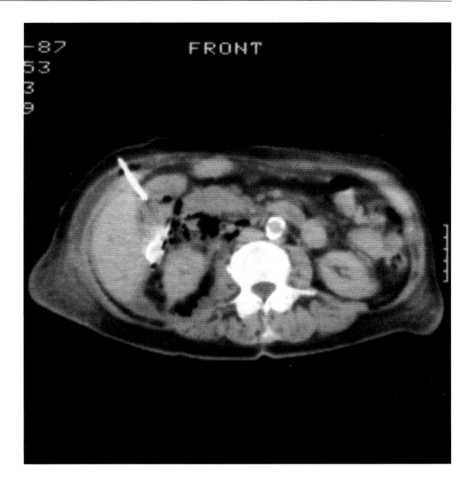

Fig. 25.26. A drainage catheter is placed at the lower liver margin. A liquefied infected hematoma is aspirated.

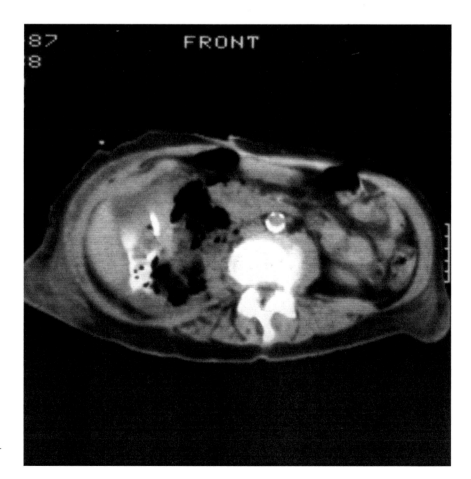

Fig. 25.27. After contrast-medium injection, solid components can be identified in the drained area.

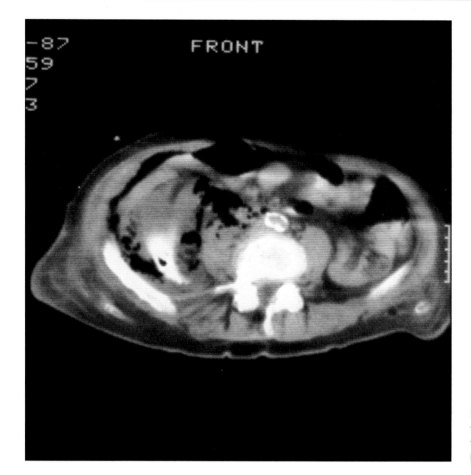

Fig. 25.28. CT scan inferior to Fig. 21.57. demonstrates the contrast-medium distribution caudally.

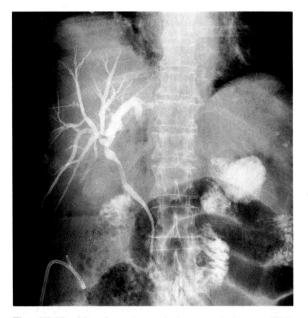

Fig. 25.29. After four days of abscess drainage, PTC was performed. Free outflow of the contrast medium is seen through a normal-calibrated bile duct system. At the right lower corner of the picture, the drainage catheter can be identified.

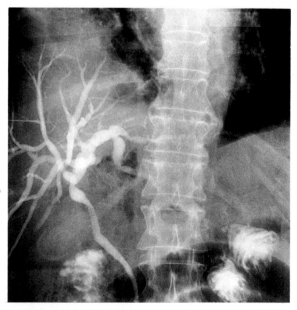

Fig. 25.30. The pneumoretroperitoneum is still recognizable, especially in the region of the right upper pole of the kidney.

Figs. 25.31.–25.40.
59-year old patient after a Wertheim-Meigs operation. Eight days after surgery, an increase of creatinine and sepsis was observed. Additionally, a pelvic vein thrombosis occurred on the left. CT shows evidence of cystic masses in the pelvis, which have led to a massive compression and displacement of the urinary bladder to the right (Fig. 25.31.). The urinary bladder can be identified by the contrast medium and air after catheterization.

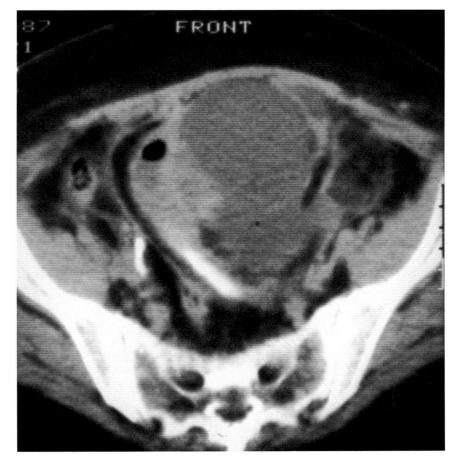

Fig. 25.31

Fig. 25.32. At a lower level (above acetabulum roof), a slit-like constriction of the urinary bladder (filled with contrast medium) is observed. The causes of these impressions are an inhomogenous fluid density structure on the left and another cystic mass with a maximum diameter of 7 cm on the right.

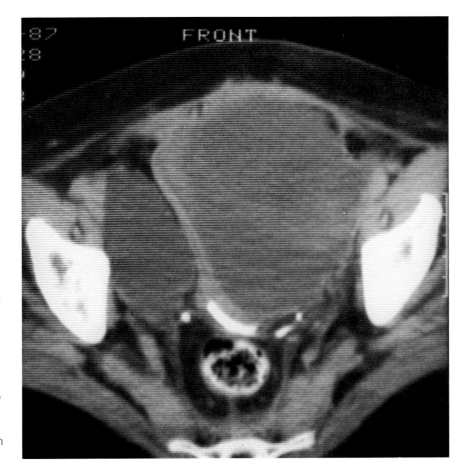

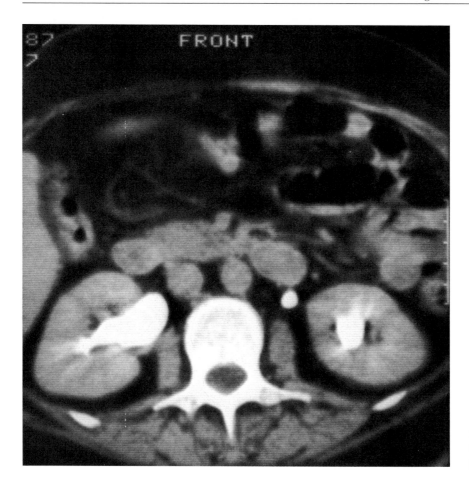

Fig. 25.33. Hydronephrosis with bilateral dilation of the pelvo-caliyceal system.

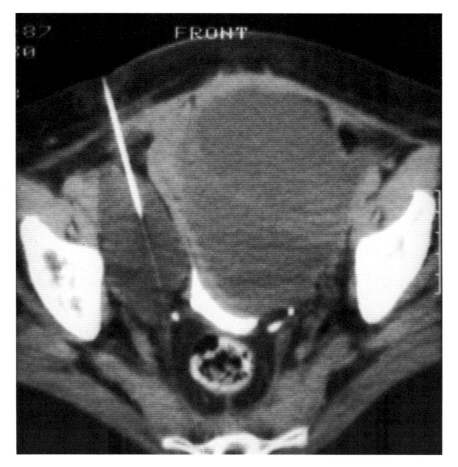

Fig. 25.34. Puncture of the right retroperitoneal fluid collection. Injury to the iliac vessels, which are located lateral to the needle, can be avoided with CT guidance.

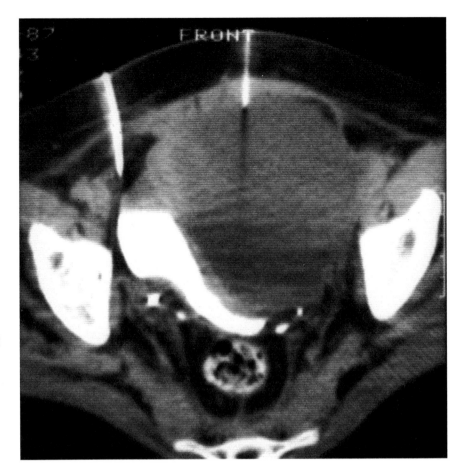

Fig. 25.35. After aspiration of 150 ml of amber-colored fluid, the urinary bladder is now better expanded and extends to the right. The puncture of the other large fluid cavity is performed by a midline approach. A septation in the fluid collection is identified.

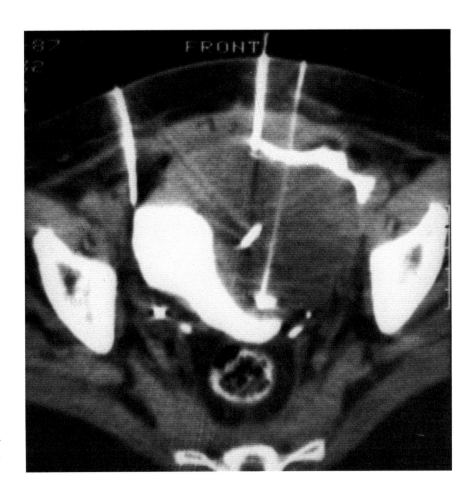

Fig. 25.36. After the puncture, a liquefied hematoma is aspirated.

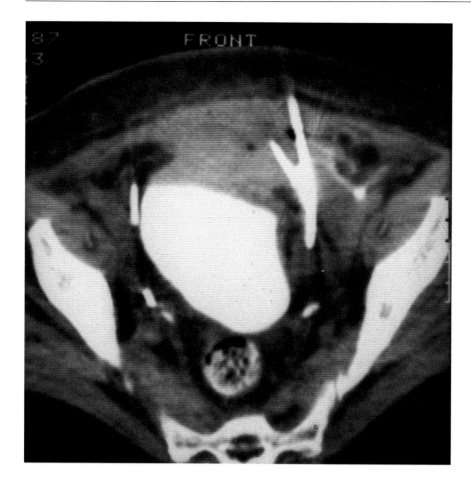

Fig. 25.37. After the hematoma has been removed via two 10-F pigtail drains, the urinary bladder is even more expanded.

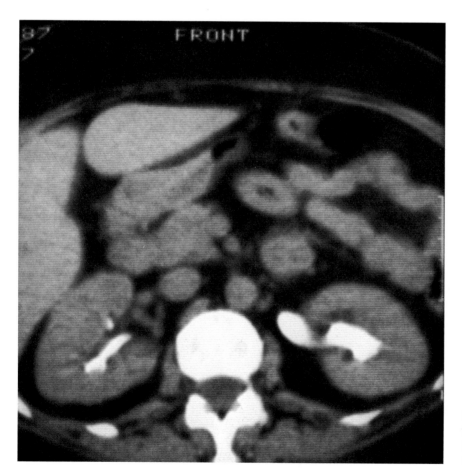

Fig. 25.38. After completion of the drainage therapy, the urinary retention resolved.

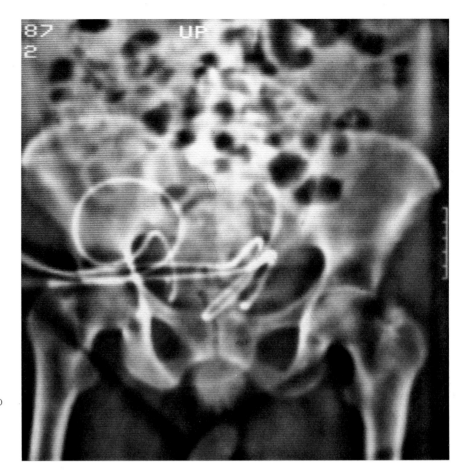

Fig. 25.39. A-P CT-topogram for documentation of the three pigtail drains. Two drains are in the midline hematoma and the third drain is in a retroperitoneal seroma.

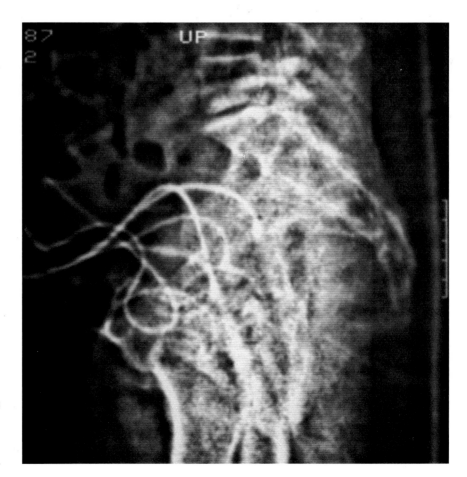

Fig. 25.40. Lateral topogram of the drains. Afebricity of the patient has taken place. A further operative revision of the hematoma and/or the seroma was not necessary.

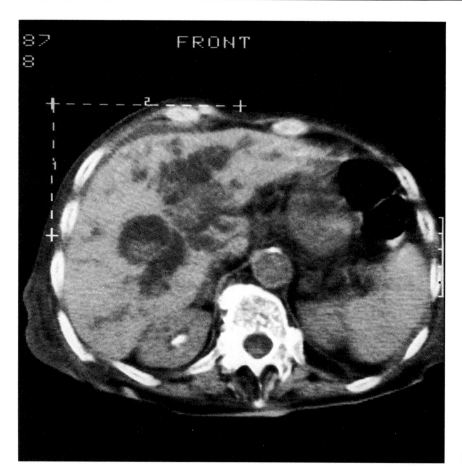

Figs. 25.41. and 25.42.
Posthepatitic icterus in a 78-year old female patient with metastasizing pancreatic carcinoma. Massively dilated intra-hepatic bile ducts are identified in all liver segments (Fig. 25.41.).

Fig. 25.41

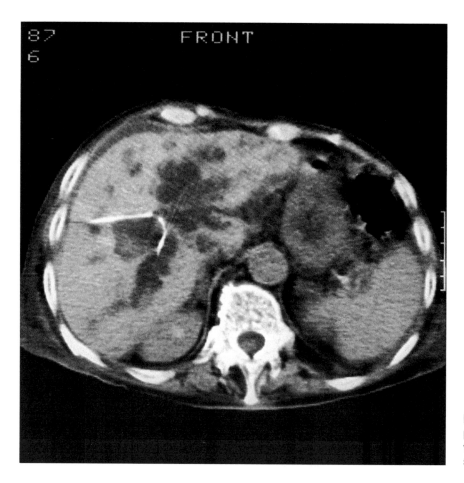

Fig. 25.42. After CT-guided puncture, a pigtail drain was placed for decompression.

Figs. 25.43.–25.46.
54-year old patient with sepsis and elevated temperature. A pancreatic pseudocyst extending from the pancreatic body to the left lobe of the liver is seen. From a caudal approach, a 10-F pigtail drainage was placed in the infected pseudocyst from below the left lobe of the liver (Fig. 25.44.).

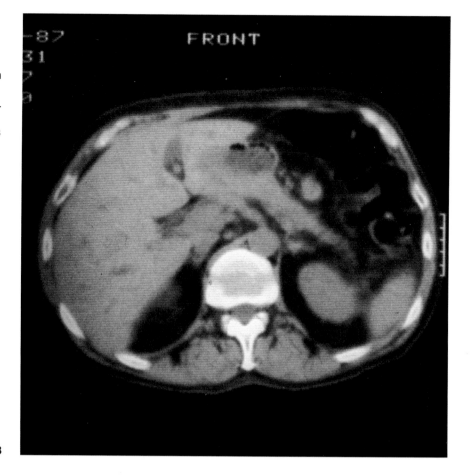

Fig. 25.43

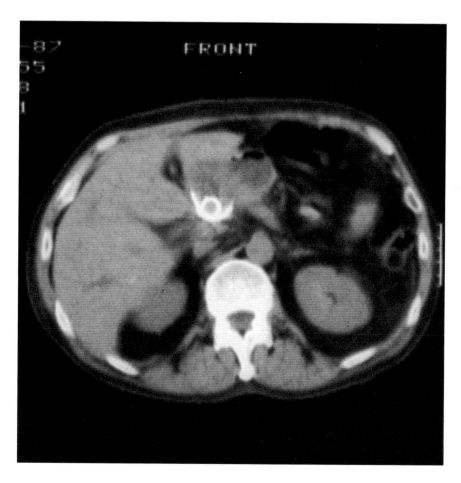

Fig. 25.44

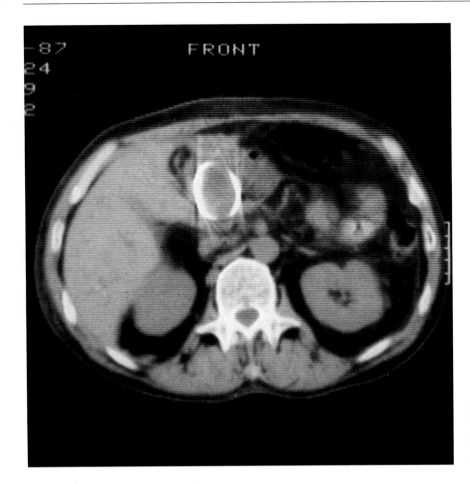

Fig. 25.45. CT-scan at the level of the largest diameter of the pseudocyst. The drain is identified along the wall of the cyst.

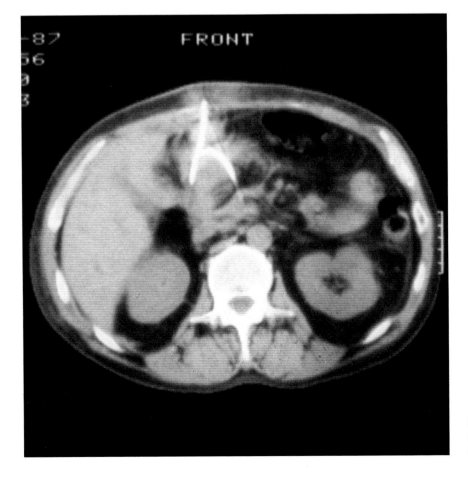

Fig. 25.46. Status post drainage of the pseudocyst.

Figs. 25.47.–25.52.
33-year old patient, admitted for sepsis. CT demonstrates an extensive retropancreatic pseudocyst. There is additional evidence of cystic changes in the spleen (Fig. 25.47.).

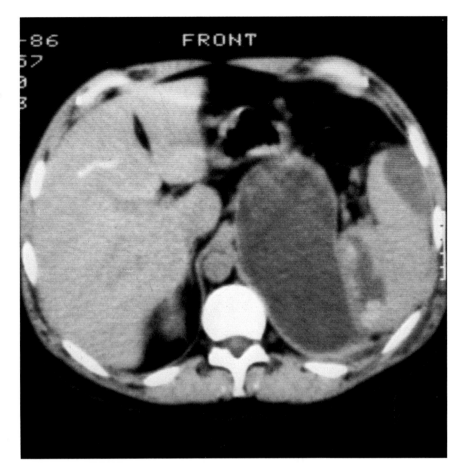

Fig. 25.47

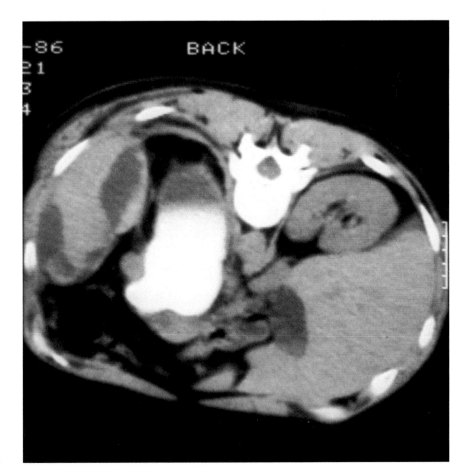

Fig. 25.48. Status post puncture of the retropancreatic pseudocyst with contrast-medium injection, from a posterior approach. Good distribution of the contrast medium is seen with the pseudocyst. Distinct thickening of the diaphragm is seen on the left.

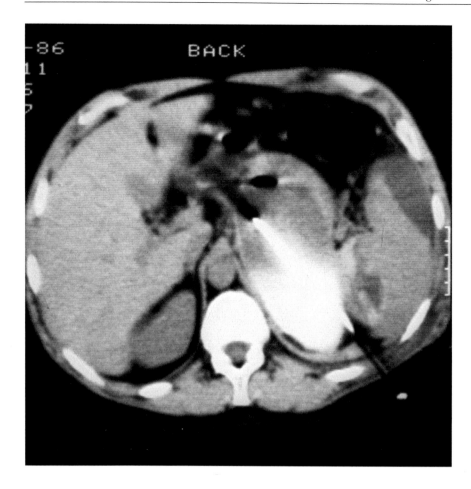

Fig. 25.49. From a posterolateral subdiaphragmatic approach, a 12-F pigtail drain (van Sonnenberg) is placed within the pseudocyst. The contrast-fluid level again appeared after changing the patient's position.

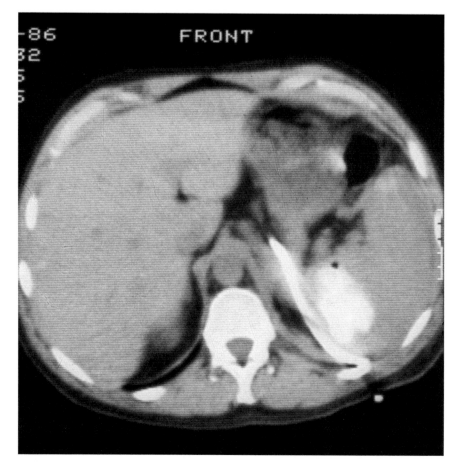

Fig. 25.50. Follow-up scan after 14 days. The pseudocyst has been completely drained. Due to kinking, the drain has to be exchanged. The second procedure was to puncture the fluid spaces in the spleen. A liquefied hematoma was found. After aspirating the hematoma, the splenic drain was removed.

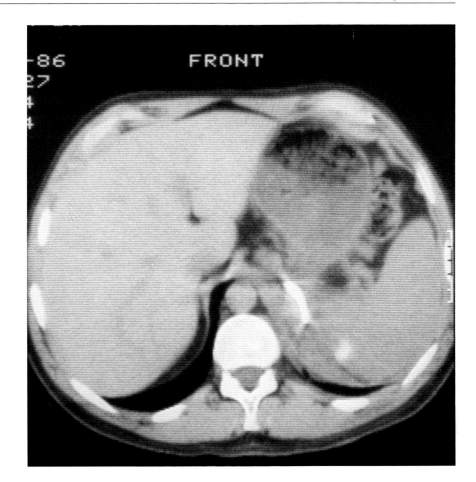

Fig. 25.51. Follow-up ten weeks after the first drainage. The pseudocyst has collapsed. No abnormal densities are identified in the spleen except for a small calcification at the medial border.

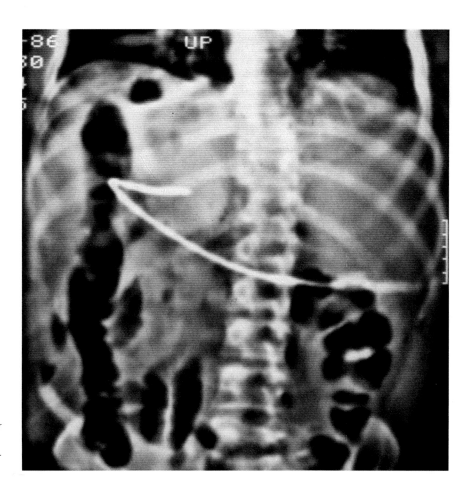

Fig. 25.52. A-P CT-topogram for documentation of the catheter position. After the injection of a diluted contrast medium, a circular cystic fluid collection can be identified in the paravertebral area on the left.

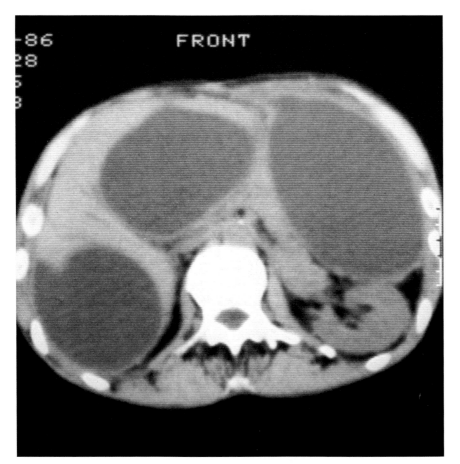

Figs. 25.53.–25.61.
40-year old patient with an extensive cachexia. The patient was hospitalized with sepsis and elevated temperature. Six months earlier, a resection of the pancreatic tail had been performed for pancreatitis. Now the prothrombin value is around 50%. Extensive perihepatic fluid accumulation is seen, reaching to the subphrenic area on the left. The stomach is completely compressed by the fluid (Fig. 25.53.).

Fig. 25.53

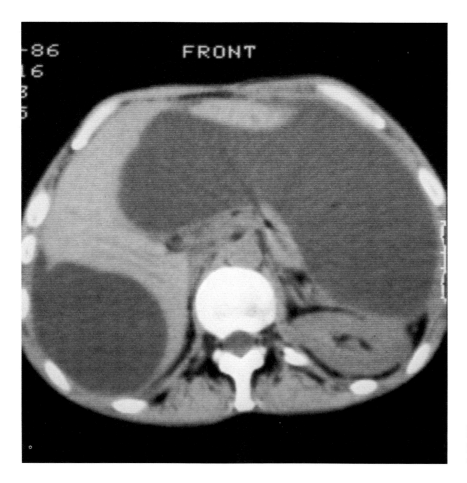

Fig. 25.54. Massive compression of the liver parenchyma by the cyst mass.

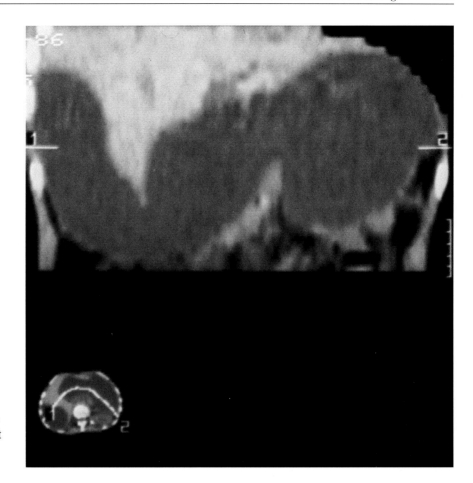

Fig. 25.55. In the curved reconstruction image, a communicating fluid cavity is found with displacement and compression of the liver.

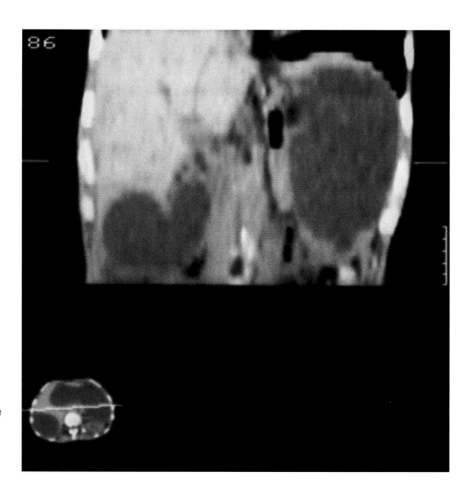

Fig. 25.56. Coronal reconstruction image through the stomach and hilus of the liver. Massive compression of the stomach with minimal air filling is seen.

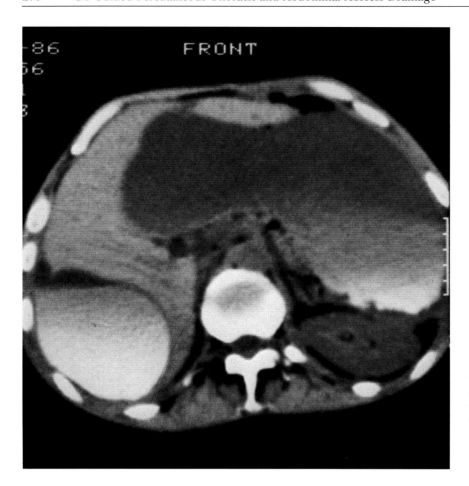

Fig. 25.57. After puncture from the left, contrast medium is injected into the fluid collection. The contrast medium was also immediately distributed to the right. This proves the free communication of the fluid.

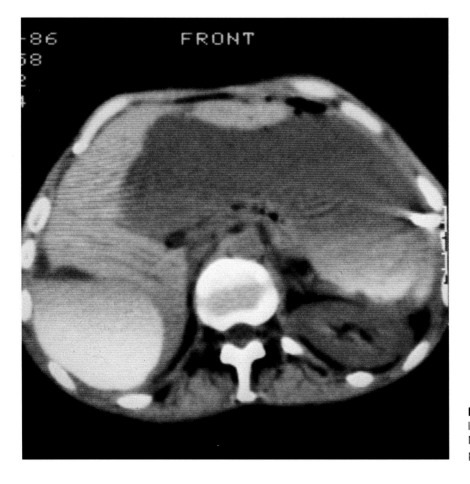

Fig. 25.58. Then, from the left lateral approach, a 14-F Mallecot drainage was placed.

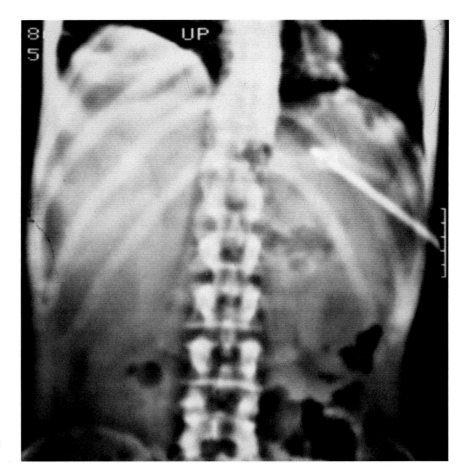

Fig. 25.59. A-P CT topogram for documentation of the position of the Mallecot drain.

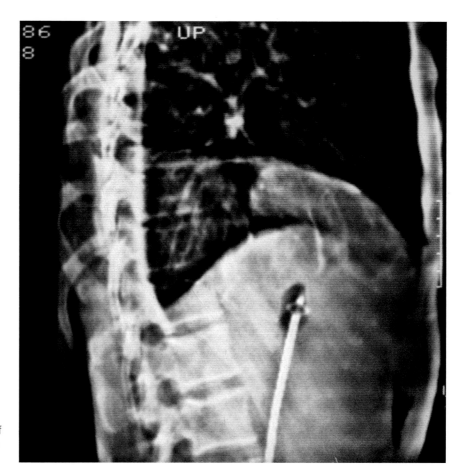

Fig. 25.60. Lateral topogram demonstrating the drain. A total of five liters of pus was removed. The patient then became afebrile.

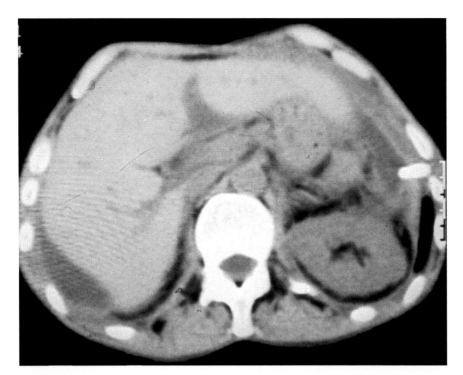

Fig. 25.61. Follow-up CT scan one week after the drainage procedure. Only a minor amount of residual fluid remained around the liver. The stomach has also re-expanded. The liver parenchyma now shows a normal structure. The prothrombin value at this time has increased to 80%.

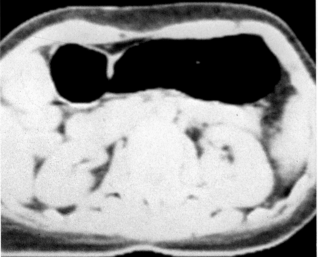 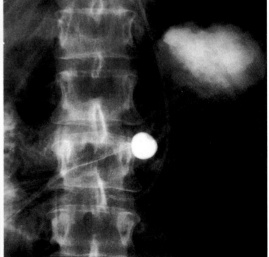

Figs. 25.62. and **25.63.** CT-guided puncture for percutaneous gastrostomy. 39-year old patient with inoperable esophageal carcinoma. With a slightly bent angiography catheter, the tumor obstruction was transversed and the stomach filled with air. This can normally be performed without difficulty under conventional fluoroscopy using a soft angiography guide wire and if required a contrast injection through the catheter. After Buscopan injection, the stomach is distended with air. Maximal filling of the stomach with gas displaces organs at risk outside the puncture area, notably the liver and colon. Further, the puncture is easier to perform because the thinner gastric wall is stretched and lies against their anterior abdominal wall over a large area. The introduction of a catheter also becomes easier because of the firm support given to the gastric wall by the air in the stomach.

For this puncture, we first use an anchor set (Cook Inc.). Along with the puncture needle, a T-like anchor is introduced with the guide wire. The needle is removed, the anchor pulled, and the anterior gastric wall is thus reliably fixed. This facilitates the safe introduction of the gastrostomy-balloon set via the guide wire. No further fluoroscopic or CT follow-ups are necessary. The gastrostomy catheter we use is the Lunderquist-gastrostomy-balloon-set. It can also be used for direct puncture. In earlier work, we used sonography for visualizing the puncture point during the procedure. But, CT has advantages, especially when puncturing directly. The position of the neighboring organs are much better documented with CT. Also the best puncture point (in the middle of or lateral to the rectus sheath, to avoid a puncture of the superior epigastric a.) is much easier to determine. Judging the puncturing depth by measuring the distance to the posterior gastric wall is not possible with sonography.

In this patient, after CT-guided puncture, a strong guide wire was introduced through the needle, and then a balloon catheter system was implanted over the wire under conventional fluoroscopic control. In this way percutaneous gastrostomy is easy to perform with CT and local anesthesia. Furthermore, it is a reliable, quick and safe procedure. Another technique for air filling of the stomach is by CT-guided puncture using a 22G-needle. This procedure is very easy to perform.

Chapter 26
Drainage Techniques in Interventional Radiology

H. Weigand

Diagnosis of abscesses and fluid accumulation was made predominantly by operative measures until the development of ultrasound and computer-tomography. These new imaging techniques especially CT, are today considered as the diagnostic procedure of choice for the documentation and description of topography, expansion, and internal structure of fluid collections.

The first step in the development of non-surgical catheter placement was CT- and US-guided fine needle punctures for diagnostic serologic and/or bacteriologic studies.

The image quality of CT is superior to that of sonography, especially for drainage placement. The access route and positioning of the catheter within the fluid collection can be determined prior to the CT procedure. The selection of a catheter depends on the amount, contents and structure of the fluid accumulation. In central, thoracic or abdominally located abscesses or fluid accumulations, it may be necessary to use a bolus CT technique at the planned puncture level to show larger vessels, so that these can be avoided during puncture. As a matter of principle, the shortest access route should be selected. However, in particular cases, it may be necessary to select a longer access route, often transhepatic, to avoid injuries to abdominal structures (i.e. intestine, stomach, kidneys, and large vessels). Also, the expected duration of drainage has to be taken into consideration in determining the access route.

A subphrenic or subhepatic abscess can heal in one to two weeks with systemic medication and drainage, whereas a pancreatic pseudocyst can take more than three months to heal completely.

The majority of these drainage cases are patients who have had one or more operations, so most are willing to tolerate a drainage catheter for an extended period of time. It is crucial that the tip of the catheter rests at the lowest area to be drained. Therefore, it must be taken into consideration whether the patient is mostly bedridden or ambulatory. In patients with infected drainage material, periodic flushes with antibiotics are performed. The appropriate antibiotics are determined by an antibiogram. These antibiotic flushes are first performed at short intervals, and at longer intervals later in the treatment. For non-necrotic fluid accumulations, a simple drainage bag without suction can be used. After a short period in hospital, the patients can return home under the care of the family doctor for continued treatment. Plain films, with contrast medium if needed, and CT are often useful for follow-up in a long-term drainage.

Materials

Catheters suitable for drainage should have the following properties: A Sliding capability, relatively sturdy, and made of X-ray dense material. B A row of holes with a large lumen along the inner curve of a pigtail or curved catheter. A terminal lumen with additional mushroom configuration is also possible. C At least one large interior lumen and, if needed, a second thinner lumen in tandem position for flushing. D Luer-Lok nozzle for connection with the drainage bag. E Availability in 6–24 French.

Drainage Technique

First, the puncture depth and angle are determined on the CT-monitor. Then, after local anesthesia, with CT guidance a relatively thin teflon-coated cannula is inserted into the area to be drained. After removal of the mandrin and aspiration of a few millimeters of fluid for serology, bacteriology and possible cytology, a guide wire is inserted without removal of large amounts of fluid. Only fluoroscopy is necessary for the remainder of the procedure. With the guide wire in place under a sterile cover, the patient can be moved from CT to a conventional fluoroscopy room.

After dilation of the tract to the desired lumen under fluoroscopy-control at multiple angles, the final catheter can be inserted using the Seldinger technique. Small amounts of a diluted contrast medium are injected into the abscesses or fluid collections to help visualize their extent. After final positioning, the drainage catheter is fixed to the skin and covered with sterile dressing.

The following examples will explain the use of drainage catheters in the thoracic and abdominal region for different indications.

First Example

This patient has chronic recurring attacks of a necrotizing pancreatitis and is status post three surgical procedures. With the drains from the third operation still in place, the patient developed over a three-month period a large pseudocyst in the pancreatic body-tail region with a central hypodense area (Fig. 26.1a,b,c.). The follow-up scans at this time show an increase in thickening of the pseudocyst wall and a further increase in the central necrosis (Fig. 26.1c.). Additionally, extensive necrotic stranding is seen along the vessel inferiorly and along the left psoas muscle into the posterior abdominal wall to the back musculature. The danger of an external abscess perforation exists (Fig. 26.2.). Two van Sonnenberg drains are inserted in exchange for the operatively placed drains. The tips of the van Sonnenberg drains are placed into the main branches of the abscess cavities using fluoroscopy-guidance at several angles (Fig. 26.3a,b.).

The central cavity, located in the body-tail area, is drained by an open-end soft silicone drain with a large lumen, using the same tract as the previously placed drains (Figs. 26.4a,b.). The total drainage time was 13 weeks. During the last part of this time, the drains were drawn back step by step so that, in a final follow-up film immediately prior to the removal of the drains, only a small residual canal can be seen after contrast injection (Fig. 26.5.).

Second Example

After an operation for a trauma-induced liver rupture, this female patient developed an intrahepatic abscess in the lower right lobe. This resulted in a second operation being necessary. The second operation was followed by a recurrence of the intrahepatic abscess and the development of a subphrenic abscess. The patient then developed an extensive pleural effusion

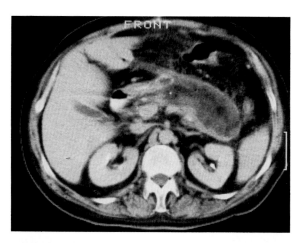

Fig. 26.1b

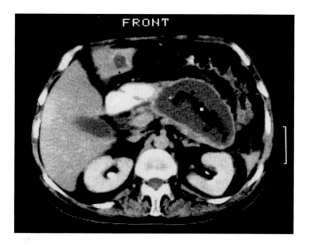

Fig. 26.1c

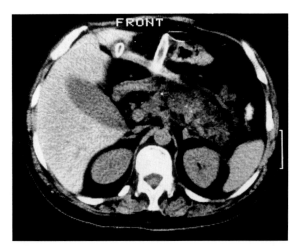

Fig. 26.1a

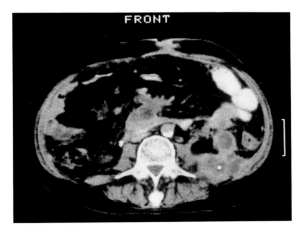

Fig. 26.2

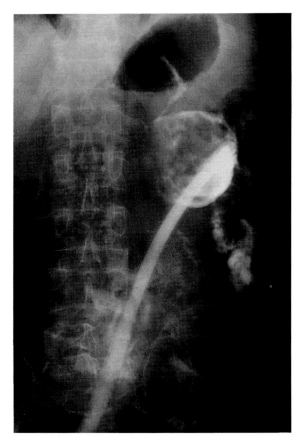

Fig. 26.3a

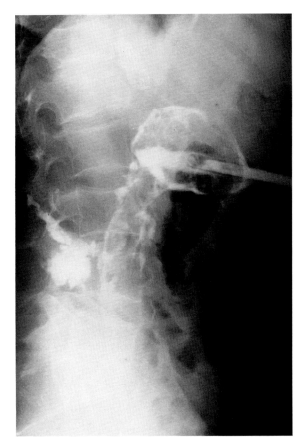

Fig. 26.3b

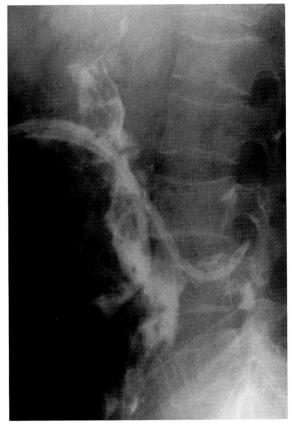

Fig. 26.4a

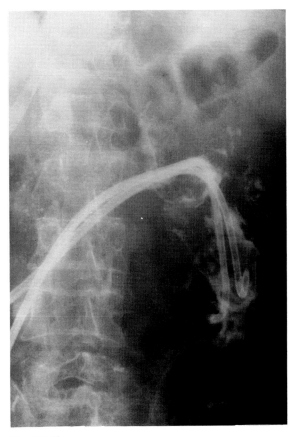

Fig. 26.4b

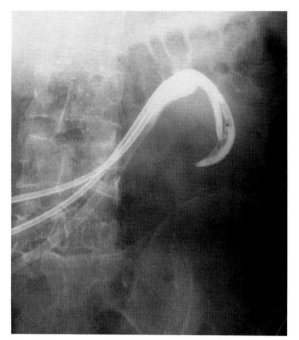

Fig. 26.5

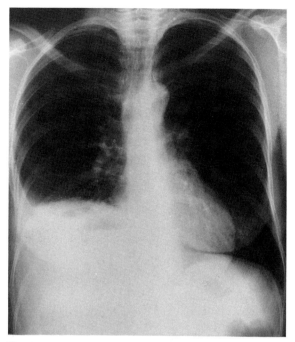

Fig. 26.6a

and progressive deterioration. CT at this time shows a subphrenic and an intrahepatic pneumatized abscess (Fig. 26.6a, b, c). A van Sonnenberg drain was placed percutaneously to drain the subphrenic abscess, and in exchange for the operatively placed intrahepatic abscess drain another van Sonnenberg drain was inserted into the intrahepatic abscess (Fig. 26.7 a, b.).

After frequent initial flushing with antibiotic solution following an antibiogram, later planning film follow-ups using contrast medium were obtained and flushes performed at greater time intervals. After a rapid regression of the abscesses, the subphrenic and intrahepatic abscess catheters were removed in a step-by-step fashion. At the time of the final catheter removal, after approximately eight weeks, there was only a minor residual canal without any purulent secretion (Fig. 26.8.).

Since that time, the patient has been symptom-free and does not show any extensive scarring in the region of the diaphragm.

With proper drainage technique and close follow-ups, a high rate of success without serious complications can be obtained. In the authors' experience over several years, no secondary infection or major bleeding has been observed and subsequent emergency operations were not required.

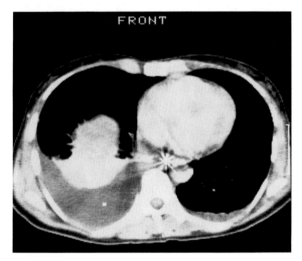

Fig. 26.6b

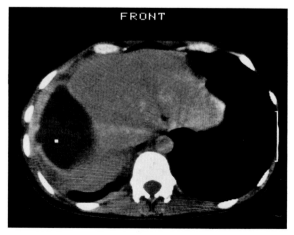

Fig. 26.6c

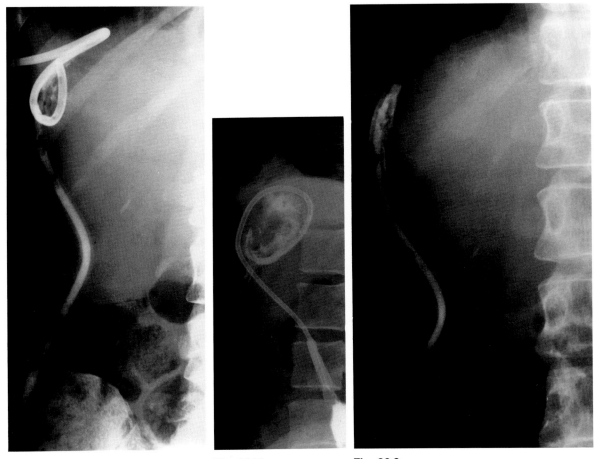

Fig. 26.7a   **Fig. 26.7b**   **Fig. 26.8**

Chapter 27
CT-Guided Therapeutic Liver Procedures

G.M. Richter, H.-J. Brambs, G.W. Kauffmann

Since the beginning of the eighties there has been an increase in CT-guided punctures of the liver performed by radiologists. The reasons for this increase in liver procedures are many, such as a greater demand for a preoperative pathologic diagnosis, closer tumor monitoring in cancer patients, the increased findings of sonographic indistinct liver processes, and also improved needles and instrumentation enabling a more reliable procedure.

Therapeutic Puncture and Drainage

In the radiologic literature, CT-guided diagnostic liver punctures far outnumber ultrasound-guided liver punctures for obtaining a pathologic diagnosis. However, the ratio is reversed for therapeutic procedures such as acute decompression of the bile ducts or for liver abscess drainage. In the majority of these cases ultrasound is sufficient to visualize a suitable access route. Furthermore, these drainage procedures most often use a larger gauge needle which is easier to visualize on ultrasound. However, the authors' experience shows that, there are situations where a CT-guided approach is better and safer. This is especially true for liver lesions deep and central in the right lobe, in the caudate lobe, in the hilar area, or lesions which are both extra- and intrahepatic in the region of the hilus. Also, highly septated lesions which can possibly be drained through several access routes are better suited for CT guidance because the septa are more easily visualized with CT than US.
Indications for interventional radiologic drainage of the liver are:
1. Pyogenic liver abscess (portalvenous, systemic);
2. abscess of the biliary system;
3. infected biloma (i.e. post-operative or post-percutaneous transhepathic procedure complication);
4. amebic abscess (complete or ruptured);
5. infected hematomas (i.e. post-traumatic or after liver transplantation).

A controversial indication for interventional drainage is that of a hydatid cyst (echinococcus

hydiatidosus). There are reports in the literature of using this procedure, but there are also reports about the danger of anaphylactic reactions and of peritoneal disseminations of the parasites.
The technique of the therapeutic liver puncture deviates in several aspects from the purely diagnostic puncture. The localization of the lesion is performed in the same way. For all interventional procedures, a "Unidwell" needle (Angiomed) with an outside radius of 4-F (= 1.32 mm) and of medium length (17 cm) is used for initial puncture. This needle consists of a trocar with a stylet, diagonally cut, tightly fitted into a teflon catheter. After verification that the needle tip is positioned within the lesion (this can most often be recognized by spontaneous reflux of purulent material), as much fluid as possible is aspirated and sent for bacteriologic and, if required, cytologic analysis. For the simplest liver abscess a one-time decompression is sufficient. After decompression, contrast is injected into the abscess cavity. Because CT is used for documentation, a highly diluted contrast medium is adequate. In all cases in which a long term drainage is to be used (such as complicated liver abscesses and points 2 to 5 of the above indication list), treatment should be performed under fluoroscopy-control. After careful contrast injection into the abscess cavity (Caution: high injection pressure can lead to sepsis) through the teflon catheter, previously fixed to the skin, an exchange for another drainage system is performed using the Seldinger technique. An important principle in abscess drainage is that the more viscous the fluid to be drained, the larger the lumen of the drainage catheter must be. Loop-catheters between 7- and 9-F that can be arrested are used for low viscous fluids, but for fluids with a high viscosity the insertion of 14-F wash-suction systems (i.e. van Sonnenberg sump catheter, from BSIC) is necessary. Each drainage system has to be installed in such a way that all the side holes are located within the lesion. The drainage procedure is considered to be successful when the following results are obtained:
– Reflux of clear fluid after injection into the abscess cavity;
– significant reduction in abscess cavity size;

– clinical improvement, especially in fever, for more than two days;
– stable condition after functional test (i.e. clamping of the catheter for at least 48 hours);
– improvement in laboratory tests, especially the CBC.

After the drainage system is no longer needed, it can be removed in one step. This is true even for large lumen catheters. Own experience as well as that of other authors has demonstrated a success rate which greatly depends on the indication for the procedure. The overall success rate is between 70% and at least 90%. The best results are found for the drainage of solitary liver abscesses, with an almost 100% chance of clinical improvement after percutaneous decompression. Results with complex abscesses which are insufficiently drained or form sequestration are much worse. An example is the drainage of infected post-traumatic abscesses which often can be maintained through hematogenous and/or biliary spread. In conclusion, CT-guided therapeutic liver procedures have a high clinical effectiveness combined with a low morbidity and mortality rate which almost always justifies an interventional radiologic drainage attempt prior to surgical decompression.

Future Outlook

Chapter 28
Interventional Magnetic Resonance Imaging

D.H.W. Grönemeyer, R.M.M. Seibel, M. Busch, A.M. Schmidt, J. Plassmann, P.A. Rothschild, L. Kaufman, D. Kramer

Interventional procedures in the past were performed with either fluoroscopic, sonographic or CT guidance, but at present MRI-guided interventional procedures are being developed. The excellent tissue differentiation provided by magnetic resonance imaging (MRI) in comparison with other techniques can be very beneficial for interventional procedures. In 1986, Thomas [17] was the first to describe MRI-guided biopsies in the brain, which was then followed by reports in 1987 by Bradford, Grunert, and Kelly [4, 7, 10]. So far, the possibilities for interventional procedures using MRI had been limited by the narrow tube-like design of the magnet and the long acquisition time, when compared with other guidance methods. Therefore, up to now, MRI interventions have been rather complicated and difficult to perform. Furthermore, only a few MRI-compatible instruments were available, since most surgical devices are made from ferro-magnetic material [14]. These ferro-magnetic instruments produce large artifacts that can make discrimination of tissue structures and visualization of the interventional instrument possible. Recently, special puncture needles have been developed. In 1986, Mueller and Stark [13] reported the successful construction of an MRI-compatible needle. Using this instrument the first liver biopsies were performed and also in the same year a series of prostate biopsies were reported [9]. Additionally, in 1986, van Sonnenberg [18] reported the clinical use of MRI-compatible interventional materials, specifically plastic catheters and stents for drainage procedures. In 1987, Lufkin, Teresi, and Hanafee [11] developed puncture needles for head and neck biopsies. After the installation of an open MRI at the authors' institute, they explored the possibilities of using the system for interventional procedures.

Open MRI

Low-field MRI, developed by the Radiologic Imaging Laboratory of the University of California at San Francisco [15], was the first open MRI-system (Fig. 28.1.). This MRI (ACCESS, Toshiba America MRI, Inc.) uses a permanent magnet with a field strength of 0.064 Tesla. The low-field system complements mid- and high-field systems for clinical-diagnostic-interventional use. The prerequisite for precise interventional localization of good tissue differentiation is accomplished by this open MR-system.

In the past, the diagnostic possibilities of low-field MRI were underestimated. Therefore, in order to assess this MR, the authors will explain in detail the physical and technical aspects, as well as the image quality. The efficiency and problems of permanent magnets have been the subject of extensive research [2, 5], so will only be mentioned briefly here.

The advantages of permanent magnets in comparison with other types of magnetic include: no cryogens or electricity required to maintain the magnetic field; relatively low maintenance cost; and a small fringe-field. Furthermore, solenoidal RF-coils can be used to improve the signal-to-noise ratio [1, 15]. Previously, the major disadvantages of these permanent magnet systems were their heavy weight (approximately 100 tons for the highest available field strength), temperature sensitivity, and a maximum practical field strength of about 0.3 Tesla [2, 5, 6, 16]. Furthermore, for interventional procedures, problems arose because of the narrow distance between the poles of the magnets.

The permanent magnet low-field system has a weight of only 7 tons. This serves to decrease both transport and installation difficulties. Also, this vertical field magnet is open on all four sides. The distance between the poles is 60 cm and the 5-Gauss line is approximately 60 cm from the edge of the magnet. The minimum size of the RF room is 15 m². Since a separate transmitter coil is a permanent part of the system, multiple simpler and less expensive receive-only type coils are used. The receive coils have a unique solenoid design providing an increased S/N ratio (Fig. 28.2.). Another advantage is the minimal gradient noise because of the low magnetic field and flat gradient coils.

When compared with the enclosed tube-like design superconductive magnets, the patient lying in the open design low-field system is gen-

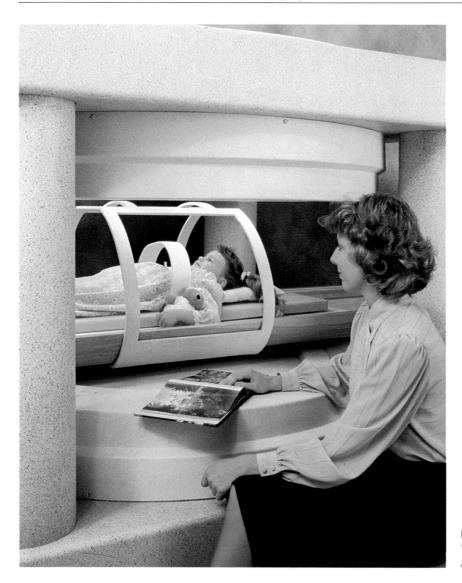

Fig. 28.1. The open "ACCESS" MRI (Toshiba America MRI, Inc.).

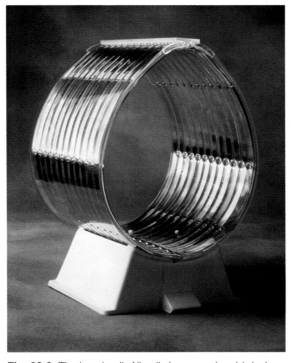

Fig. 28.2. The head coil. All coils have a solenoid design.

erally more comfortable and relaxed. As a result, patients tend to be more cooperative and amenable to percutaneous procedures. Additionally, claustrophobic as well as frightened patients can be examined in a more cooperative and relatively less upsetting manner. Therefore, sedation can be avoided or significantly reduced in many cases. Also, children and seriously ill patients can be accompanied and cared for during the scanning with continuous observation and, if necessary, life-support systems. Additionally, MRI of trauma-related injuries can be performed very readily.

In essence, percutaneous procedures using this low-field system may be approached in much the same manner as with either fluoroscopy- or sonography-guided techniques (Fig. 28.3.). After imaging, the patient can be easily removed from the center of the magnet to perform major interventional procedures where greater access is needed.

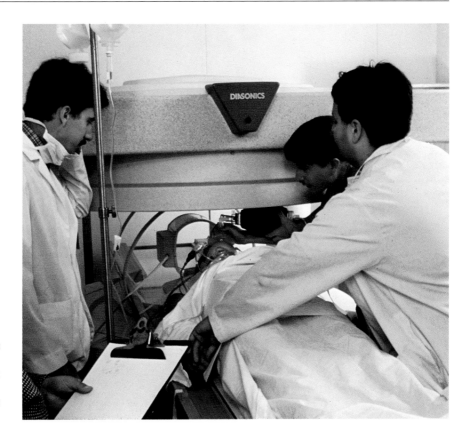

Fig. 28.3. The open design of the MRI system allows for ventilation of the patient and/or for therapeutic procedures to be performed in the magnet.

Safety Aspects of Low-Field MRI

The projectile effect of the low-field system is minimal in comparison with higher-field MR. This significantly reduces the principal and most immediate health risk of MR imaging. Additionally, it is possible to use emergency life-support equipment in close proximity with even an oxygen cylinder and a ventilator positioned next to the magnet. At the University of New Mexico in Albuquerque, small oxygen cylinders are often placed on the patient table during the MRI examination of intubated children. Furthermore, there is sufficient room inside the magnet to ventilate a patient (Fig. 28.3.). A further safety aspect is the very low RF power deposition, which permits highly efficient imaging sequences without discomfort or hazard to the patient from the RF heating.

The almost complete absence of gradient acoustic noise, permits communication with the patient at all times. The open structure of the system allows for continuous observation with the ability to give medication during the procedure. Since ionizing radiation is not used and due to the fact that to date no serious side-effects have been reported from currently used MR-systems, exposure hazards probably do not exist for patient or doctor, even for long periods. For the future developments of interventional procedures this will be a crucial factor.

Physical and Technical Aspects

The main disadvantages of the low-field system compared with higher field MR are the lower signal-to-noise ratio per unit time, the fewer number of slices per TR, and often longer examination times for the patient. On the other hand, the low-field has an approximately three times higher absolute homogeneity in comparison with high-field systems. Additional advantages of the low-field imaging system are the shortening of the T1-time and the reduction in motion and flow-related artifacts. These shorter T1-times serve to increase the signal for a given TR. Also, special techniques have been developed such as extreme bandwidth reduction, which is combined with asymmetrical echoes to provide improved S/N (Fig. 28.4.). This extreme bandwidth reduction is rarely used at high-field because of a considerable increase of susceptibility and chemical-shift artifacts. The improved signal-to-noise ratio for this technique is far beyond expectations based on the concept of linear dependency of field strength to signal-to-noise ratio. Another advantage of the vertical field magnet is the simple solenoidal structure of the receiver coils which allows for relatively quick development of special interventional coils (Fig. 28.2.).

The sequences used at low-field are significantly different from those used at higher-field

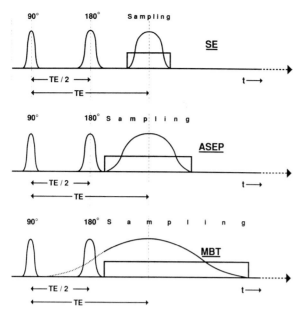

Fig. 28.4. Development steps from early spin-echo technique (SE) to more advanced techniques such as narrow-bandwidth with symmetrical echo-sampling and asymmetrical echo-sampling (matched-bandwidth technique (MBT).

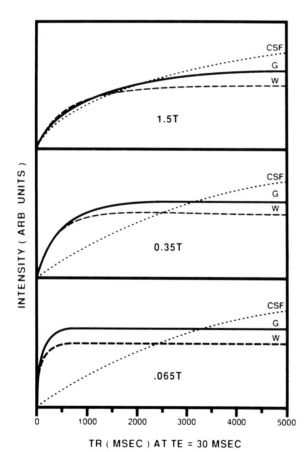

Fig. 28.5. The signal intensity of CSF, gray (G) and white (W) matter in relation to repetition time (TR) using a constant echo-time (TE) and at different field strengths (0.064, 0.35, and 1.5 Tesla). The curves for CSF are similar at all field strengths, but the differentiation between gray and white matter at short repetition time (TR) is superior at low-field.

strength MR. This is mainly due to the shortening of the T1-relaxation time at the lower-side strength. The shortened T1-time of the soft tissue allows for good contrast at short TR-time (700-1000 msec) and so called heavily T2-weighted images at TR-times between 1000 and 1500 msec with a long TE [15]. The differentiation between gray (G) and white (W) matter on a long TR image at higher-field strength is only possible at a repetition time (TR) of 2000 to 3000 msec (Fig. 28.5.). The low-field imaging has the further advantage that, with one sequence, the anatomic information of a so-called T1 weighted image and the contrast differentiation of a T2 weighted sequence can be produced, because the CSF will have a similar dark appearance at all field strengths for a given TR (1000-2000) (Fig. 28.6.). This kind of situation emphasizes the inappropriateness of characterizing sequences as T1 weighted or T2 weighted. All sequences are weighted by hydrogen density and T2. To avoid T1 weighting one needs to be at least at a TR of 3 T1 times. For CSF at low fields, this requires a TR of 10 seconds or more. It is important to understand the above for interventional procedures using MRI because not only are short imaging times valuable, but also good tissue contrast is essential. Tissue contrast is good at the low-field when using shorter TRs (750-2000) (Fig. 28.7.).

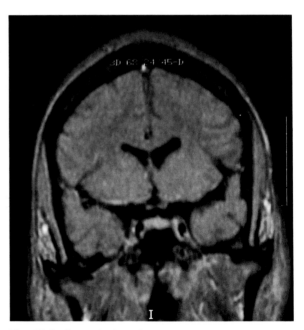

Fig. 28.6. Coronal slice of the pituitary. With a short TR of 70 msec and short echo-time (TE) of 28 msec and 3.5 mm slice thickness with 3-DFT, a differentiation between gray and white matter is possible. This examination technique gives the anatomic information of T1-weighted images and the contrast differentiation of T2-weighted sequences in one sequence (resolution: 1.1 × 1.1, matrix 256 × 256, 1 average).

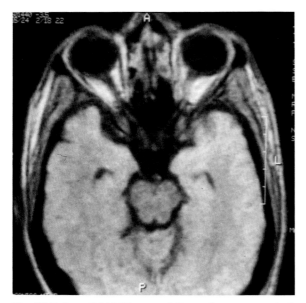

Fig. 28.7. Low-field MR scan of the optic nerves and of the chiasm. 3-DFT technique (TR 68 msec, TE 24 msec, flip-angle 45 degrees, 1 average, 32 scans in 8 minutes, 4.5 mm).

Comparative and Experimental Work

For the development of the first interventional procedures using open MRI, it was important to test in general how reliable low-field MRI is in the diagnosis of normal or pathological conditions. Therefore, a small pilot study was performed, comparing low-field with different high- and mid-field systems as well as CT. Following this, in a second phase, material for the interventional procedures were tested, and then the first experimental interventional procedures using a phantom phase (phase 3) were performed. Finally, in phase 4, further refinements of MRI interventional techniques were accomplished and the first interventional procedures were performed on patients.

Table 28.1. Development phases of interventional procedures using low-field MRI-systems.

Phase 1	Comparison of low-, mid-, high-field MR, CT
Phase 2	Material development and testing
Phase 3	Experimental interventional procedures
Phase 4	Interventional procedures in patients

Phase 1

Comparison of Different Systems

During the period from August 1988 until March 1989, comparison examinations were performed on 120 patients on several different diagnostic imaging systems. A clinical comparison was made between the ACCESS system (Toshiba America MRI, Inc.) and either, a General Electric 1.5 Tesla MRI, a Picker 0.5 Tesla system, a Siemens 0.5 Tesla system, or a Toshiba America 0.35 Tesla system.

The study population was divided into four groups of 30 patients each. Each group consisted of patients with a pathologic abnormality in either the brain, spinal column, abdomen/pelvis, or knees (Table 28.2.). A significant number of patients were also imaged with CT.

Table 28.2. Examinations (n = 120).

Skull	30 patients
Spinal column	30 patients
Abdomen/pelvis	30 patients
Knee	30 patients

A consistent finding in this small study was that the low-field, in comparison with high-field, needed longer acquisition times and several repetitions (averages), due to the lower signal-to-noise ratio per unit time. Also, fewer slices for the same TR- and TE-time were obtained compared with higher-field strength systems, so the slice thickness or TR had to be increased for the same degree of coverage. As with the other systems, spin echo technique as well as inversion recovery technique, partial flip, or 3-D sequences [12, 15, 19] were routinely used. Additionally, an average examination time of up to 1.5 hours per patient can be expected with the low-field.

Cranial Examinations

For low-field brain examinations, double-echo sequences (e.g., 30/105 msec) with a TR-time from 1000 to 2000 msec are performed with 14 sec and 2 averages. This resulted in an acquisition time of approximately 17 minutes (Fig. 28.8.). Following this, other techniques such as 3-D techniques (Fig. 28.9.) at 3.5 or 4.5 mm slice thickness, or SE/IR techniques at 5 or 10 mm thickness, can be selected in the desired plane (Fig. 28.8.). Images with good signal-to-noise ratio and thin slices can be obtained with the 3-D partial flip technique (Figs. 28.6. and 28.7.) with an acquisition time of approximately 8 minutes for 32 slices (3-D).

Images with any TE can be mathematically reconstructed from the double-echo data. Comparison with the 1.5 Tesla-GE system and the 0.5 Tesla Picker and Siemens systems, showed that in most cases at the same TR and TE a better contrast between gray and white matter

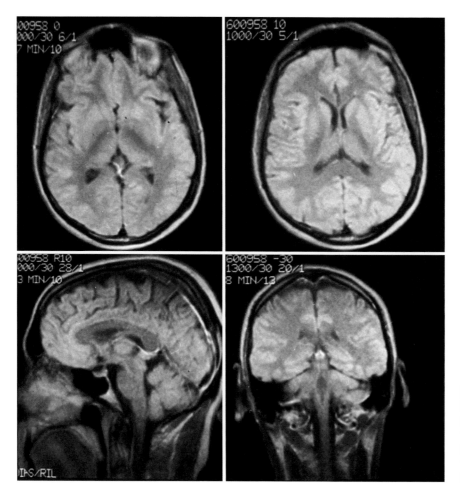

Fig. 28.8. MRI of head in transverse, sagittal and coronary plane (TR 1000 or 1300 msec, TE 30 msec, 0.064 Tesla, 5 mm thick, 17 minutes acqusition time).

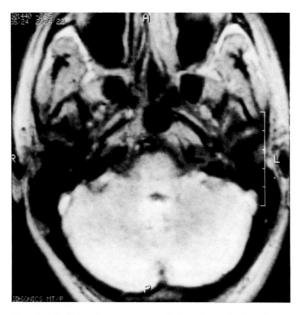

Fig. 28.9. 3-DFT acquisition at 0.064 Tesla for documentation of the acoustic nerve.

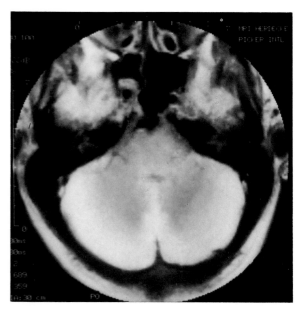

Fig. 28.10. The acoustic nerve imaged with a 0.5 Tesla in the same patient as in Fig. 28.9.

was seen with the low-field system. Cerebral infarcts, tumors, and inflammatory lesions all had a similar appearance at all field strengths. However, low-field has a lower signal-to-noise ratio, a lower resolution, and longer acquisition time. Also, the edges of pathologic lesions were better defined at higher fields, but contrast sequences with gadolinium in low-field give equally good information as higher field strength in tumor tissue (Figs. 28.11.–28.14.).

A comparison between low-field and mid-field (0.5 T-systems from Picker and Siemens) did not show remarkable differences in fine structures such as the 7th and 8th cranial nerve, with the exception of a slightly lower resolution and lower S/N in the low-field system. Comparison was made between a 4.5 mm thickness by 0.064 Tesla (Fig. 28.9.) and a 5 mm slice thickness in a 0.5 Tesla MR (Fig. 28.10.). The gray-white matter and CSF contrast in a TR-time of 65 msec, TE-time of 24 msec, and a flip angle of 20 degrees in the 3-D technique are similar to an image in 0.5 Tesla (2500 msec/30 msec). A flip-angle of 60 degrees with this 3-D technique corresponds to a T1 weighted image at low field.

It was observed in a small number of patients that areas of contusion and infarcts showed up early (within the first ten hours) in low-field MRI. Therefore, it may complement CT for early diagnosis in trauma cases, but further research is needed in this area.

Spinal Column Examinations

For evaluation of the spinal column with low-field imaging, normally 3.5 mm, 5 mm or 10 mm thick slices are used. Spin-echo technique, partial flip sequences (also called FLASH, GRASS, or gradient-recalled echo technique), and 3-D techniques are also possible with this system [12, 15, 19] (Fig. 28.13.). The 2-DFT partial-flip sequence can be used for a myelographic effect. In comparison with 0.5 Tesla (Fig. 28.14.), the examination time is longer, but the morphology differentiation is almost identical. The lower signal-to-noise ratio makes diagnosis of small lateral protrusions, small spinal lesions, or bone narrow defects somewhat more difficult. However, contrary to expectations, the ventral and dorsal nerve roots can be visualized by 3-DFT scans with only one average and an acquisition time of 4.5 minutes (Fig. 28.15.). In comparison with the 0.35 and 0.5 Tesla systems, the low-field produces diagnostic images of intervertebral disc lesions, alterations of vertebral bodies, and end-plate fractures (Figs. 28.16. and 28.17.). However, here also a lower signal-to-noise ratio and discrimination of very small (1–2 mm) structures must be tolerated. Interest-

ingly, scar tissue seems to be better differentiated from recurrent intervertebral disc herniations without contrast medium at low-field.

Examination of Joints

A strong point of low-field MRI is the high quality images of joint anatomy and pathology, especially with the 3-DFT technique. 32 images at 3.5 mm thickness can be achieved in 9 minutes (TR 65 msec, TE 24 msec, flip-angle 45 degrees, pixel resolution 0.7 × 0.7, field of view 18 × 18 cm with a matrix of 256 × 256 and 1 average). Torn menisci and crucial ligaments were well evaluated when compared with a 0.5 Tesla-Picker system (Figs. 28.18. and 28.19.). Also, good images of degenerated menisci and traumatic alterations can be obtained with the low-field system. The major differences with higher-field strength in the examination of extremities were the slightly longer acquisition time and a slightly different contrast.

Imaging of pathologic alterations of the upper ankle joint (Fig. 28.20.) and the elbow (Fig. 28.21.) using 3-DFT technique holds considerable potential. The articular cartilage of the joint can be evaluated in its entire circumference, as can the tendon, ligament, and joint capsule. This may open up new aspects for joint biopsy and therapy with MRI-guided interventional procedures.

Abdominal Examinations

Due to the physical characteristics at low-field, fewer motion artifacts are seen in abdominal scans. This may incrase the usefulness of the low-field MRI when compared with higher-field MR, especially in abdominal MRI interventional procedures. When compared with CT, a more exact differentiation of metastases, cysts or hemangiomas is often possible with MRI without using contrast media (Fig. 28.25.).

Phase 2

Testing and Development of Interventional Material

Phase 3

Experimental Models

In the development of interventional procedures for MRI, extensive experimentation with different material was necessary. These experiments were performed in a water bath with a

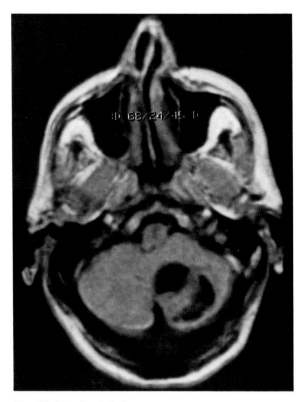

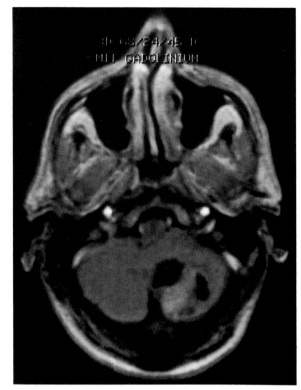

Fig. 28.11a. Sagital plane

Fig. 28.11b. Transversal plane

Figs. 28.11a,b. and **28.12.** Contrast-sequences with gadolinum (Fig. 28.11b). It is remarkable that contrast enhancement in low-field gives the same information as higher-fild strength. (Metastasis of bronchial carcinomas: TR 68 msec, TE 24 msec, FA 45°, slice 4.5 mm, NEX 2).

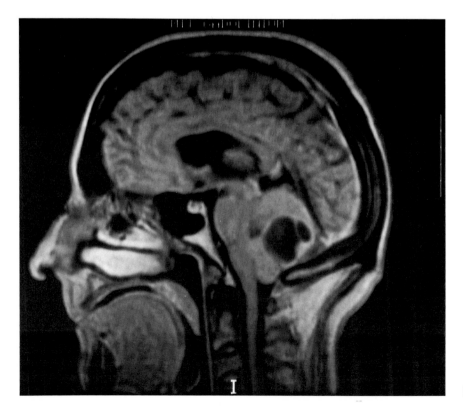

Fig. 28.12

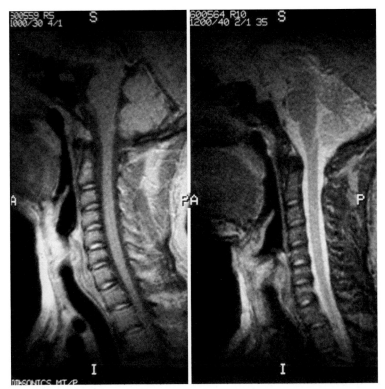

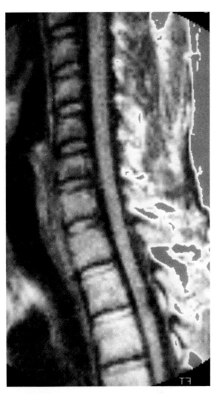

Fig. 28.13. MRI examination of cervical spine with a 0.064 Tesla MR-system. Left: Spin-echo technique (TR 1000 msec, TE 30 msec). Right: Myelography effect with a partial-flip examination (TR 1200 msec, TE 40 msec, flip-angle 35 degrees).

Fig. 28.14. MRI examination of cervical spine with a 0.5 Tesla MR. Same patient as in Fig. 28.13. (TR 6000 msec, TE 40 msec).

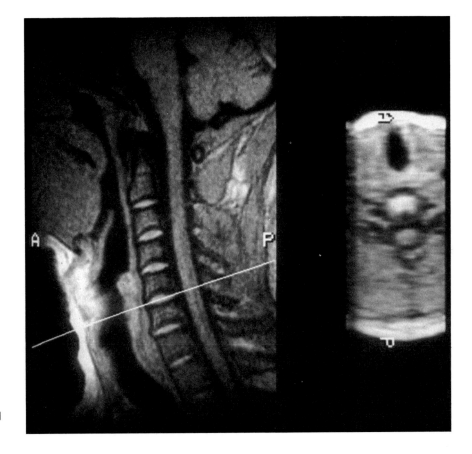

Fig. 28.15. 3-DFT scans with two averages (0.064 Tesla, oblique reconstruction 3.5 mm thick). The ventral and dorsal nerve roots and the intervertebral foramen are clearly seen.

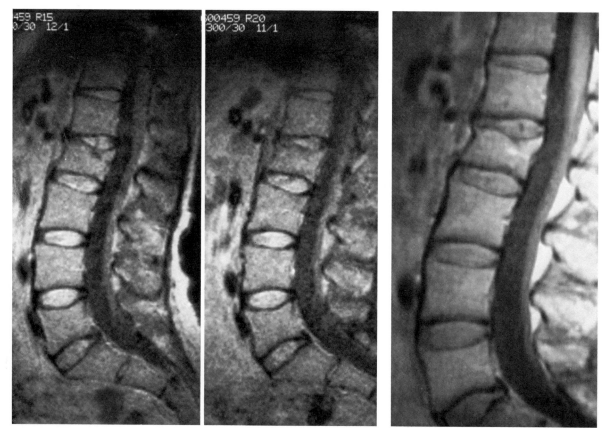

Figs. 28.16. and **28.17.** Lumbar spine examination with a 0.064 Tesla and a 0.35 Tesla MRI. In both examination techniques, the fracture of the 2nd lumbar vertebral body is well documented (left: 0.064 Tesla MRI (Toshiba America MRI, Inc.): TR 1300 msec, TE 30 msec, 5 mm thickness, 4 averages, matrix: 256 × 256, resolution: 1.25 × 1.25, acqusition time: 22 minutes; right: 0.35 Tesla-MRI (Toshiba America MRI, Inc.): TR 1000 msec, TE 22 msec, 5 mm thickness, 4 averages, matrix: 256 × 256, resolution: 0.95 × 0.95, acquisition time: 17 minutes).

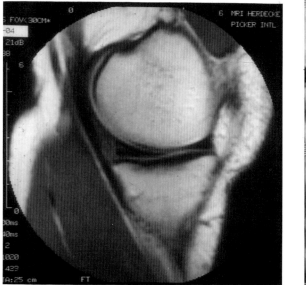
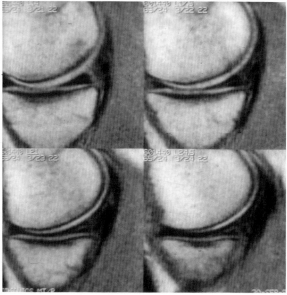

Figs. 28.18. and **28.19.** Comparing the posterior horn of the medial meniscus with a 0.064 Tesla and a 0.5 Tesla system (left: 0.064 Tesla MRI, right: 0.5 Tesla MRI).

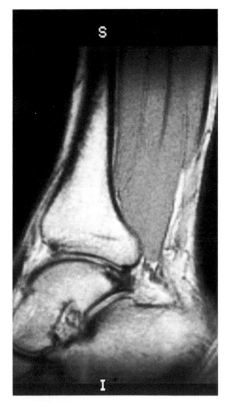

Fig. 28.20. Ankle joint with a 0.064 Tesla. Degenerative changes are visualized at the ventral and dorsal tibia articular surface.

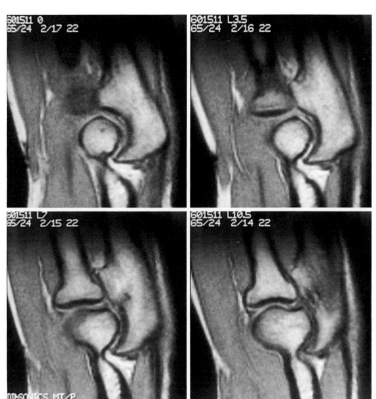

Fig. 28.21. Elbow joint (0.064 Tesla).

NaCl solution and also in different types of animal tissues. It was found that beef steak and axial slices of cow leg were especially well suited to testing different needles and tubular materials. The authors then tested acquisitions with different TR and TE combinations in all three planes; here special consideration was given to the use of short acquisition times. Also, from these experiments they obtained a general idea of how much time would be needed for the interventional MRI procedures and of the accuracy to which the procedures could be performed. Especially well suited was the sequence listed in Table 28.3.

Lufkin et al. [11] used for their material studies a 0.3 Tesla permanent magnet (Fonar) with a TR of 400 msec, a TE of 14 msec, and a 256 × 256 matrix with a 1.0 × 1.0 mm pixel.

Table 28.3. Sequence for MRI punctures.

– TR	300 msec
– TE	30 msec
– Matrix	256 × 256
– Voxel	1.1 × 1.1 × 10 mm
– Acquisition time	1 min. and 16 sec/3 scans
– Averages	1

Extensive work on artifacts after placement of surgical and dental implants was performed by Bellon et al. [3], Heindel et al. [8] and New et al. [14].

The following substances and alloys were tested:
1. Endoprosthesis material;
2. pure titanium 98%;
3. titanium 96%;
4. titanium-nickel alloy;
5. aluminium;
6. aluminium-titanium alloy (+ 5% impurity);
7. aluminium-titanium alloy (+ 15% impurity);
8. Becton-Dickinson needle and tubing;
9. Abbocath needle and tubing

In these tests, aluminium and pure titanium were found to be particularly suitable for MR procedures because there were no artifacts detectable around these materials. Furthermore, the needle tip made from these materials could be localized precisely in the sagittal, coronal, and axial planes. As shown in Figs. 28.26. and 28.27., the advancement of the needle can be checked step by step.

Titanium-nickel alloys can also be used for interventional procedures at low-field. However, a moderate artifact formation due to nickel, is seen with this material. This effect has already been described by Lufkin et al. [11]. The authors also observed artifacts from titan-

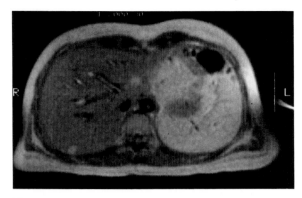
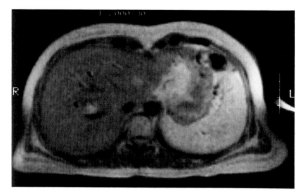

Figs. 28.22. and **28.23.** Liver-sequence without breathhold: hemangioma (spin-echo: TR 2000 msec, TE 30 msec, matrix 256 × 128, resolution: 2.2 × 2.2, slice: 10 mm, 4 averages).

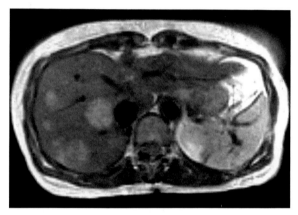
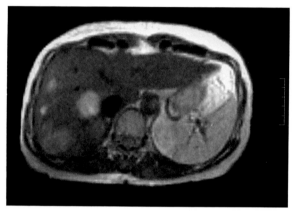

Fig. 28.24. Access 0.064 Tesla. (Toshiba America MRI, Inc): TR 2000 m sec, TE 30 m sec, matrix 256 × 128, resolution 2.2 × 2.2, slice 10 mm, 4 averages, acquisition time: 17 minutes, without breathhold). Diagnosis: adenocarcinoma of colon, metastatic to liver.

Fig. 28.25. The same patient. Toshiba America MRI-System (0.35 Tesla): TR 2000 msec, TE 30 msec, matrix 256 × 128, resolution 2.0 × 2.0, slice 10 mm, 2 averages, acquisition time: 8 minutes, breathhold. Diagnosis: adenocarcinoma of colon, metastatic to liver.

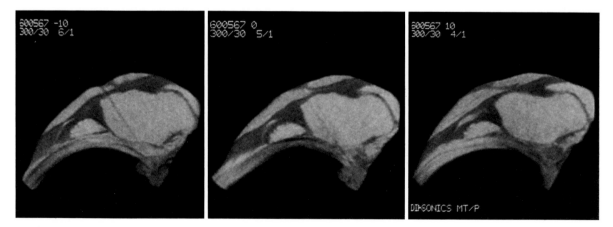

Figs. 28.26. and **28.27.** Interventional test punctures at three different levels with an experimental puncture material. The needle tip can be differentiated from the soft tissue without interference from artifacts. The slightly slanted course of the needle and the position of the tip in front of the spine are documented in the transverse scans. (TR 300 msec, TE 30 msec, 1 average, matrix: 256 × 256, resolution: 1.1 × 1.1, acqusition time: 1 minute, 16 seconds).

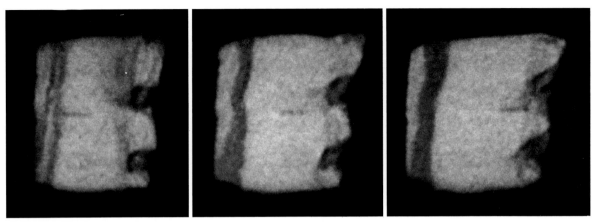

Fig. 28.27. Sagittal scan of a 3-D puncture with the same acquisition sequence as in Fig. 28.26. The course of the needle tip can be seen next to the ribs.

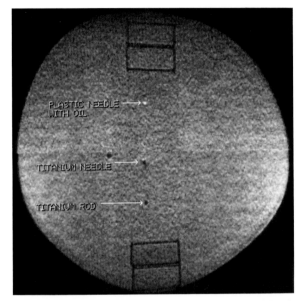

Fig. 28.28. Interventional test with different materials. A puncture was performed in sponge. An oil-filled plastic needle, a titanium needle, and a titanium rod are seen. The needles themselves are sharply demarcated from the sponge on the transverse scan. Only the titanium needle shows any artifacts.

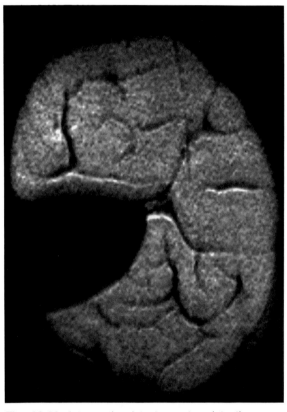

Fig. 28.29. Interventional test puncture into the cross section of a cow leg with a needle developed at MKI. The entire needle is documented free of artifacts.

ium impurities (Fig. 28.28.). Unfavorable results were obtained from different aluminium-titanium-alloys with considerable artifacts which were caused by ferromagnetic impurities.

The use of interventional instruments such as the Becton-Dickinson and Abbocath-needle catheters proved to be particularly well suited for these interventional procedures. The use of plastic material for MRI interventions has been known through the work of van Sonnenberg [18]. The ferromagnetic guide needle from the above-named interventional needles caused considerable artifacts. The catheter material can not be detected in the image with the short TR- and TE-sequences used in our studies. Only by filling the catheters with oil does it become visi-ble. For the test procedure itself, the oily mixture of Lipiodol-Ultrafluid (Byk Gulden) was found to be suitable. The catheters had experimentally been placed into sponges which were fully saturated with water, in order to avoid bulk magnetic susceptibility artifacts. The entire length of the catheters as well as its tip can be discriminated in this way. Filling the catheter after positioning with a titanium-nickel guidance wire is a further refinement of this method. A puncture needle with a special alloy developed at MKI is shown in Fig. 28.29.

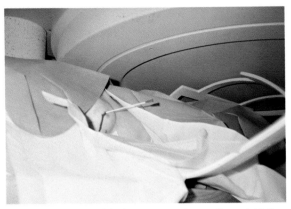

Fig. 28.30. MRI-guided puncture of a malignant histiocytoma with a Becton-Dickinson needle. The puncture is performed with the patient directly in front of the magnet. The small belt-like coil is opened for better access.

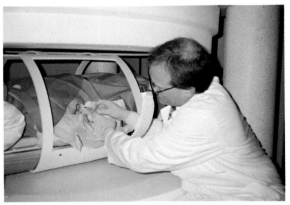

Fig. 28.31. MRI-guided interventional procedure. Correction of the needle position, if needed, and injection of any treatment medication can be performed in the open MRI without moving the patient.

Phase 4

Interventional MRI Procedures

Technique

Following the above experimental phases, we performed abdominal interventions using MRI guidance at our clinic in Mülheim. In the supine position, the patients were placed in a belt coil in the same way as for a diagnostic study, but with the area of pathology not under the coil. Then, MRI scans with short and long TR- and TE- times are performed in order to differentiate the pathologic structure from the surrounding tissue. The puncture path is defined and information such as distance of the puncture level to the center slice, distance from the puncture point to the area of interest, anatomic landmarks, puncture angle and puncture depth is obtained on the monitor. The intervention level and the puncture point are then marked on the skin.

Table 28.4. MRI-guided intervention technique.

---

1. Positions of the belt coil
2. Marking the center slice on the body next to the edge of the coil
3. Diagnostic sequences (short and long TR/TE)
4. Determining on the monitor the intervention level, the puncture point and the puncture angle
5. Measuring distances
6. Marking on body
7. Beginning of puncture outside the magnet
8. Three-axis locator for needle position
9. Correction and/or further advancement of the instruments with the patient inside the MRI
10. Follow-up scans in a fast single-slice technique
11. Three-axis locator (in case of complications or unclear conditions)
12. No breath-holding needed in abdominal interventions

At present, the needle is inserted outside the magnet (Fig. 28.30.). The puncture should be performed exactly as for CT-guided interventions, with the entire needle contained in the 10 mm slice. Less desirable, but also possible with an increase in slices and scan time, are the slanted 3-D puncture techniques (previously described in this text). The patients are then placed back into the MRI and three slices are obtained. After localizing the tip, the needle position or the puncture angle can be changed with the patient inside the MRI. Then, once the needle is in the correct position, the biopsy and/or therapy is performed (Fig. 28.31.). Abdominal interventions, even close to the diaphragm, can be performed without respiratory gating (Table 28.4.).

For difficult cases and for a more accurate localization the 40 seconds 3-axis scan is used to obtain 10 mm slices in each of the three projections (axial, coronal and sagittal). A so-called footprint, i.e. a 10 or 20 mm wide marking strip in each of the three images, makes localization of the other slices possible and can be helpful for 3-D visualization (Figs. 28.32.–28.34.).

Interventional Procedures and Instruments

During the period from November 1988 to April 1989, thirteen interventional procedures were performed on the same patient at MKI using this technique. Three separate liver biopsies were obtained for pathologic diagnosis in this patient with a known metastasis from primary tumor (malignant histiocytoma). Also, 10 intratumoral therapies with 96% alcohol were performed. The tumor size at the beginning of the treatment was approximately 15 cm × 12 cm × 8 cm and it was located close to the diaphragm in the right lobe of the liver with infiltration to the lung and soft tissue with rib de-

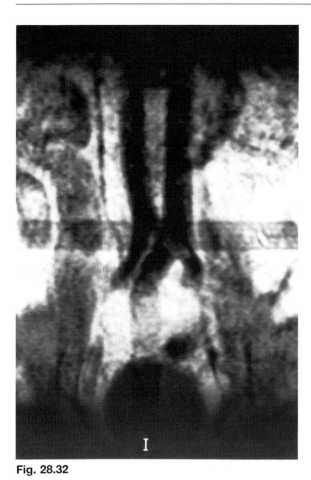

Fig. 28.32

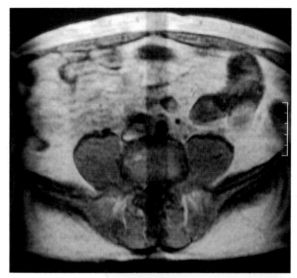

Fig. 28.33

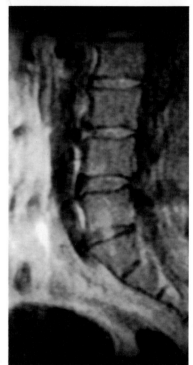

Fig. 28.34

Figs. 28.32.–28.34. Specially developed 3-axis scan for interventional procedures. Within 40 seconds a scan in each of the three planes can be obtained at 10 or 20 mm slice thickness. For interventional procedures, this 3-axis locator is of great value because the interventional instruments can be immediately demonstrated in all three planes.

struction. The patient's major complaint was severe pain.

Punctures were performed with an Abbocath or Becton-Dickinson needle. The catheter tip was visualized after the insertion of a titanium-nickel guide wire (Figs. 28.35. and 28.36.). Following local anesthesia with 10–15 ml Scandicaine (1%), either a 20–22–G Seibel-Grönemeyer needle (Cook) was inserted via a guide wire in the catheter for biopsy and/or 5 ml of alcohol (96%) was injected into the center of the tumor for therapy. The distribution of the medication mixture inside the tumor tissue was then checked with computed-tomography.

The biopsies were taken from the edge and center of the tumor. Due to the lack of a significant projectile effect, ferromagnetic items such as puncture needles can be used in the low-field MRI, but must be removed before imaging. Intratumoral therapy was performed in the central region of the tumor and in an area close to the rib (Figs. 28.35. and 28.36.). Intervals between treatments were two to three weeks. Prior

Instruments for interventional MRI
Abbocath or Becton-Dickinson puncture plastic tube
Titanium-nickel guide wire
Seibel-Grönemeyer biopsy needle (Cook)
Lipiodol Ultrafluid (Byk Gulden)
1-10 ml 96% alcohol (Pfrimmer)
1-10 ml 1% Scandicaine (Astra Chemie)

to the second and following treatments up to 20 ml of liquefied and necrotic tissue was aspirated. Each treatment was checked with CT (Fig. 28.36.). At the end of treatment the tumor had

Figs. 28.35. and **28.36.** MRI-guided tumor therapy for a malignant histiocytoma. The wire is located in the same area in MRI and CT.

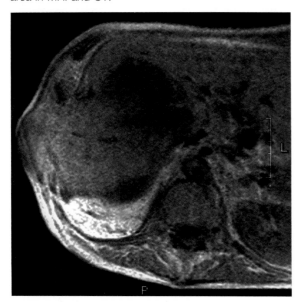

Fig. 28.35. MRI-guided puncture. Identified in the liver tumor is a small linear low-signal structure (tube with guide wire). Examination was made without breath-holding.

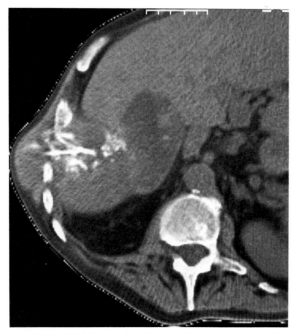

Fig. 28.38. CT Scan after interventional treatment with contrast media.

been reduced in size by 20% and the patient had a reduction in pain of 80%. Tumor pain therapy is also well done in this MRI-technique as described in chapter 15. The advantage is three dimensional view and lack of X-ray as well as contrast media (Figs. 28.37. and 28.38.).

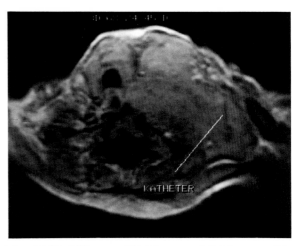

Fig. 28.37. MRI-scan: TR 68 msec, TE 24 msec, FA 45°.

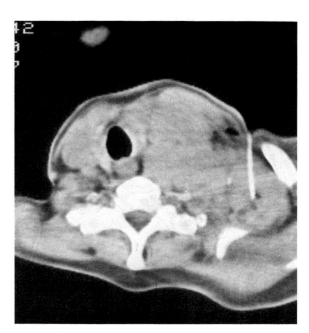

Fig. 28.38. CT-Scan after interventional treatment with contrast media.

Discussion

In interventional radiology there is a promising future ahead for MRI. The absence of ionizing radiation and the precise morphologic tissue differentiation in all three planes offer significant advantages for the patient as well as for the physician performing the procedure. The possibility of acquiring angled slices as with sonography is also of considerable help. However, MRI-interventions are time-consuming and at least 30 minutes must be added to the time of the procedure compared with CT. Also, the positioning of the patient is more difficult than in CT. For seriously ill patients it can be difficult to remain still in the MR during the scan.

The advantages of the MR method are based on the possibility of performing three-dimensional interventions in which the entering axis can be chosen as either axial, sagittal or coronal and then angled. The high morphologic contrast of MRI is much superior to that of CT. Vessels, edema etc. can normally be differentiated without contrast medium administration. Low-field MRI allows for interventions in the abdomen close to the diaphragm without respiratory gating. However, for further development of interventional MRI, many more research and development projects are necessary.

Open MRI with sufficient space for physicians and assistants is optimal for interventional MRI. Furthermore, special intervention coils and positioning aids need to be developed including three-dimensional localization light and an extensive assortment of instruments which will not produce artifacts. Additionally, the development of interventional MRI depends on new ultrafast sequences.

The comparison with high- and mid-field systems in 120 patients demonstrates that a differential diagnosis of pathologic alterations is possible with low-field MRI, but a lower signal-to-noise ratio per unit time and longer examination times are a drawback. However, the high acceptance of open MRI by patients, no disturbing gradient noise, and a relatively low start-up and maintenance cost can somewhat offset its disadvantages. Finally, it remains to be seen if there are diagnostic advantages with contrast media like Gadolinium-DTPA in interventional procedures.

Summary

The open 0.064T ACCESS system is well suited for interventional MRI. After experimental studies in the area of material research and extensive experiments, the first interventions were performed in patients, partially with instruments developed at MKI. These first interventions were performed by us in the abdomen with MRI localization and documentation of the positioning of the needle tip. More research is necessary for the further development of ultrafast sequences as well as special instruments for MRI intervention.

In conclusion, developments in the area of low-field MRI will lead in the foreseeable future to a greater utilization of MRI and expansion of the interventional possibilities.

References

1. Arakawa M., Crooks L.E., McCarten B., Hoenninger J.C., Kaufman L.: Comparison of S/N Levels in Solenoidal and Saddle-Shaped RF Coils. in: Abstracts of the Society of Magnetic Resonance in Medicine Meeting. Aug. 13–17, New York 1984, 10
2. Bell R.H.: Magnetic Resonance Instrumentation in: Brant-Zawadzki M., Norman D. (eds.): Magnetic Resonance Imaging of the central nervous system. New York 1987, 13–21
3. Bellon E.M., Haacke E.M., Coleman P.E., Sacco D.C., Steiger D.A., Gangarosa R.E.: MR Artifacts: A Review. Amer. J. Roentgenol. 147 (1986) 1271–1281
4. Bradford R., Thomas D.G., Bydder G.M.: MRI directed stereotactic biopsy of cerebral lesions. Acta Neurochir. [Suppl] Wien 39 (1987) 25–27
5. Crooks L.E., Kaufmann L.: Instrumentation and Techniques in: Higgins Ch.B., Hricak H. (eds.): Magnetic Resonance Imaging of the body T. New York 1984, 11–21
6. Ganssen A.: Planung und Kosten einer Anlage. In: Zeitler E. (Hrsg.): Kernspintomographie. Köln 1984, 85–95
7. Grunert P., Koos W., Ungersboeck K., Kitz K.: Stereotaktische Biopsie von Hirntumoren. Wien, Klin. Wochenschr. 99 (1987) 672–674
8. Heindel W., Friedmann G., Bunke J., Thomas B., Firsching R., Ernestus R.-I.: Artifacts in MR Imaging after surgical intervention. J. Comput. Assist. Tomogra. 10 (1986) 596–599
9. Herman S.D., Friedmann A.C., Radecki P.D., Caroline D.F.: Incidential prostatic carcinoma detected by MRI and diagnosed by MRI/CT-guided biopsy. Amer. J. Roentgenol. 146 (1986) 351–352
10. Kelly P.J., Daumas-Duport C., Kispert D.B., Kall B.A., Scheithauer B.W., Illig J.J.: Imaging-based stereotaxic serial biopsies in untreated intracranial glial neoplasma. J. Neurosurg. 66 (1987) 865–874
11. Lufkin R., Teresi L., Hanafee W.: New needle for MR-guided aspiration cytology of the head and neck. Amer. J. Roentgenol. 149 (1987) 380–382
12. Mills T.C., Ortendahl D.A., Hylton N.M., Crooks L.E., Carlson J.W., Kaufman L.: Partial flip angle MR Imaging. Radiology 162 (1987) 531–539
13. Mueller P.R., Stark D.D., Simeone J.F., Saini S., Butch R.J., Edelman R.R., Wittenberg J., Ferrucci J.T. Jr.: MR-guided aspiration biopsy: needle design and clinical trials. Radiology 161 (1986) 605–609
14. New P.F.J., Rosen B.R., Brady T.J., Buonanno F.S., Kistler J.P., Burt C.T., Hinshaw W.S., Newhouse J.H., Pohost G.M., Taveras J.M.: Nuclear magnetic resonance. Potential hazards and artifacts of ferromagnetic and nonferromagnetic surgical and dental materials and devices in nuclear magnetic resonance imaging. Radiology 147 (1983) 139–148
15. Rothschild P.A., Winkler M.L., Grönemeyer D.H.W., Kaufman L., D'Amour P.: Mid-Field and Low-Field-Magnetic Resonance Imaging of the spine. Top. Magn. Reson. Imag. 1 (1) (1988) 11–23
16. Seiderer M.: Technische Komponenten. In: Lissner J., Seiderer M. (Hrsg.): Klinische Kernspintomographie. Stuttgart 1987, 71–82
17. Thomas D.G., Davis C.H., Ingram S., Olney J.S., Bydder G.M., Young I.R.: Stereotaxic biopsy of the brain under MR imaging control. Amer. J. Roentgenol. 7 (1986) 161–163
18. van Sonnenberg E., Hajek P., Baker L. et al.: Materials for MR-guided interventional radiology procedures: laboratory and clinical experience (actr). Radiology 161 (1986) 121
19. Winkler M.L., Ortendahl D.A., Mills T.C., Crooks L.E., Sheldon P.E., Kaufman L., Kramer D.M.: Characteristics of partial flip angle and gradient reversal MR Imaging. Radiology 166 (1988) 17–26

Chapter 29
Aspects of CT-Guided Puncture Techniques Using Ultra-Fast Cine-CT

W. Jaschke, D.H.W. Grönemeyer, R.M.M. Seibel, D.P. Boyd

Computer-tomography has developed quickly to become the preferred localization aid for percutaneous punctures of organs and fluid accumulations. Geometrically accurate imaging of organic structures at one level allows for the safe placing of biopsy needles and drainage catheters. However, at this time, there is no CT available, which provides optimum conditions for CT-guided interventional procedures. A machine that can image a larger body volume in a Real-Time Technique would be desirable. This would have the advantages not only of localization of the target volume but also insertion of the puncture needles could take place under "CT-vision". Also, with these circumstances smaller structures that undergo movement from breathing, could be punctured more safely and faster. The retention time of the relatively rigid biopsy needles in tissue would be shortened and shear injuries to the surrounding tissue could be reduced to a minimum. The concept of the recently introduced Cine-CT (Fig. 29.1.) fulfils some of the above conditions and will be briefly discussed as a part of this book.

Equipment technique

Cine-CT consists of a relatively large, evacuated metal receptacle in which an electronic accelerator and four half-moon shaped material rings are mounted (Figs. 29.2. and 29.3.).

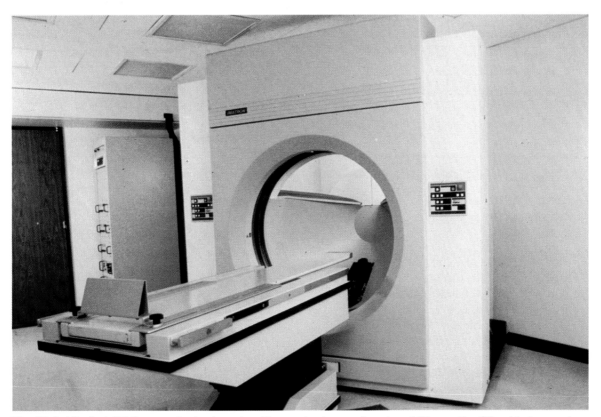

Fig. 29.1. Ultrafast CT Scanner by Imatron, Inc. The gantry has a diameter of 90 cm. For CT-guided procedures, especially with long interventional instruments, the gantry is optimal because it has space even for obese patients. The procedures can be performed conventionally in front of the gantry or for the first time also behind the gantry. In the rear of the gantry, there is a platform with a rail attached to it. The slant of the patient's couch can be varied by up to 25 degrees. Also, at the same angle the patient's couch can be turned sideways.

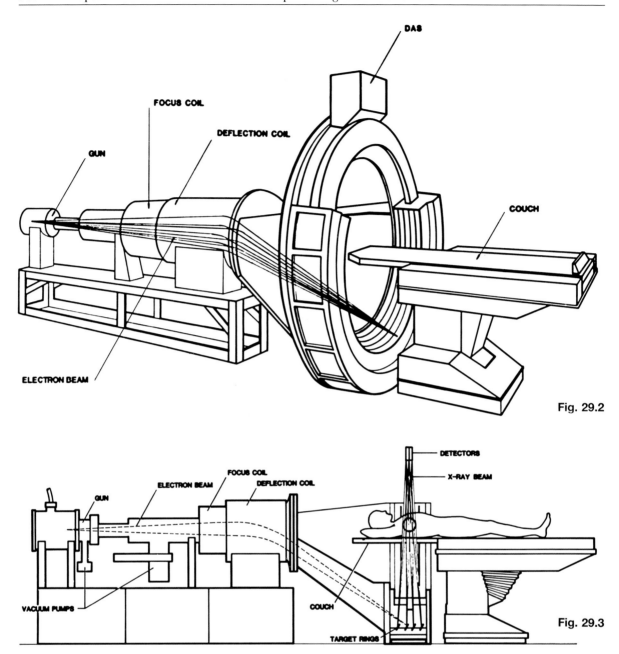

Figs. 29.2. and **29.3.** Technical illustration of the ultra fast scanner with schematic illustration of the course of the electronic beam and its deflection. Fig. 23.3 shows the splitting of the electronic beam to the different targets. The acceleration unit, the largest and longest part of the instrument, is mounted in a room next door and is connected with the gantry through a wall.

On each water-cooled metal ring are mounted several relatively thin tungsten targets for production of X-rays. During the scan process, an electronic beam is accelerated along the direction of the longitudinal axis of the apparatus and focused through magnetic coils. Additional magnetic coils steer the electronic beam to one of the four metal rings. Thereby, the beam performs a quick 210 degree movement alongside the target; this swivel movement lasts 50 or 100 milliseconds (operator-dependent). When the electronic beam hits the metal ring, X-rays are generated which are changed to the desired thickness through collimators. The intensity of this radiation is measured by a stationary detec-

tor system with 432 (detector ring A) and 864 (detector ring B) semiconductor detectors (Fig. 29.1.).

In the 50 millisecond scan time, there are 432 detectors used on each detector ring, so that two 10 mm thick images can be calculated for each scan. To increase the scan volume, the electronic beam can additionally be steered from metal ring to metal ring in 8 milliseconds. In this way, cross-section pictures with a frequency of up to 17 images per second can be taken at a total of eight different localizations without moving the table.

The 864 detectors of ring B have so far only been used for the 100 millisecond scan. With this scan speed, the Cine-CT can only be run in the single-scan method (thickness of scan 3, 6 or 10 mm).

Operational Alternatives

The computer programs of the Cine-CT allow a flexible combination of short scanning times, high image frequency, and volume scans. The result application possibilities are explained in more detail below.

The *localization of the scan level* takes place with the help of a digital survey radiograph as well as with the use of a survey scan at eight different positions. The survey radiogram is taken simultaneously at two levels perpendicular to each other. The combination of both scan types makes a rapid localization of the target volume in the region of interest possible. With the help of the examination table, movable at all three levels, the patient can be positioned in such a way that slant images can be taken at all three levels. Thereby, the puncture can be performed in most cases parallel to the scan level, which makes documentation of the needle position and also the puncture itself much easier. Therefore, extracorporally fixed puncture aids which do not run perpendicular to the body axis become unnecessary.

In the *Cine-Mode*, the scanner produces cross-section images in real time. In this mode, one can choose to direct the beam to either one or all of the metal rings so that at least two and a maximum of eight cross-sectional images can be obtained with a speed of 17 images/sec. The reconstructed images can be viewed on a TV monitor either as single slices or endless film strip. With this modus operandi, in the near future it may be possible to position the puncture needles under CT vision, thereby making the follow-up scans for checking needle position unnecessary.

The so-called *Flow-Mode* is mainly used in first-pass examinations. Thereby, the passage of a contrastmedium bolus can be followed with any scan frequency up to three pictures/sec. Then, after the manual start of the picture sequence, the subsequent images are automatically obtained (Fig. 29.4.). The scanning process can be triggered either by an internal timer or ECG. The time between acquiring the images can be programmed at will, e.g., 2 slices/sec for 3 sec or 1 slice/sec for 10 sec, or 1 slice/heart action etc. The passage of the contrast medium can – as with the Cine-Mode – be viewed in the form of single slices or in an endless strip.

For quantitative analyses, presentation in the form of a density/time diagram has proven to be successful. With this method, important data with reference to the blood circulation and blood volume of the target organ can be obtained prior to the puncture.

Since the administered dose is relatively small because of the short display times compared with those of common CT scanners, the manufacturer offers another operation mode to

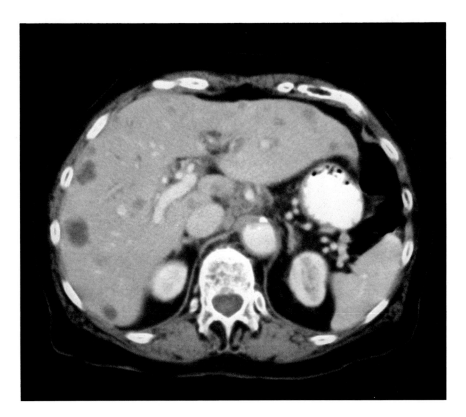

Fig. 29.4. Bolus-CT of liver metastases from a colorectal carcinoma. Even the small vessels are reproduced sharply (scantime 0.8 sec.) In this way great possibilities are created for on-line procedures with millimeter accuracy due to the vessels discrimination.

improve the signal-noise ratio, the so-called *Averaged-Volume Mode*. This mode uses fast multiple scanning of the metal ring as with the Cine-Mode. However, several single slices are not calculated from the rough data but two averaged cross-section slices (1 slice/detector ring). Typically, the data from four to six scans are averaged so that the scan time is increased from 50 to 200 or 300 msec. With the help of a rapid table movement (< 1 sec) a larger body volume can be scanned with this mode. Due to the better signal-to-noise ratio, the Averaged-Volume Mode is best suited for good contrast in soft-tissue organs, e.g. a tumor in the region of the liver.

With the so-called *High-Resolution Mode*, high resolution single slices can be obtained. This is achieved by utilizing the 864 detectors of ring B and simultaneously increasing scan time to 100 msec. In this way a quadruple amount of data is available for slice reconstruction. To obtain an optimal image quality, the High-Resolution Mode is frequently combined with the Averaged-Volume Mode. This mode is preferred for scanning of the vertebral column and brain (Tables 29.1. and 29.2.).

retroperitoneum (Fig. 29.6.) and lung (Fig. 29.5.). Scan times were 0.4-0.8 sec/slice. Due to the large diameter of the gantry (90 cm), after insertion of the puncture needle, the patients do not require to be moved out of the gantry. This is a considerable advantage compared with conventional CT. Furthermore, not moving the patient during the interventional procedure, means higher precision for the interventional procedure and reduces the procedure time by at least 50%.

On-line observation during the procedure is not possible at the present time. For this reason, prior to each scan one must leave the room to check the procedure on the monitor.

As soon as this problem is solved, the positioning of interventional instruments can be performed under CT observation. Especially for procedures in areas that undergo movement such as the mediastinum, regions close to the diaphragm, etc. Ultra-Fast-Cine-CT holds great promise. With this technique, it will be possible to obtain tissue and perform therapeutic procedures less traumatically.

Table 29.1. Ultra-Fast-CT in anatomic imaging.

1. **Multi-slice technique**
   50 msec scan-time
   8 scans in 224 msec.

2. **Single-slice technique**
   100 msec scan-time
   0.1-1.2 seconds per scan
   fast table movement (up to 17 cm/sec)

Table 29.2. Ultra-Fast-CT for function imaging.

1	Continuous scan operation	
2	Multi-slice technique	17 scans/sec
3	Single-slice technique	9 scans/sec

Ultra-Fast-CT-Guided Interventional Procedures

Within the context of the scientific cooperation which exists between the Physics Reasearch Laboratory of the University of California (Prof. Douglas Boyd) and the Institute for Diagnostic and Interventional Radiology, Medical Computer Sciences of the Witten-Herdecke University in Mülheim (MKI), it was possible to perform interventional biopsy procedures of the

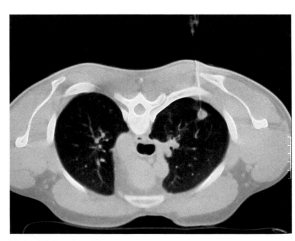

Fig. 29.5. Ultra-Fast-CT-guided biopsy of a peripheral circular mass (6 mm slice thickness and 0.4 sec scan time).

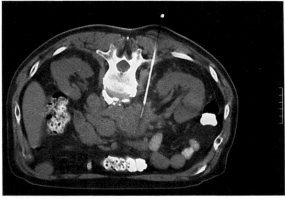

Fig. 29.6. Ultra-Fast-CT-guided biopsy of a retroperitoneal lymphoma compressing the vena cava (6 mm slice thickness, 0.8 sec scan time).

By using Cine-CT in interventional radiology, it is possible for the first time to differentiate even small vessels from the surrounding organic structures during the procedure (Fig. 29.4.).

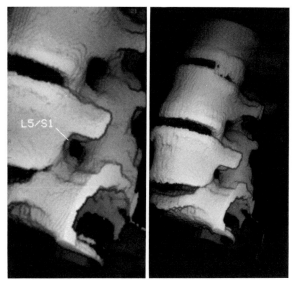

Fig. 29.7. 3-D reconstruction of the vertebral column. Note the excellent detail of the intervertebral foramina. By reconstructing the segmental nerves and segmental vessels, an accurate interventional procedure preparation will be possible, e.g. for a CT-guided percutaneous nucleotomy.

This is due to the high speed of Cine-CT and a simultaneously performed contrast bolus (angio-CT). This combination technique is especially important for further development of CT-guided intra-tumorous therapy and for diagnostic punctures of tumors located in the vicinity of vessels such as carotid or vertebral artery. Furthermore, the 3-D reconstruction together with a workstation will be of enormous value for interventional procedure planning (Fig. 29.7.; see Chapter 3-D techniques).

In future, Ultra-fast-CT should become an indispensable part of an interventional radiologic department.

Further reading

Boyd D.P., Lipton M.J.: Cardiac computed tomography. Proc. IEEE 71 (1983) 298

Lipton M.J., Higgins Ch.B.: Evaluation of ischemic heart disease by computerized transmission tomography. Radiol. Clin. North. Am. 18 (1980) 557

Ritman E.I., Kinsey J.H., Robb R.A., Harris I.D., Gilbert B.K.: Physics and technical considerations in the design of the DSR: a hightemporal resolution volume scanner. Amer. J. Roentgenol. 134 (1984) 369

Chapter 30
Combination of CT and Fluoroscopy; Workstation for 3-D Image Processing

D.H.W. Grönemeyer, R.M.M. Seibel, J. Plassmann

Interventional procedures have been known since the first therapeutic bile duct drainage in 1953 and percutaneous nephrostomy in 1955. Then in the sixties, interventional radiology with fluoroscopy-guided fine-needle punctures (e.g. of the lung) and percutaneous vessel recanalisations (Dotter) experienced rapid development. The fluoroscopy- and sonography-guided methods for diagnosis and therapy are today indispensable in the majority of radiology departments. In addition, CT-guided interventional procedures are being performed with increasing frequency.

Almost all interventional procedures have been performed with a single imaging method (sonography, computed-tomography, or fluoroscopy). Sometimes computed-tomography has been used for planning fluoro-guided interventions.

Since 1988, the authors have used in their clinic a simultaneous combination of compute-tomography and fluoroscopy for interventional procedures (3-D procedure). The major advantage of this combined method is the possibility of visualizing the region of interest in all three dimensions. Furthermore, it allows for more precise instrument placement (Fig. 30.1.).

In addition, they have found the 3-D workstation to be invaluable in planning these combined three-dimensional procedures.

Technical Process

Directly in front of the CT-gantry a mobile C-arm is positioned. The C-arm can be rotated through 180 degrees and angled at 180 degrees.

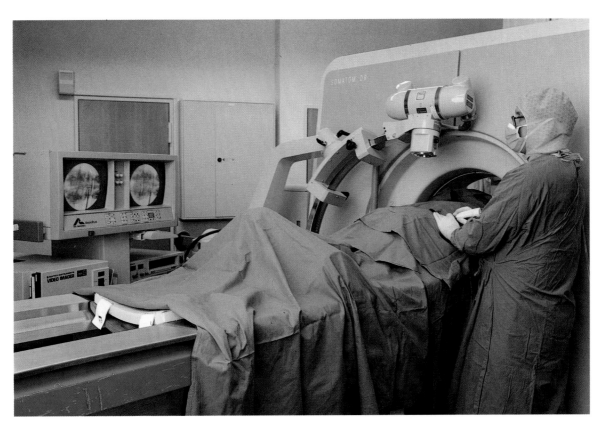

Fig. 30.1. For the combination of CT and fluoroscopy (or digital subtraction radiography), a C-arm system is installed in front of the CT. With this technique a combination of fluoroscopy and CT is possible without changing the patient's position.

Routinely, the C-arm is positioned in the anterior-posterior (A-P) direction. Two mobile monitors can be placed in the CT room. The examiner should always face the C-arm and the monitors. Positioning is carried out in such a way that the region of interest and the monitors are lined up, so that the region of interest and one monitor can be seen by the treating doctor (Fig. 30.1.).

In order to keep the radiation dose as low as possible, coning-in must be done optimally and fluoro-time kept to a minimum. Additionally, gonadal shielding should be used when possible. After a diagnostic CT in the region of interest, the treatment level is defined. The interventional procedure begins with fluoroscopy guidance. Then, in single steps, fluoroscopy and computed-tomography are performed alternately.

Because of the high morphologic resolution, most of the imaging is clearly performed by computed-tomography – especially in the case of pathologic findings. Fluoroscopy is considered as merely an aid to help form a three-dimensional picture of the area to be treated.

At each step the CT and fluoroscopy should be documented – at least for medico-legal reasons. The entire fluoroscopy is recorded on video tape at MKI.

Equipment

For fluoroscopy the clinic uses a SIEMENS SIRE-MOBIL as well as an OEC-Diasonics Angioplus C-arm. This combined mobile fluoroscopy and DSA unit consists of an X-ray system controlled by a micro-processor with two monitors and an integrated digital real-time image-processor, making real-time subtraction possible at 30 images per second. The images can be stored on a magnetic disk or on a video cassette recorder (O-Matic or VHS). Adjustments of between 40 and 120 kV and 0.5 to 5 mA are possible with a 20 mA boost.

Two monitors are available, one displaying the last stored image and the other displaying the fluoroscopic image. Furthermore, up to 60 single images can be stored on a hard disk and reviewed on the monitor. Also, all patient data including statistical evaluation are processed and displayed by one of the monitors.

In addition, a CT from Siemens is used. This has a gantry diameter of 70 cm which is adequate for interventional procedures. The gantry can be angled up to 50 degrees. The longest distance from the edge of the gantry to the CT-table base is 30 cm. Only in this space can A-P or angled fluoroscopy be performed.

Indications

The possibilities for these combined interventional techniques are almost unlimited. The following areas have been found to be optimal for combined interventional procedures:
1. Percutaneous nucleotomy;
2. complicated interventions in or near organs filled with air or contrast medium, hollow systems, and/or vessels;
3. pain therapy at a plexus and for evaluation of medication distribution;
4. 3-D drainage techniques;
5. local tumor therapy.

Workstation and 3-D Image Processing

With the significant increase of CT-, MRI- and fluoroscopy-guided interventional procedures at the institute, including combination methods (at present 4000 procedures per year), precise and systematic planning and follow-up procedures are necessary. This is the reason why the authors installed the image-processing workstation Siemens Lite-Box in their institute (Fig. 30.2., Tables 30.1. and 30.2.).

Table 30.1. High-speed network technique.

Topology	Tree (extended star)
Maximum nodes in local net	62
Maximum distances between adjacent nodes	1000 m (for fiber optics)
Total distance within network	Unlimited
Transfer medium	Double fiber-optic cable 100/140 μ
Size of signal frames	16 bits
Bit rate	16 MBits/s
Wave length	820 nm

All computer-based equipment including various PCs, MRI ACCESS (Toshiba America MRI, Inc.), DRG computed-tomograph (Siemens), Multiskop/Polytron digital angiography unit (Siemens), mobile DSA/radioscopy C-arm (OEC-Diasonics, Inc and SIEMENS SIRE MOBIL), two laser printers 100 (Kodak), and two multi-format cameras are interlinked with fiberoptic cables.

The major advantage of a workstation is the fact that prior to the interventional procedure the region of interest can be presented in all planes and an optimum access route can be determined. Also, the use of different interventional instruments and their position in relationship to adjacent organs can be simulated. Literature on this subject is presented at the end of the chapter.

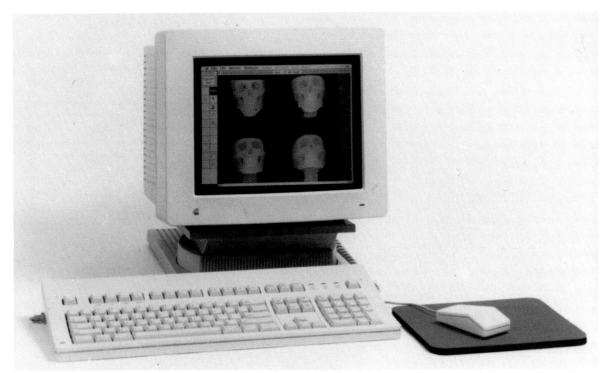

Fig. 30.2. As a central work place, the workstation is used for planning interventional procedures. Here the optimum access route can be three-dimensionally calculated and interventional procedures can be reviewed (Lite Box, Siemens).

An example of the use of the workstation in the planning of a combination procedure is prior to nucleotomies. In these cases, it can be determined, using the workstation, in which way the segmental spinal nerve can be shifted away from the instrument or which puncture angle is best in order to achieve the greatest possible aspiration of the prolapsed tissue. Furthermore, in soft tissue tumors, skeleton pathology and tumor therapy, the normal and pathologic tissue structures must be discriminated under 3-D guided procedures (Figs. 30.3.–30.5.). In many cases, three or four imaging methods have to be used pre-operatively in order to obtain as much information as possible about the differentiated morphology and three-dimensional extension. For example, the skeleton information obtained with computer-tomography has to be combined with the detailed tissue information which is seen by MRI. Also, required for preprocedure planning is detailed information about the location of tumor vessels. This information is obtained from the angiogram.

The different data concerning the patient can be brought together at the workstation. Important also will be the further processing in order to combine the different image information after geometric size correction and to construct a synthetic picture consisting of CT, MRI and angiography. Here the authors have started pilot projects.

The method for the post-procedure evaluation is similar to the above. Here, for example, the success or failure of intervention can be determined and a possible repeat procedure

planned. Also helpful is the post-interventional 3-D reconstruction for evaluating the specific distribution of contrast media and medications.

Future Outlook

Combined interventions with CT and fluoroscopy (DSA) were developed at MKI. A major advantage of this combination is the accurate appraisal and the ability to view the interventional area inside the patient in three-dimensions. The methods used in interventional radiology until now worked with one imaging method only, with the disadvantage of only a two-dimensional representation of the examination or treatment area. The major disadvan-

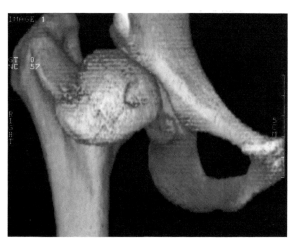

Fig. 30.3. Three-dimensional presentation of a hip.

Table 30.2. Technical specifications.

Hardware

The CPU includes the 68030 microprocessor, 68882 floating-point co-processor, 4 megabytes of RAM, 1.4 megabyte floppy disk drive, and 160 megabyte internal hard disk drive.

68030 Processor:
- The 32-bit 68030 processor runs at 15.667 MHz.
- The 32-bit address bus provides a total addressable space of 4 gigabytes.
- Separate instruction and data caches provide fast processing.
- This processor provides power and performance.

68882 Floating-Point Math Coprocessor:
- The 68882 performs complex mathematical calculations such as logarithmic and trigonometric functions.

RAM:
- The CPU is delivered standard with 4 megabytes of RAM memory.
- Optionally, 4 megabytes may be added for larger software applications.
- This RAM memory configuration provides growth flexibility and the ability to manage large amounts of data.

Accelerator Board (OPUS):
- A Siemens RISC-based 9 megabyte image accelerator board for image display and management.

NuBus Expansion Slots:
- NuBus provides a multiplexed 32-bit address bus and data on a single 96-pin connector.
- The NuBus architecture can support data transfer rates of up to 37.5 megabytes per second.
- Expansion, flexibility and custom configurations are provided with this architecture.

SCSI (Small Computer Systems Interface):
- SCSI is a high-performance interface for connecting the CPU to hard disks and other peripherals. Up to seven SCSI peripherals (including the internal hard disk) can be connected.
- SCSI provides data transfer rates of up to 1 megabyte per second.

Interfaces:
- Two mini-8 serial (RS-232/RS-422) ports
- SCSI interface: uses a 50-pin connector (internal) and a DB-25 connector (external)
- Two Desktop Bus ports will allow daisy-chaining of multiple peripheral devices
- Sound jack for stereo output

Sound Generator:
- A custom digital sound chip provides 8-bit stereo sampling at 44.1 kilohertz and includes fourvoice wave-table synthesis. Capable of driving stereo headphones or other stereo equipment through the sound jack
- Provides audible warnings and other applications.

3Mouse:
- Mechanical tracking: optical shaft encoding at 3.94 ± 0.39 pulses per mm (100 ± 10 pulses per inch) of travel.

Extended Keyboard:
- Includes 15 function keys, a numeric keypad, standard cursor arrow keys in a T-style layout and 6 cursor-control keys. It is ideal for running terminal emulation and related data communications programs, and other commercially available software applications.

Software

Operating System Software:
- System 6.03 or greater (the standard operating system)
- Printer disk (the printer drivers for all compatible printers)
- Utility disk, which includes utilities such as File exchange, HD SC Setup, CloseView, Disk First Aid, and the Font/DA Mover

Siemens LiteBox Application Software:
- Desktop which covers entire screen providing tool palette and standard interaction

● Menu bar	● Database access
● Folder windows	● Image folder display
● Shortcuts	● Zoom
● Standard menu	● Pan/Roam
● File menu	● Window/Level
● Edit menu	● Invert
● Display menu	● Flip/Rotate
● Image menu	● Token View
● Process menu	● Stack View
● Macros menu	● Cine View
● Tools	● Magic glass

Dimensions

CPU:

Height:	5.5 in.	(14.0 cm)
Width:	18.7 in.	(47.4 cm)
Depth:	14.4 in.	(36.5 cm)
Weight:	24 lb.	(10.9 kg)

Mouse:

Height:	1.1 in.	(2.8 cm)
Width:	2.1 in.	(5.3 cm)
Depth:	3.8 in.	(9.7 cm)
Weight:	6 oz.	(0.7 kg)

Extended keyboard:

Height:	2.25 in.	(56.4 mm)
Width:	19.13 in.	(486 mm)
Depth:	7.4 in.	(188 mm)
Weight:	3.63 lbs	(1.6 kg)

Monitor:*

---

* See separate data sheet

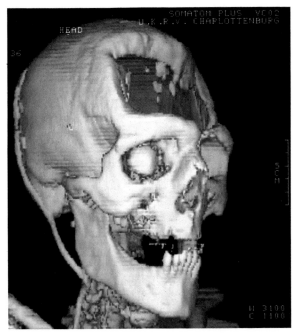

Fig. 30.4a. Three-dimensional presentation of a patient's skull for planning a surgical reconstruction.

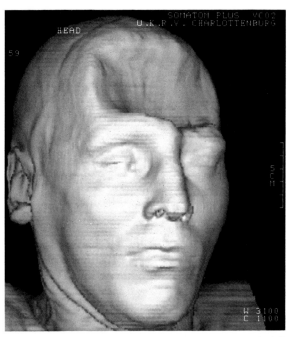

Fig. 30.4b. Three-dimensional presentation of the facial soft tissue of the same patient as in Fig. 30.4a. This reconstruction was performed using the same program as in Fig. 30.4a.

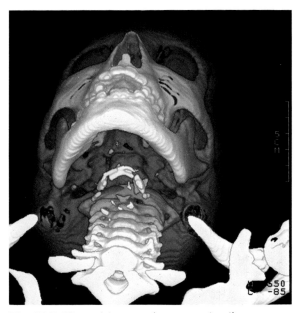

Fig. 30.5. The quick secondary reconstructions are an important aid for the exact planning of the intervention.

tages of these combined methods: extensive equipment (including the workstation), prolonged time-expenditure, and a highly specialized radiologic and operative training, are countered by the possibility of less invasive and traumatic procedures. The fact that these therapeutic methods are to a large extent replacing more invasive operative procedures and increasing the accuracy and success of other interventions such as in pain therapy (Figs. 30.6.–30.23.),

weakens the argument that these procedures increase medical costs due to the expenditure for the equipment. It is hoped that hospitalized procedures can be shifted to out-patient centers by interdisciplinary cooperation. Therefore, the use of these methods can reduce costs and make the treatment more agreeable to the patient.

The possibility of combining in a network the slices from different methods at a workstation and evaluating the pre- and post-procedure, adds considerable support for the future development of new dimensions in interventional radiology.

Further reading

Axel L., Herma G., Udupa J.K., et al.: Three-dimensional display of nuclear magnetic resonance (NMR) cardiovascular images. JCAT 7 (1983) 172–174

Dotter C.T., Judkins M.P.: Transluminal treatment of arterosclerotic obstruction. Description of a new technique and a preliminary report of its application. Circulation 30 (1964) 654 in: Günther R.W., Thelen M.: Interventionelle Radiologie. Stuttgart, New York 1988

Hohne K.H., Bernstein R.: Shading 3 D-images from CT using gray level gradients. IEEE Trans. Med. Imag. 5 (1986) 45-47

Klaue K., Wallin A., Ganz R.: CT evaluation of coverage and congruency of the hip prior to osteotomy. Clin. Orthop. Rel. Res. (1988) 23215–23225

Lang Ph., Steiger P., Genant H. et al.: Three-Dimensional CT and MR imaging in congenital dislocation of the hip: clinical and technical considerations Comp. Ass. Tomogr. 12 (1988) 459–464

Lang Ph., Genant H.K., Steiger P., et al.: 3-D reformating asserts clinical potential in MRI

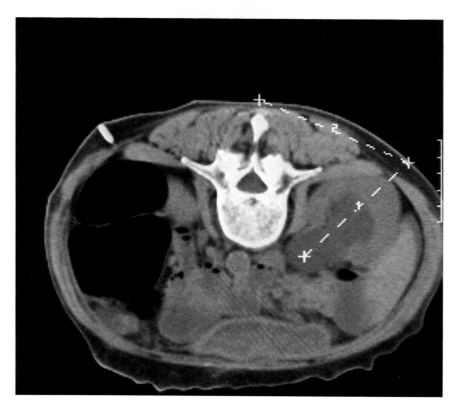

Figs. 30.6.–30.23. Example of a combination intervention.

Fig. 30.6. 53-year old patient with bilateral hydronephrosis due to an extensive cervix carcinoma with infiltration of the posterior wall of the bladder. The left nephrostomy catheter is already in place. Measurements to determine the appropriate access route for the right nephrostomy are performed at the monitor. The spinosus process serves as an anatomic landmark.

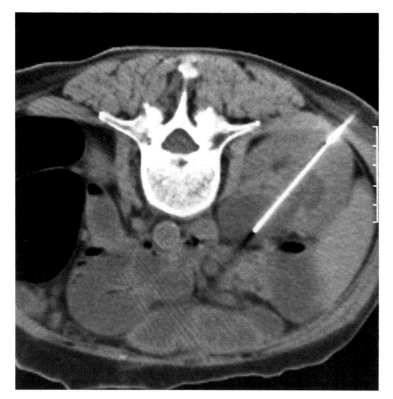

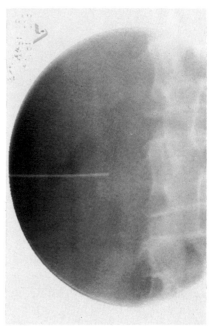

Figs. 30.7. and **30.8.** With a coaxial needle system the renal pelvis is punctured under CT control. The fine needle within the renal pelvis is seen under fluoroscopy without contrast medium injection.

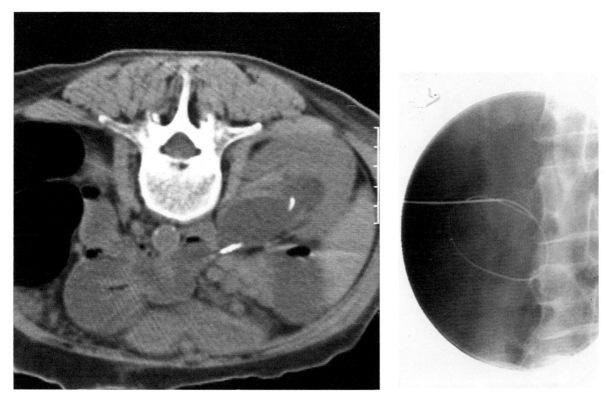

Figs. 30.9. and **30.10.** An 18-G wire is advanced through the fine needle into the renal pelvis and can be documented with CT as well as with fluoroscopy.

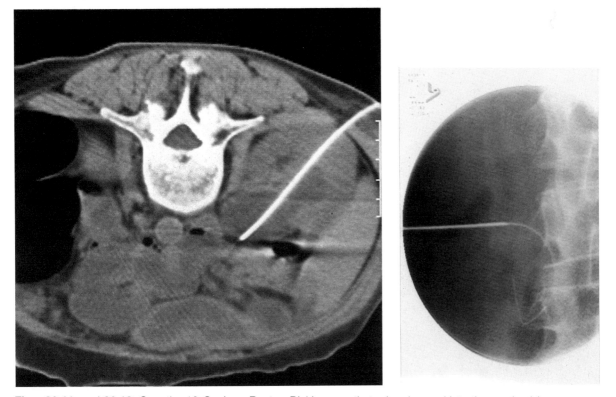

Figs. 30.11. and **30.12.** Over the 18-G wire a Becton-Dickinson catheter is advanced into the renal pelvis.

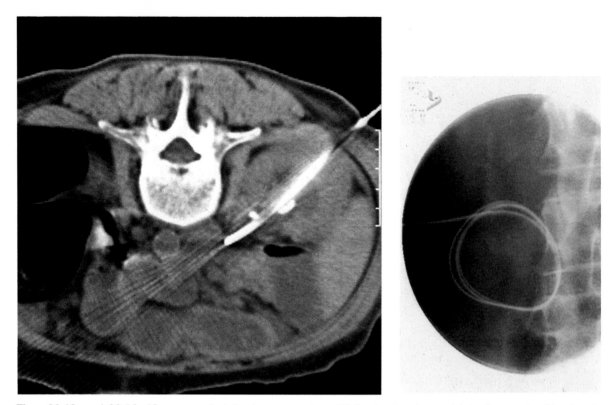

Figs. 30.13. and **30.14.** After removal of the inner cannula a 38-G wire is advanced into the renal pelvis. Stable positioning of the wire is important.

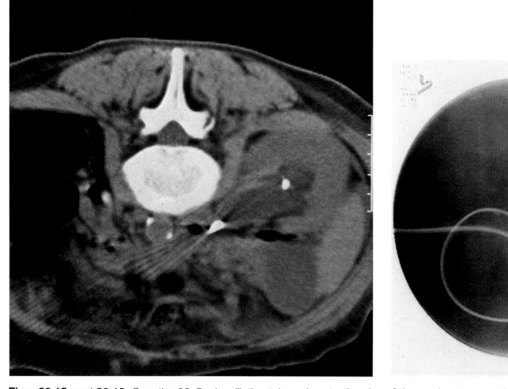

Figs. 30.15. and **30.16.** Over the 38-G wire dilation takes place to the size of the nephrostomy catheter.

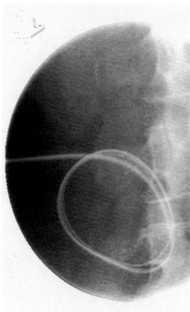
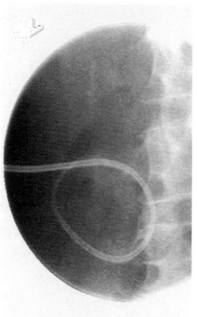
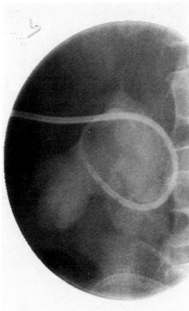

Fig. 30.17. In this case a 7-F pigtail-catheter is inserted over the wire for short-term decompression of the renal pelvis.

Fig. 30.18. Stable positioning of the catheter at the renal pelvis is shown. The insertion wire is removed.

Fig. 30.19. For exact position diluted contrast medium is injected. A massive dilated renal pelvis is visualized.

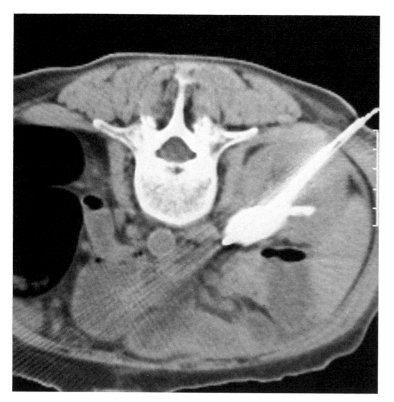
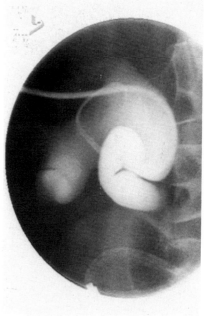

Figs. 30.20. and **30.21.** With CT the exclusion of extra-luminal contrast medium is possible and perirenal hematomas can be excluded. For further diagnosis and planning for a ureter prosthesis, the ureter must be visualized. In this case, there is a massive dilation with a distinct kinking of the ureter.

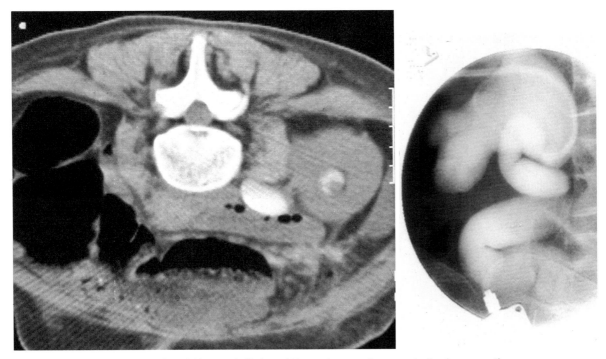

Figs. 30.22. and **30.23.** Massive kinking and dilation of the ureter are also seen in the lower portion.

Lang Ph., Genant H.K., Chafetz N.I., et al.: Three-dimensional computed tomography and multiplaner reformations in the assessment of pseudarthrosis in posterior lumbar fusion patients. Spine 13 (1988) 69–75

Lang Ph., Genant H.K., Steiger P., et al.: Three-dimensional MR imaging of the brain: technical considerations. Radiology 165 (1987) 345

Lang Ph., Hedtmann A., Steiger P., et al.: Dreidimensionale Computertomographie bei Erkrankungen der Knochen und Gelenke. Z. Orthop. 125 (1987) 418–31

Marrett S., Evans A.C., Collins L., Peters T.M.: Three-dimensional MR-PET imaging in the human brain. Radiology 169 (1988) 369

Pate D., Resnick D., Andre M., et al.: Perspective: three-dimensional imaging of the musculoskeletal system. AJR 147 (1986) 545–51

Peterson H.A., Klassen R.A., McLeod R.A., Hoffman A.D.: The use of computerised tomography in dislocation of the hip and femoral neck anteversion in children. J. Bone Joint Surg. 63 (1981) 198–208

Scott W.W., Fishman E.K., Magid D., Riley L.H., Brooker A.F., Johnson C.A.: Three-dimensional evaluation of acetabular trauma. Radiology 161 (1986) 122

Scott W.W., Fishman E.K., Magid D.: Acetabular fractures: optimal imaging. Radiology 165 (1987) 537–539

Vannier M.W., March J.L., Warren J.O.: Three-dimensional CT reconstruction images for craniofacial surgical planning and evaluation. Radiology 150 (1984) 179–184

Vannier M.W., Marsh J.L., Gado M.H., et al.: Clinical applications of three-dimensional surface reconstruction from CT scans: Experience with 250 patient studies. Electromedica 51 (1983) 122–131

Vannier M.W., Grönemeyer S., Gutierrez F.R., et al.: Three-dimensional MRI of congenital heart disease. RadioGraphics 8 (1988) 857–871

Woolson S.T.: Three-dimensional imaging and preoperative planning of reconstructive hip surgery. Contemp. Orthop 12 (1986) 13–22

Woolson S.T., Dev P., Fellingham L.L.: Three-dimensional imaging of the ankle joint from computerized tomography. Foot Ankle 6 (1983) 2–6

Electric Stimulation

Chapter 31
Electric Stimulation Methods in Interventional Radiology

D.H.W. Grönemeyer, R. Schliffke, R.M.M. Seibel, M. ten Hompel

History of Electrostimulation for the Alleviation of Pain

Claudius Galen was the first to report the use of electric stimuli for pain therapy. He did this by laying electric fishes (which emit electric shocks up to 150 volt) on the skin surface. Electrotherapeutic methods with electric stingrays have been known from ancient times. In 2500 BC, in Egypt, the malapterus electricus was used for treating pain. Illustrations of the malapterus electricus, which lives in the Nile, have been found on Egyptian murals [4].

In 47 AD, it was reported that patients with arthritic and gout pain were healed by Scribonius Largus with skin stimulations from an electric stingray [8]. Electroshock therapy became increasingly interesting for medical science since the invention of the Leyden flask (1745). With this condenser bottle, the storage of electric charge was possible. Successful treatments of paralysis, sciatica and kidney stones using this condenser bottle were published. A comprehensive publication on electrotherapy at acupuncture points was written in 1825 by Salandière [6]. In 1850, W.G. Oliver achieved local anesthesia with electricity. In 1855 a thesis by Duchenne de Boulogne was published about the use of electricity in physiology, pathology and therapy, and in 1952 the first electric stereotaxic treatments of deep brain structures were performed by Heath and Mickle [7].

In 1978, Dickhaus, Pauser and Zimmermann [3] published their results on inhibition of noxic information at spinal level by repeated 50 Hz electric stimulation of A-fibers. The peripheral effect of the electric stimulation in a model was shown by the work of Wall and Gutnick [10] in 1974 and by Devor and Wall [2] in 1976. Both publications clearly demonstrate that A-Delta-fiber activity is suppressed after peripheral electrostimulation. The frequency dependency of the effects of electric nerve stimulation and the influence of endorphins and central inhibition mechanisms were elaborated by other authors [1, 5, 9, 11]. They documented a pain-inhibiting effect of 2 Hz stimulation, which is antagonized

Table 31.1. History of electrostimulation for alleviation of pain after [7].

2500 BC	Pain therapy in Egypt with electric stingray
47 AD	The Roman physician Scribonius Largus performed and reported the first electrotherapy
1745	Invention of the Leyden flask making storage of electric charge possible
1825	Thesis by Salandière on electro acupuncture
1850	W.G. Oliver in Buffalo, New York: Local anesthesia by means of electricity
1855	Thesis by Duchenne du Boulogne on application of electricity in physiology, pathology, and therapy
1952	First stereotaxic implantation of electrodes for stimulation of deep brain structures by Heath and Mickle
1965	"Gate-control theory" of Melzack and Wall
1967/1968	Shealy, Mortimer, Reswick, Sweet and Wepsic produced clinical proof of pain alleviation with electrostimulation
1974/1976	Wall, Gutnick, Devor, Wall: Proof of a peripheral effect of electrostimulation
1978	Dickhaus, Pauser, Zimmermann. Fundamental research into the effect of 50 Hz electrostimulation of an A-fiber.

by Naloxon, but between 80 and 100 Hz, there is no antagonistic effect (Table 31.1.).

During the past ten years, transcutaneous electric nerve stimulation (TENS) again renewed medical interest in treating pain with electric therapy. With transcutaneous electric nerve stimulation, electric impulses can be applied through the skin to the painful area by surface electrodes.

In the percutaneous electric nerve stimulation (PENS), electrodes are placed deep into the areas to be stimulated. So far, implantable indwelling electrodes have been placed only in nerve roots lesions and areas of spinal cord damage. The stimulation of intracerebral structures by means of stereotaxic implantable electrodes has also been attempted (DBS = Deep brain stimulation, Table 31.2). The possibilities of a CT-guided electrical pain therapy are discussed later in this chapter.

Table 31.2. Types of electro-stimulation (for pain) (from [11]).

External systems	Internal systems (implanted)	
Transcutaneous and percutaneous nerve stimulation	Spinal Cord stimulation	Brain stimulation
TENS (Transcutaneous Electrical Nerve Stimulation)	**SCS** (Spinal Cord Stimulation)	**DBS** (Deep Brain Stimulation)
PENS (Percutaneous Electrical Nerve Stimulation) **IPENS** (Interventional Percutaneous Electrical Nerve Stimulation)	**DCS** (Dorsal Column Stimulation)	

References

1. Chapmann C.R. and Benedetti C.: Analgesia following transcutaneous electrical stimulation and its partial reversal by a narcotic antagonist. Life Sci. 21 (1977) 1645–1648
2. Devor M. and Wall P.D.: Type of sensory fibre sprouting to form a neuroma. Nature (Lond.) 262 (1976) 705–708
3. Dickhaus H., Pauser G. und Zimmermann M.: Hemmung im Rückenmark, ein neuro-physiologischer Wirkungsmechanismus bei der Hypalgesie durch Stimulationsakupunktur. Wien. Klin. Wochenschr. 90 (1978) 59–64
4. Kellaway P.: The part played by electric fish in the early history of bioelectricity. Bull. hist. med. 20 (1946) 130
5. Pomeranz B. and Chiu D.: Naloxone blockade of acupuncture analgesia: Endorphin implicated. Life Sci. 19 (1976) 1757–1762
6. Salandière J.B.: Memoires sur l'électropuncture. Paris, 1825
7. Schmerzbekämpfung durch Elektrostimulation. Medtronic Handbuch 1983, 4-5
8. Scribonius Largus: De compositione medicamentorum liber CLXII
9. Sjölund B.H., Eriksson M.: Endorphins and analgesia produced by peripheral conditioning stimulation. Adv. Pain and Th., Vol. 3 (1979) 587–591
10. Wall P.D. and Gutnick M.: Ongoing activity in peripheral nerves: the physiology and pharmacology of impulses orginating from a neuroma. Exp. Neurol. 43 (1974) 580–593
11. Woolf C.J., Barrett G.D., Mitchell D., Myers R.A.: Naloxone reversibel peripheral electroanalgesia in intact and spinal rats. Eur. J. Pharmacol. 45 (1977) 311–314

Theoretical Background

Maximum Points

Maximum zones and points have been known since the work of Head. The British neurologist Head wrote about these zones in 1898. He found reproducible pain regions on the body surface in patients with disease of the internal organs, which are only partially equivalent to the appropriate dermatomes. These areas respond to internal diseases with a hyperalgesic or hyperpathic effect. Within these zones are located centers, called maximum points, which are frequently identical to the trigger points. A pathologic reaction can be triggered with mechanical stimulation of a trigger point (e.g., a trigeminal neuralgia). It is suspected that these trigger points are commonly found at certain sites, especially where a lot of capillaries and sympathetic neuroplexi exist.

The trigger and maximum points cause pain only in disease states; otherwise they are silent. These points are special in that they have an altered electric resistance compared with the surrounding tissue and thereby can be measured. In pathologic processes, sweat secretion can be changed in the maximum zone area and also in these zones small skin hair reaction (piloreaction) often occurs.

Histologic examinations of the maximum points so far have not shown any uniform anatomic structures. Kellner discovered that in maximum point areas, compared with other areas, there are twice as many receptors present, especially Kraus's and Meissner's corpuscles. Furthermore, he reported that special capillaries, lymph vessels and nerve fibers, are only present at maximum points. However, more important, these maximum points often correspond to trigger points. It is assumed that the stimulation effect is based on the excitation of sensory nerves [10]. Almost all maximum points are located in the vicinity of special anatomic structures such as nerves, blood vessels, and neuromuscular connecting points. Contrary to previous assumptions, it appears that most maximum points are located deep, because injection of local anesthetics in or just under the skin does not have any influence on the stimulation effect, whereas deep infiltration can effectively counteract TENS and other analgesia effect [11].

Numerous animal studies have shown that therapy at maximum points is more effective than so-called pseudo-stimulation [12]. Studies of lab-induced acute pain also showed the superiority of the "genuine" stimulation [11]. However, due the small number of patients in the studies, no statistically significant results have been achieved in the treatment of chronic pain. The above mentioned animal studies were partially performed under anesthesia to avoid a stress-induced analgesia. Furthermore, the placebo effect should not have played any role in these animal studies.

Nervous Structures

The micro-electro-lead derivation of the human median nerve demonstrates that the sensation of numbness is conveyed through type II-muscle afferents. Additionally, the sensation of heaviness, tension, and pressure is conveyed through type-III and pain through type-IV afferent nerves.

It has been shown that stimulation of type-II afferents is very well suited to triggering electric or other stimulation analgesia [12]. Also, it should be noted, that bathyesthesia (deep sensibility) cannot be triggered from all of the maximum points which are located deep in the tissue and at the skin surface. If, for example, a maximum point is stimulated, in the interosseus 1 muscle of the hand, then a lesion of the ulnar nerve will not influence stimulation analgesia, whereas lesions of the radial nerve can cancel the analgesic effect [12]. By placing a tourniquet on the arm, it can be demonstrated by the existence of bathyesthesia that circulatory products do not convey electric analgesia. On the other hand, an injection of procaine into the maximum point will cancel bathyesthesia and the sensation of pain [5].

A segmental connection [2] becomes clear if a high-frequency mild stimulation of the maximum points is used. In this way Anderson was able to show clearly that the intersegmental stimulation by a lab-induced toothache significantly raised the pain threshold, whereas an external segmental stimulation was only able to shift the previously induced stimulation analgesia [1].

Humoral Transmitters

Since the discovery of endorphins, researchers have come much closer to an explanation of stimulation analgesia. It was always suspected that stimulation analgesia was based on several different mechanisms [1], and a distinction has been made between segmental and generalized effects.

Opioids

Experiments with Naloxone, an endorphin antagonist, showed that the stimulation analgesia is transmitted by endorphins [4, 14]. However, several studies could not verify these results, such as Walker's experiment [13] using high frequency, low stimulating stimuli. Studies by Martelete [9] created no bathyesthesia, which is indispensable for the stimulation effect. In the other studies, it was unclear when the Naloxone had been administered. This is important because Naloxone can prevent stimulation analgesia, but at most only poorly [4] reverses the effect once the analgesia has been established.

With dynorphin anti-bodies, Han demonstrated that dynorphin in the spinal cord transmits stimulation analgesia. He could also only minimally influence an existing stimulation analgesia with Naloxone [6]. This could be because Naloxone does not bind well with the Kappa receptors or because the endorphin had started a cascade of other neuro-transmitters [14]. Further experiments were performed to explain the endorphin theory: Cheng and Pomeranz could stop the stimulation analgesia with four different endorphin blockers [3, 4]. They also reported that rats with congenital deficiency in the endorphin system scarcely react to stimulation. Substances such as phenylalanine prolong the stimulation analgesia because they protect the endorphins from disintegration [3]. This stimulation analgesia can be transmitted to a second animal by a transfer of cerebrospinal fluid, and yet Naloxone can block this effect.

These experiments clearly show that endorphins are involved in stimulation analgesia.

Serotonin and Other Transmitters

Serotonin serves as a transmitter of the descending inhibition system at the posterior lateral column. Methysergide (serotonin receptor blocker) I.V. can (like Naloxone) block stimulation analgesia by peripheral stimulation [8]. The same effects are achieved by parachlorophenylalanine (serotonin synsthesis blocker) [8], or by chemical or electrical destruction of the nuclei raphae, which are the origin of the descending inhibition system.

Norepinephrine antagonists have shown the involvement of descending noradrenergic fibers in the production of stimulation analgesia. Since the combination of both these antagonists (methysergide and phentolamine) showed the best cancellation of stimulation analgesia, a synergistic action mechanism of both systems is under discussion.

Spinal Cord

Pain suppression at spinal cord level by stimulation procedures appears to be based on three mechanisms:
- pre-synaptic
- post-synaptic suppression by afferents of the so-called flexor-reflex (FRA)
- by activation of the descending suppression systems which can also be triggered by the FRA.

These mechanisms act strictly segmentally and are predominantly activated by high frequency stimulation [2].
The descending suppression system appears to be mediated by serotonin and other substances, whereas pre- and postsynaptic suppression is apparently mediated by dynorphins and endorphins [6].

Midbrain

The nuclei raphae are the origin of the descending serotoninergic tracts. They are influenced by the periaqueductal gray (PAG).
The hypothalamus is connected with the PAG via axones which contain connections to the frontal lobe. These can be selectively destroyed with 5,6 dihydrotryptamin, which results in elimination of the stimulation analgesia. Cinanserinin (serotonin blocker) injections into the limbic system have the same effect.

Hypothalamus and Hypophysis

The arcuate nucleus in the ventromedial thalamus and the hypophysis contain almost all the beta-endorphinergic cells of the brain. Endorphin is transported into other brain sections via their axones (e.g. to the PAG) [7].
Lesions of the arcuate nucleus destroy the stimulation analgesia of rats, whereas injuries of the hypophysis cancel stimulation analgesia as well as stress-induced analgesia. By the different stimulation processes, there is an increase of ACTH and beta-endorphine in blood in equimolar amounts and of beta-endorphine in the cerebrospinal fluid.

Interventional Skin Resistance Measurements and Electrotherapy

For interventional pain therapy, the authors have developed electric instruments for skin resistance measurements (BioHoloTon) and electrostimulation (BioHoloTens) (BHT, Inc.). With these diagnostic instruments it is possible to find the maximum points on the skin surface by taking multiple skin measurements. The technique is to perform a relative measurement of impedance. With this procedure, the maximum point or zone for inventional therapy can be determined because the electric resistance of the maximum points is often altered in comparison with the surrounding tissue.
With the therapy instrument, it is relatively simple to administer electric impulses into the region of interest, deep in the body, and with different needles, electric impulses can be delivered to almost any structure in the body. During the procedure, these instruments function as anodes. The therapy apparatus surface is the cathode and is normally brought into contact with the skin on the opposite side of the body. The therapy frequency can be adjusted between 2 and 100 Hz. The amplitude of the stimulation current can be adjusted by the patient if necessary. A combination of both instruments (BioHoloPens) is shown in Fig. 31.1.
During the development of the instrument, it was important that the length of the single stimulation impulse was below 0.2 msec. In this way irritation and erythema of skin within the region of the anode are avoided. The effects of the electric nerve blockades are similar to those caused by local anesthetics. Symptoms similar to those created by the application of local anesthetics (e.g., Horner syndrome, minor local anesthesia, or hyperemia after LS), can be produced by using different frequencies and a long duration of therapy.

The Combined Diagnostic and Therapeutic Instrument

Technical Aspects

The authors started from the concept that (contrary to widespread opinion) it is not the voltage but the power in electric stimulation therapy that determines the effective stimulation. Therefore, they did not use a common unregulated high voltage generator while developing their combined diagnostic and therapeutic instrument but a source of electric power which allows precise regulation of the current flow into the patient at any time. This source of current is fed by a regulated source of voltage, which has an exit voltage that can be accurately regulated. The curves of the exit voltage form a square wave function with a maximum amplitude of 20 mA and an impulse range of 200 milliseconds. Three fixed frequencies (2, 50, 100 Hz) can be selected by the physician with a switch. Over the entire frequency range, the rise- and fall-time of the signal is less than 2 milliseconds (on any Ohm's capacity). The built-in regulator prevents

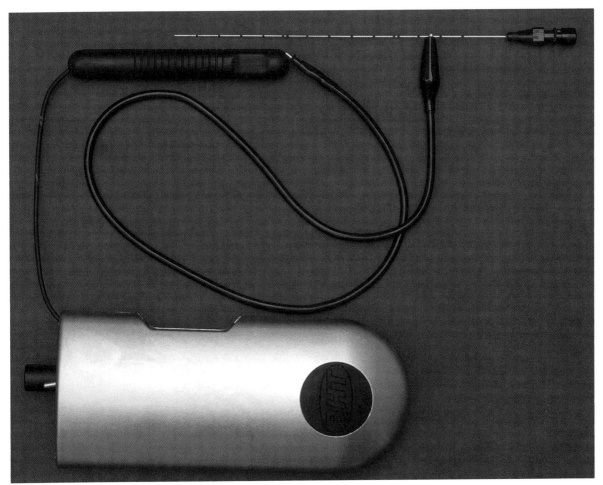

Fig. 31.1. Combined diagnostic and therapeutic instrument BioHoloPens. With this instrument it is possible to detect the maximum and trigger points on the skin surface by a measurement of impedance. At these points or zones a sterile interventional needle is advanced to the region of interest. A sterile clamp is attached to the needle and connected with the instrument. After adjusting the therapy frequency at 2 or 100 Hz, the amplitude of stimulation can be adjusted by the patient if necessary.

the otherwise normal trans-oscillation of the edges of the right angular signals and thereby undesirable short voltage increases. Fig. 31.2. shows the exit voltage of a conventional device in comparison with the new combination instrument. The improvement in the signal imaging is clearly seen.

As can be seen in Fig. 31.3., the voltage (upper curve) when connected with a complex resistance (capacity) is regulated in such a way that the therapeutically important flow of current (lower curve) does not change its form. This guarantees that, regardless of the therapy location, the set parameters will not vary.

The integrated search part makes the discovery of maximum points possible with the aid of resistance measurements. The results are demonstrated acoustically by whistling sounds of different frequencies. The reading characteristic runs logarithmically and thus the reduced inner resistance of the body at the maximum point can be localized by irregular changes in the sound frequency. The technial data are summarized in Table 31.3.

Table 31.3. Technical data.

Therapy instrument

Power	0 to 20 mA, adjustable
Voltage	max. 100 V (as function of current)
Frequency	2, 50 and 100 Hz
Impulse width	200 milliseconds
Rise time	< 2 milliseconds

Diagnosis instrument

Inner resistance	> 100 kOhm
Reading characteristic	logarithmic

Interventional Percutaneous Electric Nerve Stimulation

Interventional percutaneous electric nerve stimulation (IPENS) was used in 67 treatments; 32 stellate blocks and 35 lumbar sympathetic trunk blocks were performed. For the stellate blocks, the needle was placed on the skin and described

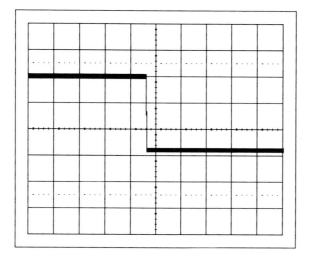

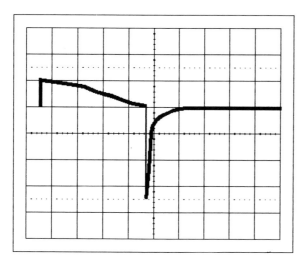

Fig. 31.2. Documentation of the exit voltage of a conventional instrument compared with the combination instrument BioHoloPens developed at MKI (bottom).

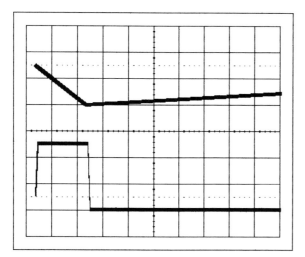

Fig. 31.3. Tension of upper curve when connected with a complex load (capacity) is regulated in such a manner that the therapeutically important current flow (lower curve) does not alter its form. In this way the set parameters are not changed during treatment, and are independent of the location.

in the Chapter Cervical blockades, then a sterile clamp was attached to the needle and connected to the stimulation instrument. After locating the stellate ganglion, the electric nerve block was started by using stimulation with 2 Hz. The duration of treatment was 20 minutes in each case. The procedure was considered to be successful when a Horner's syndrome was obtained. The results of this therapy are described in the Chapter Cervical blockades.

The lumbar IPENS sympathetic trunk blockade was performed as a pilot project using a similar technique to that described in the Chapter Lumbar Sympathectomies; however, the difference was that, prior to the puncture, the maximum point was electrically measured in the paravertebral area. Normally, the point was located 4-6 cm from the vertebral column. This point was determined as the puncture point. The puncture needle was then advanced through the maximum point to the sympathetic trunk. Here an electric stimulation of 2 Hz was given for a period of 20 minutes. The treatment was considered of be successful if an increase in the temperature of the extremity occurred. This method was performed as a pilot experiment in patients with occlusive arterial disease. After treatment, the patients were pain-free for several hours, especially on exertion, and there was a distinct increase of circulation in the extremities. However, the success of this method only lasted from several hours up to two days. The pain-free interval was prolonged with each successive treatment.

Future Outlook

By different stimulation methods on the surface or deep in the body, different nerve fibers can be activated. These fibers emit impulses to the spinal cord and, from there, the following three centers are activated. The centers involved with the analgesia are:

spinal cord: by dynorphin, encephalin and segmental connections

mesencephalon: by encephalin and endorphins and the descending inhibition system, transmitted by monoamines

hypothalamus/   by axons to the mesencephapituitary gland: lon and by direct release of beta-endorphins into the blood and in the CSF

Different types and frequencies of stimulation trigger different mechanisms. Low-frequency intense stimulation (massage, needle stimulation, low-frequency TENS/IPENS, 2-4 Hz)

appears to stimulate all three of the above-mentioned centers. Since this effect can be antagonized with Naloxone, the transmitters are thought to be endorphins. This effect appears gradually, is long lasting [1] and repeated treatments are cumulative [9, 13].

High-frequency stimulation (TENS, PENS, IPENS, 50-200 Hz) shows a rapid onset of analgesia, short duration of effect, no cumulative effect, and tolerance development. The effect is primarily segmental and can be altered by manipulation of monoamines, but Naloxone has minimal effects [1].

The IPENS method appears to be promising. A more detailed evaluation of the pilot study has not been completed until now. A controlled study is at present being prepared. First of all, it must be determined what type of combination possibilities exist with drug therapy and whether all tissue layers have to be stimulated or if an isolated stimulation of the nerve fibers close to the spinal cord will be sufficient. Furthermore, extensive examinations are necessary to define the therapeutically important current characteristics. This research is aimed at exploring the possibilities of combining injection methods with electrostimulation in order to develop a less stressful therapy for the patient.

References

1. Anderson S.A., Holmgren E.: An acupuncture analgesia and the mechanism of pain. Am. J. Chin. Med. 3 (1975) 311–334

2. Chapman C.R., Chen A.C., Bonica J.J.: Effects of intrasegmental electrical acupuncture on dental pain: evaluation by threshold estimation and sensory decision theory. Pain 3 (1977) 213–227

3. Cheng R., Pomeranz B.: Correlation of genetic differences in endorphin systems with analgesis effects of D-amino acid in mice. Brain Res. 177 (1979) 583–587

4. Cheng R., Pomeranz B.: Electroacupuncture analgesia is mediated by stereospecific opiate receptors and is reversed by antagonists of type 1 receptors. Life Sci. 25 (1979) 631–639

5. Chiang Ch.Y.: Peripheral afferent pathway for acupuncture analgesia: Sci. sinica 16 (1973) 210–217

6. Han J.S., Xie G.X.: Dynorphin: important mediator for electroacupuncture analgesia in spinal cord of the rabbit. Pain 18 (1984) 367–377

7. Herz A.: Endorphine: Körpereigene Opiate. Deutsch. Apotheker Ztg. 121 (1981) 771–774

8. Lennan Mc H., Gilfillian K., Heap Y.: Some pharmacological observations on the analgesia induced by acupuncture. Pain 3 (1977) 229–238

9. Martelete M., Fiori A.M.: Comparative study of the analgesic effect of transcutaneous nerve stimulation (TNS), electroacupuncture (EA) and meperidine in the treatment of postoperative pain. Acupunct. Electrother. Res. 10 (1985) 183–193

10. Melzack R., Stillwell D.M., Fox E.J.: Trigger points and acupuncture points for pain: correlation and implications. Pain 3 (1975) 3–23

11. Pomeranz B., Paley D.: Electroacupuncture hypalgesia is mediated by afferent nerve impulses: an electrophysiological study in mice. Exp. Neurolog. 66 (1979) 398–402

12. Toda K., Ichioka M.: Electroacupuncture: relation between forelimb afferent impulses and suppression of jaw opening reflex in the rat. Exp. Neurol. 61 (1978) 465–470

13. Walker J.B., Katz R.C.: Non opioid pathways supress pain in humans. Pain 11 (1981) 347–354

14. Watkins L.R., Mayer D.J.: Organisation of endogenous opiate and non-opiate pain control system. Sciens 216 (1984) 1185–1192

Appendix

Theory About Different Types of Pain – a General View

D.H.W. Grönemeyer, Th. Flöter, R. Schliffke, R.M.M. Seibel

Pain is the most frequent symptom prompting patients to consult a physician. Additionally, pain often serves as a warning sign for an acute or chronic pathologic condition and as a localizing symptom which helps to establish a diagnosis [2].

Often pain can be alleviated by successful treatment of the underlying etiology (especially in acute pain). In cases where the origin of pain is unknown or where the cause cannot be removed (e.g. tumor pain, migraine), there remains only symptomatic therapy [33].

When defining pain it becomes apparent that pain is not only a sensory modality, i.e. sensation of pain [27], but motivation and cognitive function are also important components [17]. The International Association for Study of Pain (IASO 1979) defines it as follows: "Pain is an unpleasant sensory and emotional experience which is associated with actual or potential tissue damage" [19].

The experience of pain is a complex phenomenon; even the word "pain" is in itself an abstract term which describes a tremendous variety of sensations. Furthermore, pain is a symptom which accompanies most diseases and can only be judged by the person experiencing it. Therefore, pain research and pain therapy require a differentiated approach which can only be mastered through an interdisciplinary process.

Pain is a multi-dimensional experience with wide individual variability. The word pain is an attempt to form a comprehensive term for innumerable individually different experiences and numerous different qualities. In every case the experience of pain is modulated by the patient's previous experiences as well as his psychosocial and socio-cultural environment.

Despite intensive pain research during the past several years, many aspects of pain have been neglected by the medical community, including tumor-related pain. Very few papers in the literature have been dedicated specifically to an understanding of the causes, etiology, and treatment of tumor-related pain. Only in recent years has there been extensive research performed in this branch of medicine. A major area of interest is at the final stage of cancer and in malignant bone processes (bone pain being

one of the most frequent oncologic symptoms), where the patient's pain is often unbearable.

Infiltration and narrowing of blood or lymphatic vessels, nerve lesions, and infections or therapeutic side-effects secondary to tumorous diseases can be further causes for pain. In 1953 Bonica documented for the first time, the different types of pain from carcinomas.

Pain Qualities

Pain, in general, is subdivided according to its location of origin and divided into the following classifications:

Somatic Pain

Somatic pain is further divided into two types (superficial and deep) depending on the location of origin. Pain is called superficial when it occurs on the surface of skin, in contrast to deep pain, which originates in the muscles, tendons, or joints. Additionally, the nature of this pain can be characterized. Superficial pain tends to be acute and well localized, in contrast to deep dull aching pain, which can be difficult for the patient to localize.

Visceral or Intestinal Pain

Visceral pain is a dull, difficult to localize pain, which can be produced by dilation spasms or ischemia of internal organs (e.g., stomach, intestine, kidneys) [26]. This visceral pain can be divided into acute and chronic types. The *acute* type of pain is normally in the area of the lesion and is diminished with the removal of the cause, whereas *chronic* type pain exists for a longer period of time or may return periodically. Interestingly, the chronic type of pain has lost its warning and protective function and can act as a disease by itself which, if chronic, can change the patient's personality [30]. Therefore, the symptoms themselves can become an independent disease. Furthermore, there are fundamental differences at a hormonal, vegetative, and psychological level in patients suffering from acute or chronic pain.

When analyzing pain in accordance with pathologic mechanisms, five currently known groups of pain mechanisms emerge.

Nociceptor Pain

In nociceptor pain it is assumed that a noxious stimulus, e.g. bacteria, ischemia, etc., triggers a chain of vascular and tissue reactions. At the final stage of these reactions, pain transmitters such as prostaglandins, bradykinin, serotonin, etc., are released [27]. These substances have both neuroactive and vasoactive functions, which act on the micro-circulation and vascular permeability [33].

The nociceptor itself is the terminal arborization of a sensory nerve fiber [5]. This receptor reacts to strong and potentially harmful sensations such as heat or mechanical irritations. There is a difference between specific (unimodal) nociceptors reacting only to a singular irritation and polymodal nociceptors reacting to several noxious stimuli [23, 31].

The threshold of these receptors can change with different influences such as inflammation mediators which lower the receptor threshold [33]. Also, a substance (substance P) can be discharged from the sensory nociceptive nerve fibers, which is felt to cause the inflammatory symptoms seen after trauma (so-called neurogenic inflammation) [32, 33].

In the case of arthritis, endogenic algetic substances are also involved. In rheumatic diseases, prostaglandins and leukotrienes are believed to be responsible for the associated pain. Additionally, in several types of headaches other chemical transmitters are felt to be responsible for pain experienced by the patient [28].

The supraliminal irritation is transformed by a receptor into an electrical receptor potential, which in the transitional zone of the afferent nerve fiber is then transformed into an action potential. The intensity of the irritation will be encoded by the frequency of the impulse pattern and in the number of involved nociceptive fibers. The localization of the irritation is thought to result from the innervation topography [26]. The exclusive involvement of the nociceptors in the pain mechanism and the function of other receptors are still controversial.

Nociceptive Afferent Fibers

Today it is believed that myelinated fibers (Group II or Delta-fibers) are the carriers of nociceptive afferent impulses. These fibers are responsible for transmission of primary pain. In contrast, the unmyelinated C-fibers (Group IV), are far greater in number and are responsible for transmitting secondary pain. The conversion of the receptor potential into the action potential is called transformation, whereas the transmitting of the nociceptive impulses from one area in the form of regenerative action potentials is called conduction. The exact details of both these mechanisms are still unclear [27].

Spinal Transmission

The afferent pain impulses reach the spinal cord at the posterior horns. Through convergence with and divergence from the different neurons, the oncoming impulses experience a multitude of transitions. The nociceptive signals are transmitted to the central nervous system via the spinothalamic tract to the thalamus. The neurons of the spinothalamic tract originate at the posterior horns, cross in the anterior commissure and pass through the anterior quadrant to the ventrobasal nucleus of the thalamus. There the oncoming signals are switched and transmitted to the cortical areas SI and SII [10, 21]. This developmentally newer area of the pain system is called "the specific system of the somato-sensory". The system is characterized by a neurophysiologically and anatomically well ordered afferent main afflux, which represents only one peripheral sensory area [26]. In contrast to this is the non-specific system which courses over the spinoreticular and paleospinothalamic tract to the reticular formation and from there to the medial nuclei of the thalamus. This system is more closely associated with the effect of perception [17, 11].

The thalamus has interconnections with many central processing areas and also emits fibers that connect with the limbic system. It is felt that in the limbic system originate the *aversive impulses* and emotions which are triggered by pain and which Melzack refers to as "the motivating component of pain" [17].

Neuropathic Pain

The function of the nerve fibers is the transmission of neuronal excitation. In order to transmit these neuronal impulses as far as possible without loss of information, extrinsic impulses must not irritate the nerve fibers en route. However, this is contrary to the case of chronic mechanical irritations like the compression of a nerve as in a disc prolapse or metastasis. The pain which radiates into the innervated area of the affected nerve is allegedly caused by the abnormal activitation of the nociceptive fibers of the nerve. This is what is called projected pain.

Furthermore, neurotoxic influences and metabolic disturbances (e.g., diabetes mellitus, paraneoplastic syndromes) can be responsible for the abnormal irritation of nerve fibers [16]. From tumor therapy cases it is now known that vinca-alkaloids interrupt the axonal transport. These trophic changes at the synapses of the spinal cord may also contribute to the origin of pain [32].

Neuroma Pain

Neuroma pain originates from the surgical or traumatic laceration of a nerve with associated regenerative changes. Following transection, the nerve fibers hypertrophy into a mass called a neuroma. Furthermore, it has been demonstrated that these fibers continuously emit nerve impulses which are considered to be the cause of the neuroma pain. This neuroma pain can also be caused by smaller nerve branches (scar pain). Additionally, it has been noticed that algetic substances such as bradykinin and histamine, injections of adrenaline or noradrenaline, and electric stimulation of the sympathetic trunk can cause an increase in pain fiber excitation [9].

Reactive Pain

Reactive pain can be the result of self-reinforcing and self-perpetuating reflex mechanisms. Therefore, it has been suspected that defective sympathetic control plays an important role in algo-dystrophia [28].

Several different mechanisms are currently being discussed:

1. One possibility is that, by a change in the micro-circulation, ischemia or vasodilation with increased capillary filtration could occur, followed by change in the local pH, which will influence the excitability of the nociceptors.
2. Another possibility is that direct electrical transmission of afferent sympathetic activities to neighboring nociceptors fibers could be the cause. In animal experiments these so-called ephapses have been demonstrated in neuromas [8].
3. A further possibility is direct excitation by neuro-transmitters of the sympathetic system [9] or indirect excitation by the contraction of local musculature [33]. By this abnormal excitation, the sympathetic system is stimulated through the spinal cord reflexes, producing a self-reinforcing and self-perpetuating reflex arch. Abnormal motor activity is believed to occur in a similar way. Thereby, an increase in muscular tone (myogelosis) can be stimu-

lated by the nociceptor in tendons and muscles, which also contribute to motor reflexes through segmental circuits. This is followed by an increase in muslce tone [5].

Pain Originating in the Central Nervous System

It is known from patients suffering from complete avulsion of posterior nerve roots in the axilla that, despite complete numbness of the extremity or an amputation, paroxysmal or permanent pain may occur. Since this type of pain (anesthesia dolorosa) cannot be caused by nociceptors, additional models for the origin of pain must be taken into consideration. The irreversible degeneration of the presynaptic afferent fibers separated from the soma has been discussed as a cause for this type of pain. In this degeneration, trophic changes at the spinal cord are common and hyperexcitability occurs (deafferentiation pain). Another explanation could be that hyperexcitability is the result of the lack of inhibition which is constantly maintained by irritation of the touch sensors [18].

It appears that a similar process occurs in thalamus pain, which can be triggered by tumors or ischemia (apoplexy). It is also felt that the sympathetic nervous system and the descending inhibiting systems play an important role in this system [22].

Transmitted Pain (Referred Pain)

Head's zones are areas of the skin where patients notice a range of feelings from increased sensitivity all the way to pain, caused by disorders of internal organs. This phenomenon can be explained by connections of the afferent impulses from internal organs to afferent impulses from the skin, which all converge at the same spinal cord neurons [5, 26]. Therefore, impulses to or from internal organs can be transferred onto the skin by processing in the brain (so-called Mackenzie zones). Another factor in transmitted pain is the segmental reflex mechanism which leads to sympathetic activity in the target areas (sweating, change in vasomotor tone of cutaneous vessels, pilo-erection, ipsilateral mydriasis, and increased muscle tone). Furthermore, it appears that an effect on internal organs can occur through skin stimulation [25].

Psychogenic Pain

Chronic pain where no organic cause can be found and where neurotic behavior is a major component, is called psychogenic pain. In many of these cases there is also a conversion neurosis present [29]. The manifestation and etiology, however, are so complex that this interesting and important aspect of pain is, unfortunately, beyond the scope of this text.

Pain Inhibition

Opioids

Endogenous opioids act as neuro-transmitters or modulators at the level of the central nervous system. There they decrease pain by either directly inhibiting the pain or indirectly activating one of the inhibiting systems. These opioids are derived from three large molecular peptide precursors by chemical processing. After being produced, they are released at the nerve ending by nerve cell excitation. The different opioids (enkephalin, endorphin, dynorphin) are distributed differently in the individual segments of the central nervous system and the point of action is determined by the opioid-receptors (mu-, delta-, kappa-receptors). The sites of action for central antinociception are predominantly the periaqueductal gray of the midbrain, the arcuate nucleus of the hypothalamus, and the Rolando's substance of the spinal cord [7]. Stress, acupuncture, or low frequency TENS (transcutaneous electric nerve stimulation) can start the endorphinergic mechanisms [4]. Depending on the localization and quality of the pain stimulus, the different opioids demonstrate varying degrees of effectiveness, which indicates that different qualities and intensities of stimuli are differently coded [6].

Descending Pain Inhibition

Important areas of function within the analgesic system are in the periaqueductal gray, the nuclei raphae magnus and the nucleus paragigantocellularis. There the descending, mainly serotoninergic tracts originate and are involved in interaction at the posterior horns of the spinal cord. Furthermore, the above named opioids apparently play a decisive role in this system [27]. Interestingly, analgesia can be produced by electric stimulation at the above-named anatomic structures [24].

Different Theories about Pain

Specificity Theory

Frey started from the assumption that a specific pain system exists which transmits information from pain receptors of the skin, to the pain center in the brain, i.e. pain originates at the receptor. Although this is the theory preferred by most physiologists, it cannot be used exclusively for the explanation of all pain phenomena (see psychogenic pain, phantom pain) [17].

Impulse Pattern Theory

Goldscheider postulated that pain is caused by specific nerve impulse patterns, which are created at the posterior horn cells by summation of the incoming sensory skin impulses. That is, pain will only result when the total number of vascular impulses has exceeded a critical limit. This may occur by an increased stimulation at the receptors or under pathologic conditions through summation of harmless tactile chemical excitations, as in tabes dorsalis [17]. However, this theory disregards the physiological aspects of pain.

Central Summation Theory

Livingston assumed that a pathologic stimulation of the sensory nerves is apparent in pain sensation (e.g., after traumas or amputation). Therefore, the feed-back mechanisms at the spinal cord will be activated which will maintain this excitation on its own. The neurons then react to this harmless stimulation with impulse bursts which are interpreted as pain at the central level.

Sensory Interaction Theory

Noordenbos postulated that a quick transmitting system exists represented by thin fibers. These fibers transmit the pain impulse to the central nervous system. The thick, slower fibers inhibit transmission, so that the proportion between thick and thin fibers is crucial for the transmission of pain. For further transmission in the spinal cord a multi-synaptic afferent system is postulated, which can be severed only by complete cross-section.

These assumptions would explain why severe pain (zonesthesia) develops after severing Gower's tract, since then the thick fibers are interrupted. The neurolysis of the sympathetic trunk (which mostly contains thin fibers), can effectively alleviate this pain [17].

Affect Theory of Pain

As an extreme proponent of this theory, Marshall has written that pain is exclusively an emotional quality which characterizes all sensory events. In his opinion, any input stimuli can trigger pain (even badly played music). Even though this point of view is rather extreme, the emotional as well as the motivating and cultural aspects of pain should be considered in any comprehensive theory of pain [17].

Diffuse Noxious Inhibitory Controls (DNIC)

The neurons that converge at the posterior horn of the spinal cord and at the caudal trigeminal nucleus receive information from almost all of the peripheral afferent nerves. If a pain signal appears, then the "background rushing" caused by these afferent impulses will be suppressed in order to better perceive the painful stimulation. This "rushing" suppression is transmitted by the descending serotoninergic tracts which are activated by a central structure (nuclei raphae). Le Bars believes to have found the basis for the counter-irritant impulses for pain suppression needed for this survey [13, 14].

The Gate-Control Theory

In 1965, Melzack and Wall assumed that part of the processing of nociceptive information takes place at the spinal level. Thereby, it is postulated that an activation of the P-cells (which project in a central direction) beyond a certain level, will stimulate the pain-processing systems. Furthermore, the authors believe that the cells in the substantia gelantinosa (SG-cells) have an inhibiting (controlling) influence on the afferent impulses of the P-cells. Also the SG-cells are stimulated by thick, non-nociceptive afferent neurons, whereas thin nociceptive afferent neurons inhibit their controlling function [18]. A main postulate of the gate-control theory is that the activation of thick afferent-neurons produces a hyper-polarization of thin afferent neurons which should be measurable as negative dorsal root potential. However, this has not been verified by later studies [27]. Nathan also could not discover a change in the level of nociception, but he pointed out that the gate-control theory of the interaction of afferent impulses was correct in principle. All of the above cited works studied only laboratory-induced pain [20].

Future Outlook

The complicated mechanisms of pain are determined by a cascade of complex interactions that occur after a local injury. The entire human being is a physical-psychic unit which affects and is affected by his/her social environment. Pain sensations and pain expression are modulated by the patient's past experiences, his/her cultural circle, and the resulting behavior. A patient-oriented or patient-centered therapy, therefore, first requires a local procedure for either resolution of the cause of the pain or symptomatic reduction of pain. However, at the same time adequate attention must be paid to the psychosomatic and psychosocial aspects of pain; therefore to improve the patient's overall condition should be the ultimate goal of all treatment.

Following the motto "Treat as gently but as effectively as possible", local pain therapy now makes use of interventional computer-tomography, which now offers innovations and many new possibilities for treating pain.

Local blocks and nerve neurolyses have been accepted forms of therapy for some time and are currently in vogue. Now with the 3-D techniques of the newer imaging and computer-supported methods like computed tomography, digital subtraction-radiography, and recently MRI, it is possible not only to make an accurate imaging diagnosis, but also to intervene percutaneously to perform FNA and treatment. With these imaging methods, structures as small as 1 mm^3 can be discriminated. Especially for interventional procedures in cases of complicated pathologic-morphologic findings, this resolving capability can be decisive for pain therapy.

In conclusion, support for general and specific pain research is absolutely necessary. The new technical possibilities with interventional computed tomography enable new therapeutic procedures requiring an extensive background (as regards pain, pathophysiology, physics, anatomy, pharmacology, etc.).

References

1. Akil H. et al.: Endogenous opioids: biology and function. Ann. Rev. Neurosci. 7 (1984) 232–255
2. Gessler M.: Was ist Schmerz. Kolloquium 22, 1985
3. Han J.S., Terenius L.: Neurochemical basis of acupunctur are analgesia. Ann. Rev. Pharmacol. Toxicol 22 (1982) 193–220
4. Handwerker H.D.: Physiologische Mechanismen des Schmerzes, Nervenheilkunde 6 (1987) 187–188
5. Hansen K., Schliack H.: Segmentale Innervation, Stuttgart 1962
6. Herz A.: Die Rolle multipler Opioidrezeptoren und ihrer Liganden bei der Schmerzmodulation. Arzneim.-Forsch./Drug Res. 34 (2), 1984
7. Herz A.: Opioide und das Schmerzgeschehen. Internist 27 (1986) 412–417
8. Hong S.K., Kniff K.D., Schmidt R.F.: Pain Abstracts Vol. 1, 2nd World Congress on Pain, Montreal 1978
9. Jäning W., Devor M.: Neurosci Lett. 1981 zit. nach: Zimmermann Triangel Bd. 20 Nr. 1/2. 1984
10. Kahle W.: Taschenatlas der Anatomie. Nervensystem und Sinnesorgane Bd. 3, Stuttgart 1976

11. Kenton B., Crue B.I., Carregal F.J.A.: The role of cutaneous mechanoreceptors in thermal sensation and pain. Pain 2 (1976) 119–140

12. König G., Wancura J.: Neue chinesische Akupunktur. Atlas und Lehrbuch. Wien 1977

13. Le Bars D., Dickenson A.H., Besson J.-M.: Diffuse noxious inhibitory controls (DNIC) 1. Effects on dorsal horn convergent neurones in the rat. Pain 6 (1979) 283–304

14. Le Bars D., Dickenson A.H., Besson J.-M.: Diffuse noxious inhibitory controls (DNIC) 2. Lack of effect on nonconvergent neurones, supraspinal involvment and theoretical implications. Pain 6 (1979) 305–327

15. Leonhardt H.: Zytologie und Mikroanatomie des Menschen. Stuttgart 6. Aufl. 1982

16. Ludin H.P., Tackmann W.: Polyneuropathien. Stuttgart 1984

17. Melzack R.: Rätsel des Schmerzes. Stuttgart. 1978

18. Mlezack R., Wall P.D.: Pain mechanism: A new theory. Science 150 (1965) 917–979

19. Merskey H.: Die Definition des Schmerzes, in: Kisker K.P., (Hrsg.), Psychiatrie der Gegenwart Bd. 2, Heidelberg 1986

20. Nathan P.W., Rudge P.: Testing the gate control theory of pain in man. J. Neurol. Neurosurg. Psych. 37 (1974) 1366–1372

21. Netter F.H.: Nervensystem I, Neuroanatomie und Physiologie, in: Farbatlanten der Medizin Band 5. Stuttgart, New York 1987

22. Pagni C.A.: Central pain due to spinal cord and brain stem damage in: Wall P.D., Melzack R. (eds.): Textbook of pain. Edinburgh 1984, 481–495

23. Perl E.R.: Pain and nociception, in: Smith J., Dorian (eds.): Sensory processes Part 1. Am. Physiological Society Washington (1984) 915–975

24. Reynolds D.V.: Surgery in the rat during electrical analgesia induced by focal brain stimulation. Science 164 (1969) 444–445

25. Richins C.A., Brizee K.: Effect of localized cutaneous stimulation on circulation in duodenal arterioles and capillary beds. J. Neurophysiology 12 (1948) 131

26. Schmidt R.: Somato-viscerale Sensibilität. Hautsinne, Tiefensensibilität, Schmerz, in: Schmidt R., Thews G. (Hrsg.), Physiologie des Menschen. Heidelberg 1983, 229–255

27. Schmidt R.: Physiologische und Pathophysiologische Aspekte, in: Wörz R., Pharmakotherapie bei Schmerz. Weinheim 1986, 1–44

28. Soyka D.: Kopfschmerz. Praktische Neurologie Bd. 1, Weinheim 1984

29. Sternbach R.A.: Acute versus chronic pain, in: Wall P.D., Melzack R. (eds.) Textbook of pain. Edinburgh 1984, 173–177

30. Uexküll v. T. (Hrsg.): Psychosomatische Medizin. München 1986

31. Wall P.D.: Mechanisms of acute and chronic pain, in: Krüger L., Liebeskind J. (eds.): Advances in pain research and therapy. Vol. 6, New York 1984, 95–104

32. Willis D.W.: The pain system. Neural basis of nociceptive transmission in the mammalion nervous system. Basel, New York 1985

33. Zimmermann M.: Pathophysiologische Mechanismen der Schmerzentstehung und Ansätze zur Schmerztherapie, in: Bergener, Herzmann (Hrsg.): Das Schmerzsyndrom – eine interdisziplinäre Aufgabe. Weinheim 1987, 37–51

34. Zimmermann M.: Physiologische Mechanismen von Schmerz und Schmerztherapie. Triangel Bd. 20 Nr. 1/2 (1981)

Further Reading

Bonica J.J.: The management of pain. Philadelphia 1953

Gross D., Thomalske G., Schmitt E.: Schmerzkonferenz. Stuttgart, New York 1984

Pongratz W.: Therapie chronischer Schmerzzustände in der Praxis. Berlin, Heidelberg, New York, Tokyo 1985

Schmidt R.F., Struppler A.: Der Schmerz, Ursachen – Diagnose – Therapie. München, Zürich 1982

Directory of Suppliers

German Abbott
Max-Planck-Ring 2
6200 Wiesbaden, Germany

Angiomed
Eisenbahnstraße 36
7500 Karlsruhe, Germany

Becton Dickinson
Tullastraße 8–12
6900 Heidelberg, Germany

BHT – Bio Holo Tronik
Bergweg 9 A
5804 Herdecke/Ruhr, Germany

Biotest Pharma
Flughafenstraße 4
6000 Frankfurt/M. 73, Germany

B. Braun Melsungen
Postfach 110
3508 Melsungen, Germany

BSIC Medizintechnik
Kölner Straße 67
4010 Hilden, Germany

Byk-Gulden
Byk-Gulden-Straße 2
7750 Konstanz, Germany

W. Cook Europe
Altmannstraße 12
4050 Mönchengladbach I, Germany

Cordis Medical Instruments
Max-Planck-Straße 20–22
4006 Erkrath 11, Germany

Toshiba American MRI, Inc.
280 Utah Avenue
So. San Francisco, CA 94080, USA

G. HUG Medical Technic
Im Kirchenhürstele
7801 Freiburg-Umkirch, Germany

IMATRON Inc.
389 Oyster Point Blvd
So. San Francisco, CA 94080, USA

KAMP-Office Organisation
Vestische Straße
4200 Oberhausen 12, Germany

Kodak
Hedelfinger Straße
7000 Stuttgart 60, Germany

A.D. Krauth
Wandsbeker Königstraße 27–29
Postfach 70 12 60
2000 Hamburg, Germany

Lederle Cyanamid
Pfaffenrieder Straße 7
8190 Wolfratshausen/Obb., Germany

Mallinckrode
Hennefer Straße 2
5206 Neunkirchen-Seelscheid, Germany

Medipha
Postfach 21
7340 Geislingen/Steige, Germany

Schering
Müllerstraße 170–178
Postfach 65 03 11
1000 Berlin 65, Germany

Schneider-Medintag
Schärenmosstraße 115
8052 Zürich, Switzerland

Dr. Sennewald Medical Technic
Augustenstraße 27
8000 München 2, Germany

Siemens Medical Technic
Henkestraße 127
8520 Erlangen, Germany

Squibb v. Heyden
Abt. Medotopcs
Volkarstraße 83
8000 München 10, Germany

Surgical Dynamics
650 Whitney Street
San Leandro
CA 94577, USA

Terumo
Lyoner Straße II A
6000 Frankfurt/M. 71, Germany

Travenol
Nymphenburger Straße 1
8000 München 2, Germany

Subject Index